Organ Preservation
Basic and Applied Aspects

Organ Preservation
Basic and Applied Aspects

A SYMPOSIUM OF THE
TRANSPLANTATION SOCIETY

edited by

D. E. Pegg
I. A. Jacobsen
and N. A. Halasz

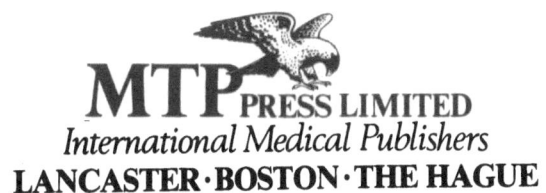

MTP PRESS LIMITED
International Medical Publishers
LANCASTER·BOSTON·THE HAGUE

Published in the UK and Europe by
MTP Press Limited
Falcon House
Lancaster, England

British Library Cataloguing in Publication Data

Organ preservation.
   1. Preservation   of   organs,   tissues,   etc.—
Congresses 2. Transplantation of organs, tissues,
etc.—Congresses
I. Pegg, D.E. II. Jacobson, I.A. III. Halasz, N.A.
IV. Transplantation Society
617'.95   RD129

ISBN 978-94-011-6269-2   ISBN 978-94-011-6267-8 (eBook)
DOI 10.1007/978-94-011-6267-8

Published in the USA by
MTP Press
A division of Kluwer Boston Inc
190 Old Derby Street
Hingham, MA 02043, USA

Library of Congress Cataloging in Publication Data

Main entry under title:

Organ preservation.

Includes index.
   1. Preservation of organs, tissues, etc. I. Pegg,
David Edward.   II. Jacobsen, I. A.   III. Halasz,
N.A.   IV.   Transplantation Society.   [DNLM: 1.
Tissue preservation—Methods—Congresses. WO
665 068 1981]
RD129.07   617'.95   82–15235
ISBN 978-94-011-6269-2   AACR2

Typesetting by Georgia Origination, Liverpool

Contents

CONTENTS

Preface

During the past 10 years, there have been many international meetings on the storage of organs prior to transplantation, and several have led to the publication of proceedings; there have also been a number of other books on this subject. Most of these publications have concentrated on practical clinical aspects of organ preservation and on empirical animal experiments directed towards well-defined clinical objectives. Progress was rapid at first, but it is now generally agreed that there has been little improvement in techniques during the past 5 years, although understanding has certainly increased.

In 1980 the Tissue Preservation and Banking Committee of the Transplantation Society decided that a fresh approach to the problem of improving preservation methods was needed: it was decided to hold a conference at which an opportunity would be provided to return to basic principles and to examine some of the advances that have occurred in recent years in areas of physiology that might be important for further improvements in preservation. The conference was held in Cambridge, UK, in April 1981 and this book is based upon the papers presented to that meeting and the work of a small discussion group that met after the main meeting. The book starts with six basic review chapters, followed by sections on the effects of ischaemia and anoxia, and on biochemical and pharmacological aspects of hypothermia. Chapters dealing with organ preservation by initial perfusion followed by hypothermia, and by continuous hypothermic perfusion, follow. The preservation of cadaver kidneys in clinical practice is dealt with in five concise contributions, and the book concludes with a section describing recent attempts to develop cryopreservation techniques for whole organs. At the conference, each of these subjects was discussed by a group of approximately forty participants in the one-and-a-half days that followed the main conference, and an edited transcript of their discussions is also included.

The meeting could not have been held without the financial support of the following: American Hospital Supply (UK) Ltd; Burroughs Wellcome Fund; Cordis Corporation; Fogarty International Center; National Institutes of Health; W. L. Gore & Associates (UK) Limited; Imperial Chemical Industries; Sandoz Limited; Smith, Kline and French; Surgical Education and Research Foundation, San Diego; Upjohn Limited; and Wellcome Research Laboratories. Gambro provided a generous donation to defray the cost of publication. To these organizations the

Transplantation Society and the Organizing Committee offers its thanks. Mr Adrian Hayes and Mr James Foreman provided invaluable help with the conference arrangements, and Mrs S. A. Harvey, Mrs C. Jackson and Miss D. Docker prepared the manuscripts for publication.

September, 1981   D.E.P.
I.A.J.
N.A.H.

List of Contributors

T. ANDRÉEN
Dept. of Clinical Research II,
Department of Urology,
University Hospital,
Uppsala, Sweden

K.-E. ARFORS
Department of Experimental
  Medicine,
Pharmacia AB,
Box 181, S-751 04 Uppsala,
Sweden

W. J. ARMITAGE
MRC Medical Cryobiology Group,
University Department of Surgery,
Douglas House,
Trumpington Road,
Cambridge, UK

G. R. ATKINS
Academic Department of Surgery,
Royal Free Hospital School of
  Medicine,
London, NW3 2QG, UK

V. D. ATTENBURROW
Academic Department of Surgery,
Royal Free Hospital School of
  Medicine,
London, NW3 2QG, UK

G. A. BALDERSON
Department of Surgery,
Princess Alexandra Hospital,
Ipswich Road,
Woolloongabba 4102,
Queensland, Australia

F. W. BALLARDIE
University Department of Surgery,
Manchester Royal Infirmary,
Oxford Road,
Manchester, M13 9WL, UK

F. O. BELZER
Clinical Science Center,
University of Wisconsin,
Department of Surgery,
600 Highland Avenue,
Madison, WI, 53792, USA

M. BEWICK
Transplant Unit,
Guy's Hospital,
London SE1 9RT, UK

H. BONDEVIK
Transplant Unit,
Surgical Department B,
Rikshospitalet, The National
  Hospital,
Oslo 1, Norway

P. BORE
Department of Biochemistry,
University of Oxford,
South Parks Road,
Oxford OX1 3QU, UK

J. BORZONE
Lady Davis Institute for Medical
  Research at the Sir Mortimer B.
  Davis Jewish General Hospital,
Montreal, Canada

J. T. BROSNAN
Nuffield Department of Clinical
  Biochemistry,
Radcliffe Infirmary,
University of Oxford,
Oxford, UK

R. Y. CALNE
Department of Surgery,
University of Cambridge,
New Addenbrooke's Hospital,
Cambridge, UK

L. CHAN
Department of Biochemistry,
University of Oxford,
South Parks Road,
Oxford OX1 3QU, UK

J. CHEMNITZ
Institute of Anatomy,
Odense University,
DK-5230 Odense M, Denmark

G. L. COHEN
University Department of Surgery,
Manchester Royal Infirmary,
Oxford Road,
Manchester, M13 9WL, UK

G. M. COLLINS
Department of Surgery,
Veterans Administration Medical
  Centre,
3350 La Jolla Village Drive,
San Diego, California 92161,
USA

R. F. DEL MAESTRO
Department of Experimental
  Medicine,
Pharmacia AB,
Box 181, S-751 04 Uppsala,
Sweden

M. P. DIAPER
MRC Medical Cryobiology Group,
University Department of Surgery,
Douglas House,
Trumpington Road,
Cambridge CB2 2AH, UK

H. G. DIETZ
Department of Paediatric Surgery,
University of Munich,
Lindwurmstr. 4,
8000 Munich 2, West Germany

R. N. DUNN
Michael Reese Hospital,
Chicago, Illinois, USA

K. ENGLISH
Rush-Presbyterian-St. Luke's
  Medical Centre,
Chicago, Illinois, USA

G. M. FAHY
Cryobiology Laboratory,
American Red Cross Blood
  Services Laboratories,
9312 Old Georgetown Road,
Bethesda, MD 20814, USA

H. FEINBERG
Department of Pharmacology,
University of Illinois at the
  Medical Centre,
PO Box 6998,
Chicago, IL 60680, USA

J. H. FISCHER
Institut für Experimentelle
  Medizin,
der Universität zu Köln,
Robert-Koch-Str. 10,
5000 Köln 41,
Federal Republic of Germany

A. FLATMARK
Surgical Department B,
Rikshospitalet, Pilestredet 32,
Oslo 1, Norway

J. FOREMAN
MRC Medical Cryobiology Group,
Department of Surgery,
Douglas House,
Trumpington Road,
Cambridge, CB2 2AH, UK

J. O. FORSBERG
Department of Surgery,
University Hospital,
Uppsala, Sweden

M. E. FRENCH
Nuffield Department of Surgery,
John Radcliffe Hospital,
Oxford, UK

L. FRÖDIN
Department of Urology,
University Hospital,
750 14 Uppsala, Sweden

M. FUHS
Institut für Experimentelle
  Medizin,
der Universität zu Köln,
Robert-Koch-Str. 10,
5000 Köln 41,
Federal Republic of Germany

K. FUKAO
Institute of Clinical Medicine,
The University of Tsukuba,
Niihari-gun, Ibaraki-ken, 305,
Japan

B. J. FULLER
Academic Department of Surgery,
Royal Free Hospital School of
  Medicine,
London, NW3 2QG, UK

D. G. GADIAN
Department of Biochemistry,
University of Oxford,
South Parks Road,
Oxford, UK

K. L. GALL
Department of Surgery,
Princess Alexandra Hospital,
Ipswich Road,
Woolloongabba 4102,
Queensland, Australia

B. GERDIN
Department of Experimental
  Medicine,
Pharmacia AB,
Box 181, S-751 04 Uppsala,
Sweden
and Department of Surgery,
  University Hospital,
Uppsala, Sweden

H. G. GOOSZEN
Department of Surgery,
University Hospital,
2333 AA Leiden,
The Netherlands

J. L. GORDON
ARC Institute of Animal
  Physiology,
Babraham,
Cambridge, CB2 4AT, UK

C. J. GREEN
Division of Comparative Medicine,
MRC Clinical Research Centre,
Northwick Park, Middlesex, UK

R. GRUNDMANN
Chirurgische Universitätsklinik
  Köln-Lindenthal,
Joseph-Stelzmann-Str. 9,
D-5000 Köln 41, Germany

F. M. GUTTMAN
The McGill University,
Montreal Children's Hospital
  Research Institute,
2300 Tupper Street,
Suite C1129, Montreal, Quebec,
  H3H 1P3,
Canada

M. HAKLIN
Rush-Presbyterian-St. Luke's
  Medical Centre,
Chicago, Illinois, USA

N. A. HALASZ
Department of Surgery,
University of California Medical
  Center,
225 Dickinson Street, San Diego,
California 92103, USA

L. B. HAMLYN
Department of Surgery,
Princess Alexandra Hospital,
Ipswich Road,
Woolloongabba 4102,
Queensland, Australia

I. HANSEN-SCHMIDT
Institut für Experimentelle
  Medizin,
der Universität zu Köln,
Robert-Koch-Str. 10,
5000 Köln 41,
Federal Republic of Germany

I. R. HARDIE
Department of Surgery,
Princess Alexandra Hospital,
Ipswich Road,
Woolloongabba 4102,
Queensland, Australia

B. HARNESS
Chemical Engineering
  Department,
University of Bradford,
Bradford BD7 1DP, UK

B. HARVIG
Dept. of Clinical Research II,
University Hospital,
Uppsala, Sweden

J. HAUSS
Department of Surgery,
University of Münster,
Jungeblodtplatz 1,
44 Münster,
West Germany

A. HIRSH
Cryobiology Laboratory,
American Red Cross Blood
  Service Laboratories,
9312 Old Georgetown Road,
Bethesda, MD 20814, USA

K. E. F. HOBBS
Academic Department of Surgery,
Royal Free Hospital School of
  Medicine,
London NW3 2QC, UK

M. HOELSCHER
Klin. fur Allgemein-Chirurgie,
Universität Göttingen,
D-3400 Göttingen,
West Germany

R. M. HOFFMANN
Clinical Science Center,
University of Wisconsin,
Department of Surgery,
600 Highland Avenue,
Madison, WI 53792, USA

B. HOWDEN
Monash University,
Department of Surgery,
Prince Henry's Hospital,
Melbourne, Victoria 3004,
Australia

L. HUNT
Department of Medical
  Computation,
Manchester Royal Infirmary and
  University of Manchester,
Manchester, UK

A. HUTCHINGS
ARC Institute of Animal
  Physiology,
Babraham,
Cambridge, CB2 4AT, UK

W. ISSELHARD
Institute für Experimentelle
  Medizin,
der Universität zu Köln,
Robert-Koch-Str. 10,
5000 Köln 41, Germany

Y. IWASAKI
Institute of Clinical Medicine,
The University of Tsukuba,
Niihari-gun, Ibaraki-ken, 305,
Japan

P. JABLONSKI
Monash University,
Department of Surgery,
Prince Henry's Hospital,
Melbourne, Victoria 3004,
Australia

I. A. JACOBSEN
Department of Nephrology,
University Hospital,
DK-5000 Odense C, Denmark

A. JAKOBSEN
Transplantation Unit,
Surgical Department B,
Rikshospitalet, Oslo 1, Norway

J. JAMART
Laboratory of Experimental
  Surgery,
University of Louvain,
Medical School, UCL 5570,
B-1200 Brussels, Belgium

R. W. G. JOHNSON
University Department of Surgery,
The Royal Infirmary,
University of Manchester,
Manchester, UK

H. E. JØRGENSEN
The Department of Nephrology B,
Herlev Hospital,
2730 Herlev, Denmark

O. KÄLLSKOG
Department of Physiology and
  Medical Biophysics,
Uppsala, Sweden

N. KAMADA
Department of Surgery,
University of Cambridge,
New Addenbrooke's Hospital,
Hills Road, Cambridge, UK

L. KARLBERG
Department of Urology,
University Hospital,
750 14 Uppsala, Sweden

A. M. KAROW
Department of Pharmacology,
Medical College of Georgia,
Augusta, Georgia 30912, USA

E. KEMP
Department of Nephrology,
University Hospital,
DK-5000 Odense C, Denmark

G. KEMP
Department of Nephrology,
University Hospital,
DK-5000 Odense C, Denmark

N. KILIAN
Department of Paediatric Surgery,
University of Munich,
Lindwurmstr. 4,
8000 Munich 2, West Germany

J. KLEMPNAUER
Department of Surgery,
University of Cambridge,
New Addenbrooke's Hospital,
Cambridge, UK

Ch.O. KÖHLER
Department of Paediatric Surgery,
University of Munich,
Lindwirmstr. 4,
8000 Munich 2, West Germany

G. KOOTSTRA
Department of Surgery,
State University of Limburg,
Maastricht, The Netherlands

J. KOSTERHON
Department of Paediatric Surgery,
University of Munich,
Lindwurmstr. 4,
8000 Munich 2, West Germany

S. KREINER
Department of Data-processing,
Herlev Hospital,
2730 Herlev, Denmark

D. KULUS
Institut für Experimentelle
  Medizin,
Robert-Koch-Str. 10,
5000 Köln 41, Germany

K. KÜRTEN
Chirurgische Universitätsklinik
  Köln-Lindenthal,
Joseph-Stelzmann-Str. 9,
D-5000 Köln 41, West Germany

L. LAMBOTTE
Laboratory of Experimental
  Surgery,
University of Louvain Medical
  School,
UCL 5570, B-1200 Brussels,
Belgium

G. LANDE
Surgical Department B,
Rikshospitalet, Pilestredet 32,
Oslo 1, Norway

M. LARSEN
Department of Data-processing,
Herlev Hospital,
2730 Herlev, Denmark

S. LARSEN
Institute of Pathology,
Herlev Hospital,
University of Copenhagen,
2730 Herlev, Denmark

E. LESLIE
Monash University Department of
  Surgery,
Prince Henry's Hospital,
Melbourne, Victoria 3004,
Australia

S. LEVITSKY
Department of Surgery,
University of Illinois College of
  Medicine,
Chicago, Illinois, USA

D. LORIEO
St. Luke's-Roosevelt Hospital
  Centre and Columbia
  University,
New York, USA

M. LOWRY
Nuffield Department of Clinical
  Biochemistry,
Radcliffe Infirmary,
University of Oxford,
Oxford, UK

S. B. LUCAS
Department of Medical
  Computation,
Manchester Royal Infirmary and
  University of Manchester,
Manchester, UK

F. N. McKENZIE
Department of Cardiovascular and
  Thoracic Surgery,
University Hospital,
London, Canada

A. MAINWARING
Department of Pathology,
University of Manchester Medical
  School,
Oxford Rd., Manchester, UK

V. MARSHALL
Monash University,
Department of Surgery,
Prince Henry's Hospital,
Melbourne, Victoria 3004,
Australia

R. McCABE
St. Luke's-Roosevelt Hospital
  Centre,
New York, USA

F. K. MERKEL
Rush-Presbyterian-St. Luke's
  Medical Centre,
Chicago, Illinois, USA

S. MONCADA
Wellcome Research Laboratories,
Langley Court,
Beckenham, Kent, UK

P. J. MORRIS
Nuffield Department of Surgery,
John Radcliffe Hospital,
Oxford, UK

A. R. MUNDY
Transplant Unit,
Guy's Hospital,
London SE1 9RT, UK

A. NIZET
Department of Internal Medicine,
University Hospital de Bavière,
Liège, Belgium

B. J. NORLÉN
Department of Urology,
University Hospital,
750 14 Uppsala, Sweden

L. H. NUTT
Academic Department of Surgery,
Royal Free Hospital School of
  Medicine,
London NW3 2QG, UK

T. OKAMURA
Institute of Clinical Medicine,
The University of Tsukuba,
Niihari-gun, Ibaraki-ken, 305,
Japan

D. R. OSBORNE
Academic Department of Surgery,
Royal Free Hospital School of
  Medicine,
London NW3 2QG, UK

A. OZAKI
Institute of Clinical Medicine,
The University of Tsukuba,
Niihari-gun, Ibaraki-ken, 305,
Japan

I. PAPATHEOFANIS
Department of Biochemistry,
University of Oxford,
South Parks Road,
Oxford OX1 3QU, UK

J. D. PEARSON
ARC Institute of Animal
  Physiology,
Babraham,
Cambridge CB2 4AT, UK

D. E. PEGG
MRC Medical Cryobiology Group,
University Department of Surgery,
Douglas House,
Trumpington Road,
Cambridge CB2 2AH, UK

L. R. POULSEN
Department of Urology,
Herlev Hospital,
2730 Herlev, Denmark

M. J. PRINGLE
Department of Cell Physiology,
Boston Biomedical Research
  Institute,
20 Staniford Street,
Boston MA 02114, USA

G.K. RADDA
Department of Biochemistry,
University of Oxford,
South Parks Road,
Oxford, OX1 3QU, UK

D. RAE
Monash University Department of
Surgery,
Prince Henry's Hospital,
Melbourne, Victoria 3004,
Australia

A.T. RAFTERY
University Department of Surgery,
Manchester Royal Infirmary,
University of Manchester,
Manchester UK

G. REIFFERSCHEIDT
Institut für Experimentelle
Medizin,
der Universität zu Köln,
Robert-Koch-Str. 10,
5000 Köln 41,
West Germany

J.M. RESTORICK
Transplant Unit,
Guy's Hospital,
London SE1 9RT, UK

B.G. RIJKMANS
Department of Surgery,
State University of Limburg,
Maastricht, The Netherlands

D. ROSEMAN
Rush-Presbyterian-St. Luke's
Medical Centre,
Chicago, Illinois, USA

B.J. ROSER
Department of Immunology,
Institute of Animal Physiology,
Cambridge, UK

B.D. ROSS
Nuffield Department of Clinical
Medicine,
John Radcliffe Hospital,
Oxford, UK

O. RULAND
Department of Surgery,
University of Münster,
Jungeblodtplatz 1,
44 Münster,
West Germany

M. SANO
Institute of Clinical Medicine,
The University of Tsukuba,
Niihari-gun, Ibaraki-ken, 305,
Japan

R. SCHOLZ
Department of Physiological
Chemistry, Physiology and Cell
Biology,
Univ. of Munich, Goethestr. 33,
West Germany

K. SCHÖNLEBEN
Department of Surgery,
University of Münster,
Jungeblodtplatz 1,
44 Münster, West Germany

D.F. SCOTT
Monash University,
Department of Surgery,
Prince Henry's Hospital,
Melbourne, Victoria 3004,
Australia

N.B. SEGAL
Lady Davis Institute for Medical
Research at the Sir Mortimer B.
Davis Jewish General Hospital,
Montreal, Canada

P. SEHR
Department of Biochemistry,
University of Oxford,
South Parks Road,
Oxford OX1 3QU, UK

E. SHOEBRIDGE
Nuffield Department of Clinical
Biochemistry,
Radcliffe Infirmary,
University of Oxford,
Oxford, UK

E. SINAGOWITZ
Urolog. Abtlg. Stadtkrankenhaus
Friedrichshafen/Bodensee,
Germany

S. SKREDE
Institute of Clinical Biochemistry,
Rikshospitalet, Pilestredet 32,
Oslo 1, Norway

O. SLAATTELID
Surgical Department B,
Rikshospitalet, Pilestredet 32,
Oslo, 1, Norway

J. H. SOUTHARD
Clinical Science Center,
University of Wisconsin,
Department of Surgery,
600 Highland Avenue,
Madison, WI 53792, USA

U. SPIEGEL
Department of Surgery,
University of Münster,
Jungeblodtaplatz,
44 Münster,
West Germany

H. STARKLINT
Laboratory of Nephropathology,
Institute of Pathology,
Odense University Hospital,
DK-5000 Odense C, Denmark

M. STUBBS
Nuffield Department of Clinical
  Biochemistry,
Radcliffe Infirmary,
University of Oxford,
Oxford, UK

P. STYLES
Department of Biochemistry,
University of Oxford,
South Parks Road,
Oxford, UK

A. SWISTEL
St. Luke's-Roosevelt Hospital
  Centre and Columbia
  University,
New York, USA

J. TANGE
Department of Pathology,
Melbourne University,
Parkville, Victoria 3052,
Australia

M. J. TAYLOR
MRC Medical Cryobiology Group,
University Department of Surgery,
Douglas House,
Trumpington Road,
Cambridge, CB2 2AH, UK

H. H. THAW
Department of Experimental
  Medicine,
Pharmacia AB, Box 181,
S-751 04 Uppsala 1, Sweden and
Department of Cardiovascular and
  Thoracic Surgery,
University Hospital,
London, Canada

H. THEMANN
Institute of Medical Cytobiology,
University of Münster,
Jungeblodtplatz 1, 44 Münster,
West Germany

G. E. THOMAS
Department of Physiology and
  Biophysics,
University of Illinois College of
  Medicine,
Chicago, Illinois, USA

K. THULBORN
Department of Biochemistry,
University of Oxford,
South Parks Road,
Oxford, OX1 3QU, UK

J. R. VANE
Wellcome Research Laboratories,
Langley Court,
Beckenham, Kent, UK

C. VOORDES
Department of Pathology,
University Hospital,
Groningen, The Netherlands

S. WALTER
Department of Urology,
Herlev Hospital,
2730 Herlev, Denmark

M. WENZEL
Institut für Pharmazie der Freien
  Universität Berlin,
Königin-Luise-Str. 2–4,
1000 Berlin 33, Germany

D. R. WHEELDON
Surgical Unit,
Papworth Hospital,
Cambridge, CB3 8RE, UK

D. G. D. WIGHT
Department of Histopathology,
University of Cambridge,
New Addenbrooke's Hospital,
Hills Road,
Cambridge, UK

J. VAN DER WIJK
Department of Urology,
University Hospital,
Groningen, The Netherlands

H. WILMS
Chirurgische-Universitatsklinik,
Hugstetterstrasse 55,
78 Freiburg Im Briesgau,
West Germany

M. WOLGAST
Department of Physiology and
Medical Biophysics,
Uppsala, Sweden

P. W. H. WOODRUFF
Department of Surgery,
Princess Alexandra Hospital,
Ipswich Road,
Woolloongabba 4102,
Queensland, Australia

R. J. WOODS
Academic Department of Surgery,
Royal Free Hospital School of
Medicine,
London NW3 2QG, UK

M. C. WUSTEMAN
MRC Medical Cryobiology Group,
University Department of Surgery,
Douglas House,
Trumpington Road,
Cambridge, CB2 2AH, UK

F. A. ZIMMERMANN
Department of Paediatric Surgery,
University of Munich,
Lindwurmastr. 4,
8000 Munich 2,
West Germany

PART I
BASIC REVIEWS

1
Energetics and mitochondria

H. FEINBERG

A recent editorial noted that kidney preservation techniques have changed
little for over a decade[1]. Storage beyond a 7–10-day period is not yet
possible. In part, this was attributed to 'lack of understanding of the
metabolic requirements of the *ex vivo* hypothermic-perfused organ,
particularly as it relates to function and pathways that are altered by
hypothermia'. The same comments are applicable to liver and heart
preservation; indeed these organs cannot be successfully stored for more
than 24 h.

Hypothermia in organ preservation constitutes an effort to reduce the
rate of energy utilization (i.e. ion pumping, contraction, etc.) in order to
minimize the rate of energy production (i.e. ATP synthesis). Implicit in this
strategy is the recognition that the two rates are coupled. The close
correlation between energy production, as measured by O_2 consumption,
and energy utilization in the form of cardiac repetitive tension
development, is well known[2], although the biochemical mechanisms that
are the basis of close coupling are only now beginning to emerge[3].

The main reactions that consume energy in functioning organs are shown
in Figure 1.1. These include maintenance of ion gradients, interaction of
contractile proteins, and synthesis of proteins and other macromolecules.
Organs may be specialized in this regard; thus, over 80% of O_2 consumed
by the kidney is associated with ion pumping[4], while tension development is
the predominant basis of O_2 utilization in the heart[2].

Two modes of energy production provide ATP for organ function
(Figure 1.1). Glycolysis involves the transduction of energy from oxidation
reactions to the formation of ATP from ADP and P_i in a process termed
substrate level phosphorylation. Glycolytic reactions take place in the
'soup' of the cytosol. Only two of a possible 36 ATPs are formed per
molecule of glucose and only 47 kilocalories are obtained of the possible
686 from the complete combustion of glucose.

The second mode of energy production is oxidative phosphorylation
wherein the remainder of the bond energy in glucose (now residing in two
pyruvate molecules) or the bond energy in fatty acids is made available
through mitochondrial respiration. The ATP utilized in the cytosol in
energy-consuming reactions is precisely resynthesized by a combination of

3

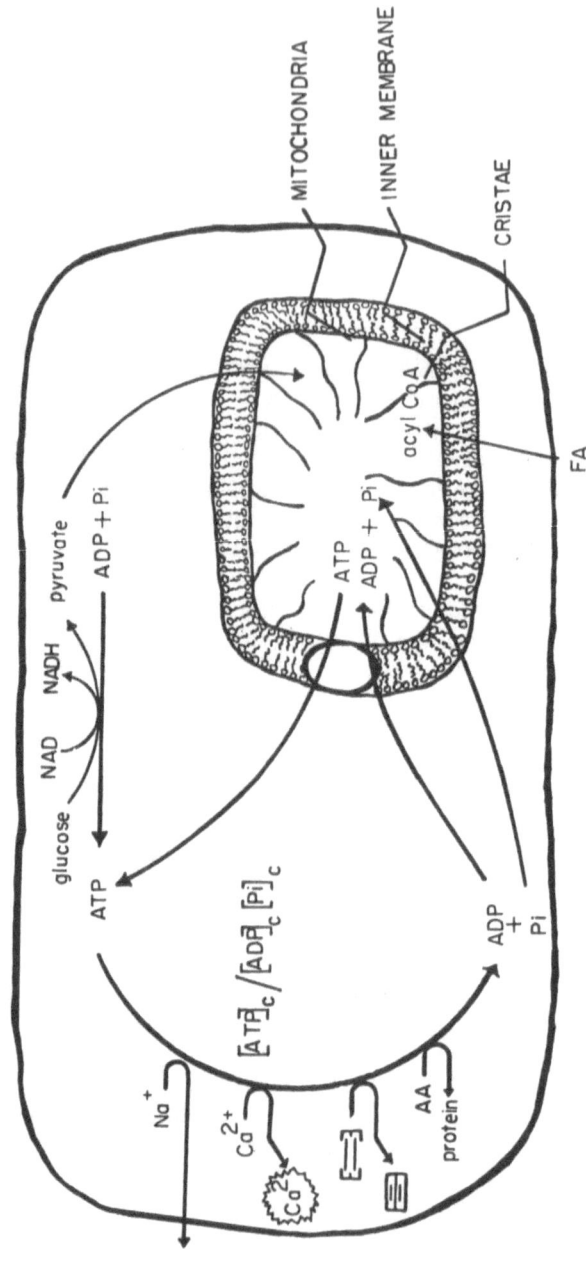

Figure 1.1 Scheme of cell energy balance. Shown are: the major energy-utilizing reactions (Na$^+$ efflux pump, Ca^{2+} sequestration, contractile protein interaction and biosynthesis) and the two energy-producing mechanisms, glycolysis and oxidative phosphorylation. [ATP]/[ADP][P$_i$] represents the cytosolic phosphorylation potential

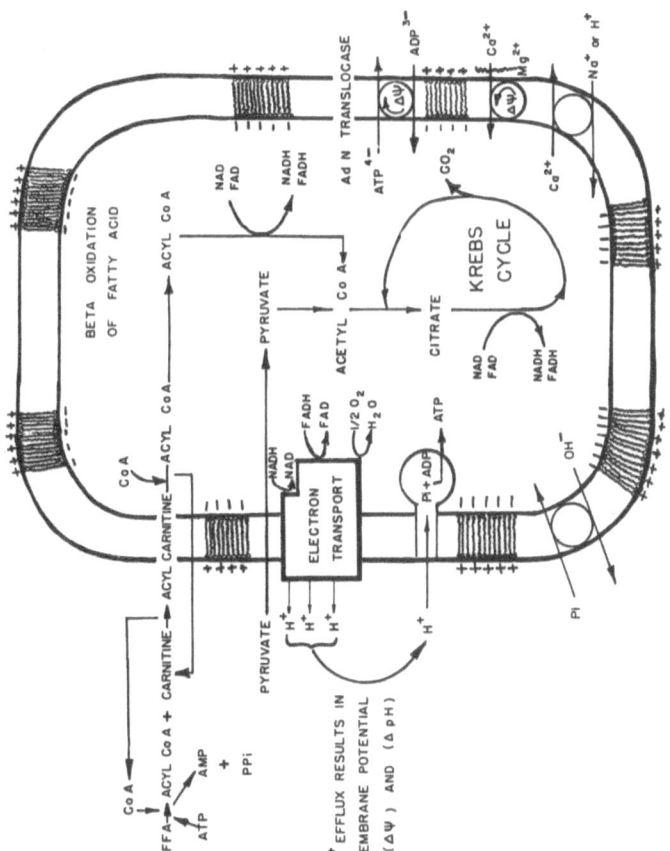

Figure 1.2 Schematic of mitochondria. Shown on the right is the adenine nucleotide (AdN) translocase carrier. The membrane potential ($\Delta\Psi$) favours the efflux of mitochondrial ATP^{4-} in exchange for cytosolic ADP^{3-}. Uptake of Ca^{2+} is also favoured by $\Delta\Psi$, except that Mg^{2+} is inhibitory. Shown on the left is the vectorial translocation of protons (H^+) and the backflow of protons through the ATPase site

these two processes of energy production such that no extra ATP is synthesized. The mechanism of energy coupling is not completely understood. However, it is apparent that integrity of energy-coupling mechanisms during organ preservation is of major importance.

Most of the cell's ATP is synthesized in mitochondria (Figure 1.2). The classic experiments of Chance and Williams[5] on isolated mitochondria showed that they utilized O_2 and substrate (i.e. succinate, β-hydroxy-butyrate, etc.) until all available ADP and P_i are converted to ATP; then, despite the continuing availability of O_2 and substrate, their O_2 utilization ceased. This condition was designated state 4, the O_2- and substrate-consuming mode being designated state 3. The ratio of O_2 utilization between states 3 and 4 is the respiratory control index (RCI). If addition of ADP and P_i to the isolated mitochondria is taken as the equivalent of energy utilization in the intact cell, then these experiments demonstrate that a part of the coupling mechanism resides in the intact mitochondria and accounts for the transition from state 3 to state 4.

Substrates (e.g. pyruvic acid, acyl-CoA, etc.) are utilized in mito-chondria by a system of dehydrogenase enzymes that catalyse the sequential dehydrogenation (i.e. oxidation) of tricarboxylic acids. Pyruvate is first decarboxylated to acetyl-CoA which then condenses with oxalacetate to form citrate. Fatty acids are converted to acetyl-CoA by β-oxidation. Thus the two carbons of acetyl-CoA are converted to CO_2, oxalacetate is regenerated and the coenzymes NAD and FAD are reduced to NADH and FADH. The reduced coenzymes are reoxidized by the respiratory carriers (cytochromes and Fe-S compounds) of the electron transport chain embedded in the inner mitochondrial membrane. Thus, the carbon–carbon bond energy intrinsic to fatty acids and pyruvate is transduced by the enzymes of the citric acid cycle to form NADH and FADH. Both of these substances have highly negative redox potentials and readily interact with oxidized cytochromes embedded in the mitochondrial inner membrane.

The energy released in the oxidation of the reduced coenzymes by the membrane-bound cytochromes was believed to be used in the formation of high-energy intermediates that interacted with ADP and P_i to form ATP[6]. However, the postulated intermediates have never been isolated. Mitchell's chemiosmotic theory[7] of energy transduction proposes that hydrogen atoms are dissociated from NADH or FADH by the respiratory chain to form protons (H^+) and electrons (e^-) (Figure 1.2). In this process the protons are translocated outwards and enter the aqueous layer surrounding the mitochondria. The electrons are translocated within the membrane in successive oxidation–reduction reactions between neighbouring components of the respiratory chain that have different redox potentials. Ultimately, O_2 accepts electrons from cytochrome aa_3 and protons from the matrix aqueous layer to form H_2O. The result of this process is a net shift of protons from inside to outside to form a pH gradient, with the inside alkaline, and an electrical charge across the membrane, with the inside negative. Thus the proton gradient ($\Delta\mu H^+$) is established with energy derived from dismutating carbon–carbon bonds and it resides in the membrane potential ($\Delta\Psi$) and the pH difference (ΔpH). The proton gradient is maintained by oxidation of reduced coenzymes, electron transport and proton efflux. However, unless the gradient is dissipated it creates a back pressure which inhibits further proton efflux[7,8]. In this condition electron transport and oxidation of reduced coenzymes slows and eventually stops. Since NAD, the product of NADH oxidation, is no longer available, flux of substrate through the citric acid cycle also stops.

Also embedded in the inner mitochondrial membrane are ATPase sites (Figure 1.2). These sites provide a pathway for proton influx back across the membrane. The accumulated energy gradient is dissipated in the synthesis of ATP from P_i and ADP. Thus the ATPase sites are proton 'sinks' which transduce the energy of the proton gradient into the high-energy bond of ATP. The flow of protons back across the membrane relieves the inhibition of forward electron transport and of NADH oxidation. Protons flow back across the ATPase sites as long as ADP and P_i are available (state 3) and this ceases when all of the ADP and P_i has been converted to ADP (state 4).

Thus, in isolated mitochondria, coupling between energy production and energy utilization is a result of the inner mitochondrial membrane impermeability to protons except at the ATPase sites, the outward vectorial translocation of protons, the establishment of a proton gradient and the transduction of energy invested in the proton gradient into synthesis of ATP from ADP and P_i[7].

Mitochondria contain only a fraction of the cell's ATP. Most ATP-utilizing reactions take place in the cytosol. Although cytosolic ATP may be regenerated locally, e.g. by creatine phosphate and creatine phos-phokinase, ultimately ADP from the cytosol must enter mitochondria to be phosphorylated. Mitochondria take up ADP in a 1:1 exchange with mitochondrial ATP (Figure 1.2) by means of the adenine nucleotide trans-locase carrier protein[9]. The highly specific translocase protein exchanges adenine nucleotides (e.g. ATP:ATP, ATP:ADP, ADP:ADP, etc.) across the mitochondrial membrane. However, the membrane potential generated by the proton gradient favours the exchange of matrix ATP^{4-} for cytosolic ADP^{3-} or the equivalent of the efflux of an anion. Thus part of the proton gradient energy is used to support the efflux of ATP (cytosolic P_i, which is also needed for ATP synthesis, enters the mitochondria independently[10] in a non-electrogenic exchange). Although ADP phosphorylation is closely coupled to redox events and the proton gradient, energy coupling in the intact cell depends on the rate of the exchange of mitochondrial ATP for cytosolic ADP, i.e. the rate of adenine nucleotide translocase. However, studies of isolated mitochondria and of intact systems show that the respiratory rate parallels changes in the cytoplasmic phosphorylation state, i.e. the ratio $[ATP]/[ADP][P_i]$, designated the cytoplasmic phosphory-lation potential[11] (Figure 1.1). This parallelism suggests that, under normal conditions, the adenine nucleotide translocase rate is not a limiting factor for ATP-requiring reactions in the cytosol[12]. On the other hand, there is evidence that there is little or no excess catalytic capacity for adenine nucleotide translocation[13]. Entry of P_i into mitochondria, in exchange for

OH^-, appears to have about a 20-fold higher activity than adenine nucleotide translocase[10]. Thus the entry of cytoplasmic ADP depends in part on the K_m for ADP and the inhibition exerted by cytoplasmic ATP (K_i ATP) and there is evidence that the respiration rate responds to [ATP]/[ADP][14]. These findings, along with evidence that there is little excess adenine nucleotide translocase catalytic capacity, and evidence of a sharp decrease (Figure 1.3) in translocase rate as temperature is lowered below 18 °C[15], suggests that the translocase rate can become limiting in energy coupling.

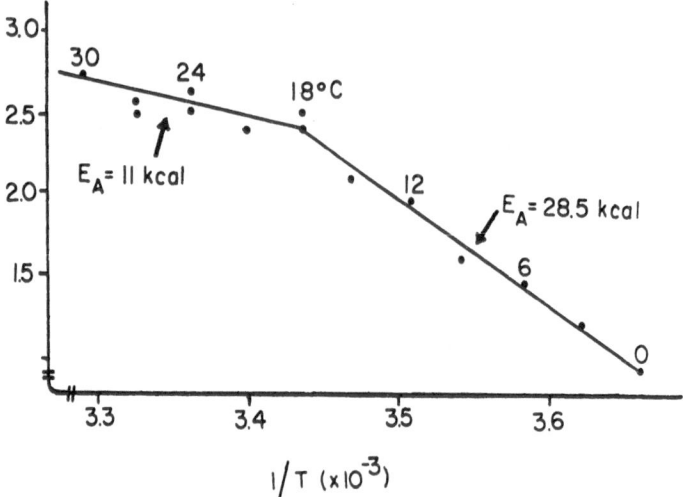

Figure 1.3 Temperature dependence of adenine nucleotide exchange as measured on rat liver mitochondria. (Modified from Pfaff *et al.*[15])

Intramitochondrial substrate flux is regulated for the most part by the oxidation–reduction state of the mitochondrial respiratory coenzymes. Substrate flux through the citric acid cycle may also be regulated by availability of acetyl-CoA from pyruvate and by disequilibrium sites in the citric acid cycle (i.e. citrate synthetase, isocitrate dehydrogenase and oxoglutarate dehydrogenase)[3]. There is evidence that Ca^{2+} entering the mitochondria in increased amounts during augmented cellular activity will increase the forward rates of these reactions; thus, in addition to cytosolic ADP the level of cytosolic Ca^{2+} may augment mitochondrial energy production[16].

Feedback control of cytosolic energy production, glycolysis, is exerted on phosphofructokinase by ATP and/or cytosolic citrate inhibition. In addition the glycolytic rate is controlled by the availability of cytosolic NAD. The mitochondrial membrane is impermeable to nicotinamide nucleotides and cytosolic NADH must be reoxidized to NAD in the cytosol or glycolysis ceases. During anaerobic glycolysis this is mediated by lactic

8

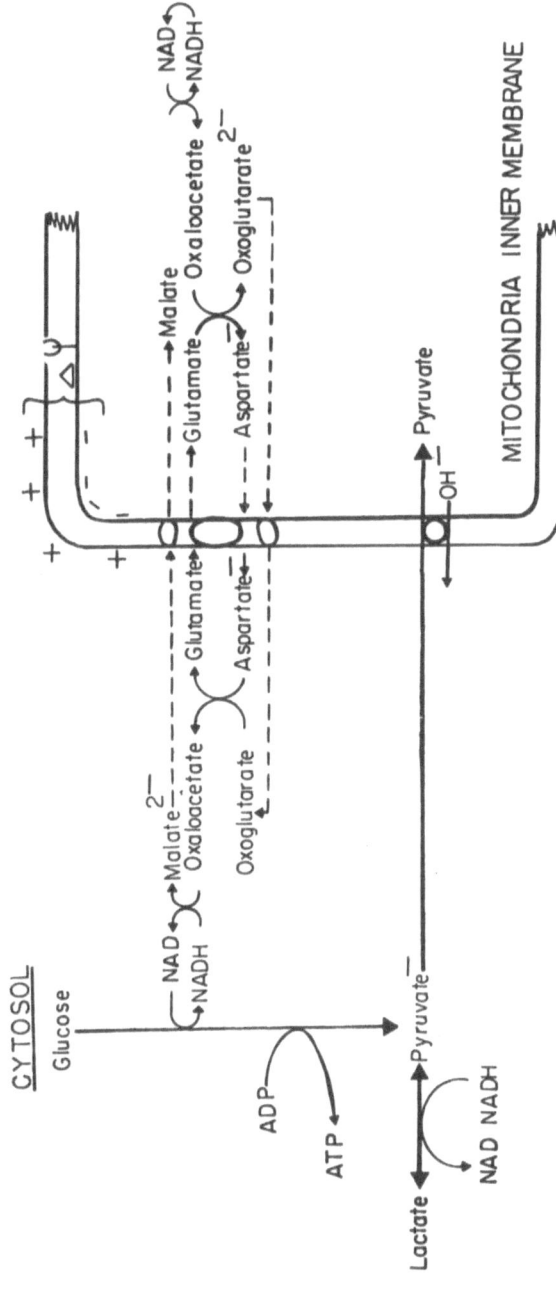

Figure 1.4 Scheme of the malate–aspartate shunt between cytosol and mitochondria. (Modified from Williamson et al.[17])

dehydrogenase which converts pyruvate to lactate. Under aerobic conditions cytosolic NADH is converted to NAD in a coupled reaction with cytosolic oxalacetate which is converted to malate (Figure 1.4). Malate enters the mitochondria in an electroneutral exchange with oxoglutarate and once inside it is reconverted to oxalacetate while intramitochondrial NAD is converted to NADH[14]. Thus malate serves as a shuttle of reducing equivalents across the mitochondrial membrane allowing glycolysis to continue[17]. Cytosolic oxalacetate used to produce malate is regenerated in a coupled reaction between aspartate and oxoglutarate. In this reaction aspartate is converted to glutamate. Cytosolic aspartate arises from mitochondrial aspartate and it is effluxed in exchange for glutamate. The exchange represents the net efflux of an anion and appears to be driven by the mitochondrial membrane potential.

The relatively impermeable inner mitochondrial membrane sustains several electroneutral exchanges that are important for cell function (Figure 1.5). Thus cytosolic P_i may enter mitochondria in exchange for OH^- and

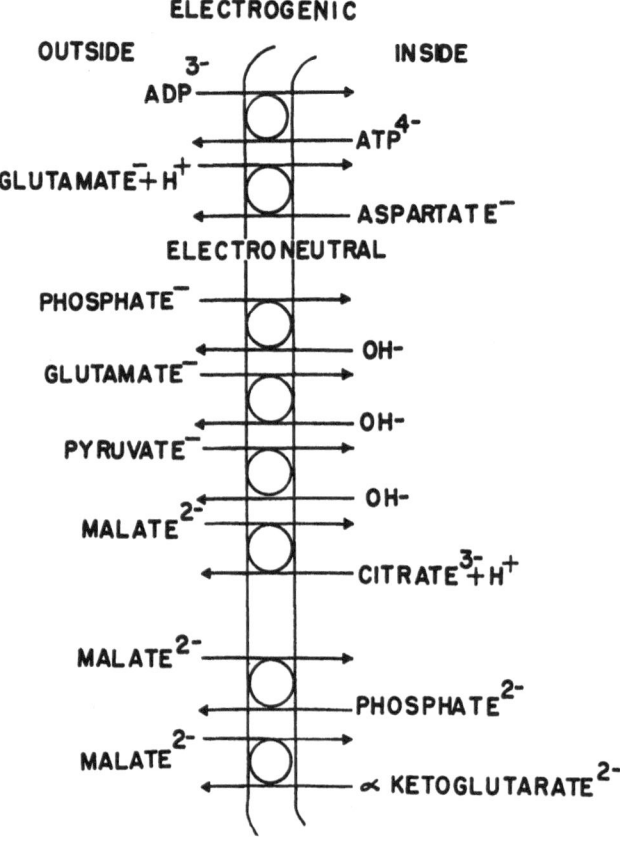

Figure 1.5 Anion translocation across the mitochondrial membrane. (Modified from Scarpa[18])

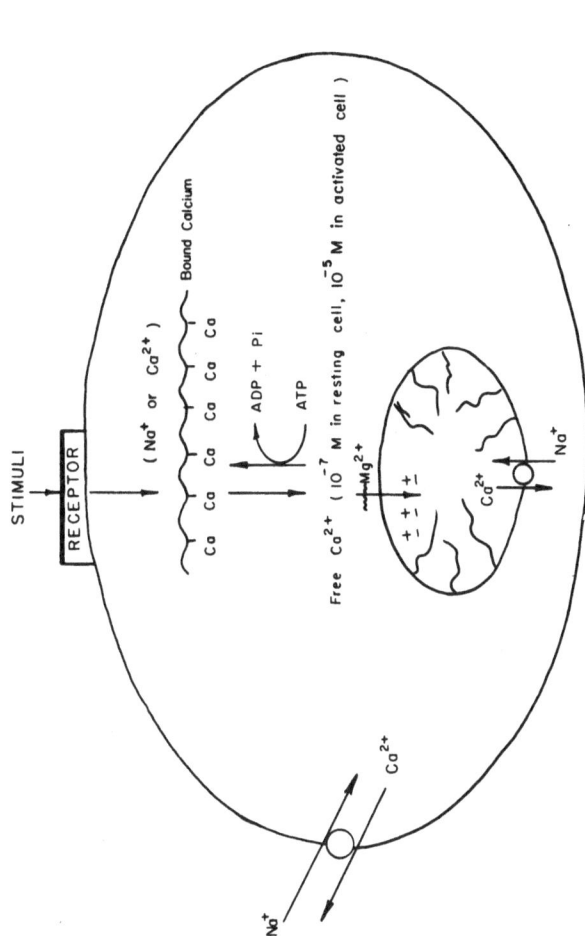

Figure 1.6 Scheme of cellular calcium movements. Shown is entry of Na^+ and/or Ca^{2+} as related to stimulation, e.g. the myocardial cell. Stimulation induces the release of calcium from bound sites (e.g. sarcoplasmic reticulum). Ca^{2+} is resequestered onto membranes or into mitochondria in an energy dependent reaction. Ca^{2+} may be effluxed in exchange for external Na^+ across the mitochondrial or plasma membrane

citrate plus a proton may exchange for malate[18]. In addition to the electrogenic exchange of ADP^{3-} for ATP^{4-} and of $glutamate^{1-}$ for $aspartate^{2-}$ mitochondria also take up Ca^{2+} on an electrogenic basis[19]. The K_m for Ca^{2+} in this process is quite low; Ca^{2+} binds to a carrier protein and enters the mitochondria on an electrical gradient due to the membrane potential[19].

Since it dissipates the membrane potential, the mitochondrial uptake of Ca^{2+} utilizes respiratory energy. The ability to sequester Ca^{2+} by mitochondria provides a means of maintaining the low cytosolic Ca^{2+} levels that are consistent with the role of Ca^{2+} as a second messenger in excitation–contraction and excitation–secretion coupling[20]. Organs appear to differ with respect to the importance of mitochondria relative to microsomal fractions (e.g. sarcoplasmic reticulum). In heart the presence of Mg^{2+} appears to play an inhibitory role in mitochondrial Ca^{2+} uptake[21]. Ca^{2+} is effluxed from mitochondria in an electroneutral exchange with Na^+. The co-ordinated mechanisms (Figure 1.6) maintaining low cytosolic Ca^{2+} allow for enzyme activation, contractile protein interaction and secretion as Ca^{2+} is increased[20]. Stimuli applied to such cells lead to Ca^{2+} entry and/or release of calcium bound to proteins. As mentioned earlier, increased Ca^{2+} associated with increased cell activity (e.g. greater contractility of cardiac muscle) may directly increase energy production reactions to balance increased energy expenditure[16].

If cells of transplanted organs are to remain normal or not be irreversibly damaged during storage, the integrity of energy coupling, the adenine nucleotide translocase activity and mechanisms regulating cytosolic Ca^{2+} must be preserved. As mentioned earlier there appears to be little spare catalytic capacity for adenine nucleotide translocation[13]. In addition nucleotide translocation exhibits a break in the Arrhenius plot of catalytic rate on temperature at $18\,°C$[15]. Hypothermic perfusion is usually carried out below $18\,°C$; therefore, the risk arises that, although oxidative phosphorylation rates are adequate to resynthesize ATP, mitochondrial exchange of cytosolic ADP for ATP becomes limiting. Provided energy utilization rates are sufficiently depressed by hypothermia a translocase limitation may not result in rapid failure of the perfused organ but rather a slow onset of failure due to loss of nucleotide from the cell.

The loss of adenine nucleotide from respiring cells depends on dephosphorylation (e.g. 5'-nucleotidase) reactions (Figure 1.7) and the high permeability of the resulting nucleosides. The 5'-nucleotidase reaction is a function of the cytosolic AMP level and it is inhibited by ADP and ATP[22]. AMP, ordinarily kept low by efficient translocase activity and oxidative phosphorylation, may increase as a result of the adenylate kinase reaction $(2ADP \leftrightarrow ATP + AMP)$. Adenosine, the product of the 5'-nucleotidase attack on AMP, is easily taken back into cells to form AMP in a reaction with adenosine kinase[23]. However, adenosine is easily and rapidly deaminated to inosine which must be degraded to hypoxanthine before it can be involved in a salvage reaction. The uptake of hypoxanthine, and the formation of ATP from it, is a much slower process than the salvage of adenosine[24]. Thus, although hypothermia may limit energy utilization, a

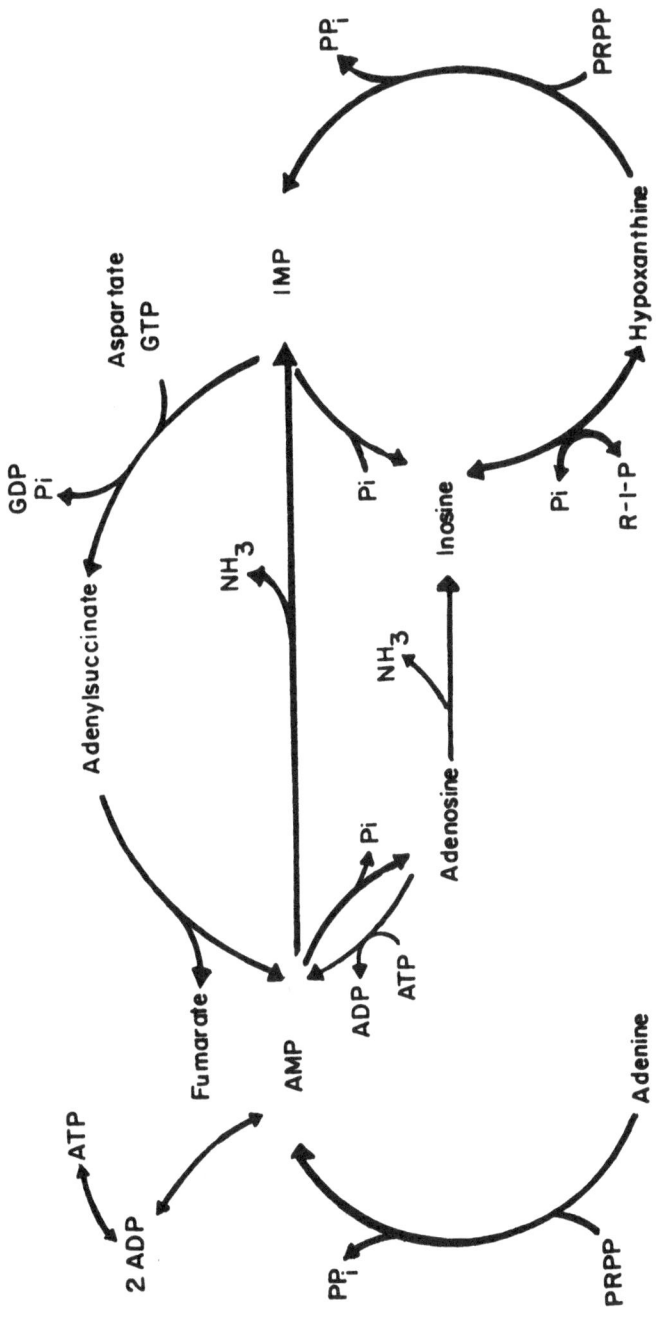

Figure 1.7 Scheme of adenine nucleotide metabolism. Shown on the left is the synthesis and catabolism of AMP. Loss of the phosphoryl group (5'-nucleotidase) leads to adenosine formation. Purine salvage of adenosine requires ATP. Purine salvage may also occur by means of the phosphoribosyl transferase reaction from adenine or hypoxanthine. (Modified from Krenitsky[27])

decrease in translocase activity could lead to loss of adenine nucleotides from the perfused organs.

Finally, a universal finding in deteriorating cells of perfused organs is increased cellular Ca^{2+}, particularly in mitochondria. The inward gradient for Ca^{2+} under most conditions of perfusion makes cells vulnerable to excessive Ca^{2+} entry or to reduced capacity to efflux Ca^{2+}. The Na/K ATPase enzyme which maintains low cellular Na^+ is indirectly the basis for Ca^{2+} efflux, as cellular Ca^{2+} is exchanged for Na^+ entering down its electrochemical gradient[25]. If ATP falls below the level needed to maintain adequate pump activity or if hypothermic perfusion decreases the capacity to pump out Na^+ then cell Ca^{2+} is likely to rise. The K_m for ATP in the Na/K ATPase reaction is quite high $(10^{-3}\,mol/l)$[26]. Thus, loss of cytoplasmic adenine nucleotides, even though the cytoplasmic phosphorylation potential is maintained, could result in an increase in cytosolic Ca^{2+} and an associated energy drain in sequestering it. In addition hypothermia reduces the rate of Na^+ efflux from cells exposed to a normal Na^+ gradient (i.e. 120–150 mmol/l) and thereby leads to an increase in cytosolic Ca^{2+}.

The challenge laid down by Belzer and Southard to extend the period during which organs can be preserved centred on the need for sound basic data. The issues raised in this cursory review, i.e. whether energy coupling, Ca^{2+} balance and adenine nucleotides are maintained by the present methodologies, seem to me among the most important and deserving in this connection.

References

1. Belzer, F.O. and Southard, J.H. (1980). The future of kidney preservation. *Transplantation,* **30,** 161
2. Feinberg, H., Gerola, A. and Katz, L.N. (1958). Effect of hypoxia on cardiac oxygen consumption and coronary flow. *Am. J. Physiol.,* **195,** 593
3. Hansford, R.G. (1980). Control of mitochondrial substrate oxidation. *Current topics of Bioenergetics,* **10,** 217
4. Weinstein, S.W. and Szyjewicz, J. (1974). Individual nephron function and renal oxygen consumption in the rat. *Am. J. Physiol.,* **227,** 171
5. Chance, B. and Williams, G.R. (1955). Respiratory enzymes in oxidative phosphorylation. III. The steady state. *J. Biol. Chem.,* **217,** 409
6. Boyer, P.D., Chance, B., Ernster, L., Mitchell, P., Racker, E. and Slater, E.C. (1977). Oxidative phosphorylation and photophosphorylation. *Annu. Rev. Biochem.,* **46,** 955
7. Mitchell, P. (1979). Compartmentation and communication in living systems. Ligand conduction: a general catalytic principle in chemical, osmotic and chemiosmotic reaction systems. *Eur. J. Biochem.,* **95,** 1
8. Williamson, J.R. (1979). Mitochondrial function in the heart. *Annu. Rev. Physiol.,* **41,** 485
9. Klingenberg, M. (1980). The ADP-ATP translocation in mitochondria, a membrane potential controlled transport. *J. Membrane Biol.,* **56,** 97
10. Coty, W.A. and Pedersen, P.L. (1975). Phosphate transport in rat liver mitochondria. *Mol. Cell. Biochem.,* **9,** 109
11. Erecinska, M., Wilson, D.F. and Nishiki, K. (1978). Homeostatic regulation of cellular energy metabolism: Experimental characterization in vivo and fit to a model. *Am. J. Physiol.: Cell Physiol.,* **3,** C82
12. Vignais, P.V. and Laugquin, G.L.M. (1979). Mitochondrial adenine nucleotide transport and its role in the economy of the cell. *Trends Biochem. Sci.,* **April,** 90

13. Lemasters, J.J. and Sowers, A.E. (1979). Phosphate-dependence and atractyloside inhibition of mitochondrial oxidative phosphorylation. The ADP–ATP carrier is rate-limiting. *J. Biol. Chem.*, **254**, 1248

14. Davis, E.J. and Lumeng, L. (1975). Relationships between the phosphorylation potentials generated by liver mitochondria and respiratory state under conditions of ADP control. *J. Biol. Chem.*, **250**, 2275

15. Pfaff, E., Heldt, H.W. and Klingenberg, M. (1969). Adenine nucleotide translocation of mitochondria, kinetics of the adenine nucleotide exchange. *Eur. J. Biochem.*, **10**, 484

16. Carafoli, E. (1980). Regulation of aerobic metabolism in muscle. In Cerretelli, P. and Whipp, B.J. (eds) *Exercise Bioenergetics and Gas Exchange*, pp. 3–12. (New York: Elsevier/North Holland Biomedical Press)

17. Williamson, J.R., Safer, B., La Noue, K.F., Smith, C.M. and Walajtys, E. (1973). Mitochondrial–cytosolic interactions in cardiac tissue: Role of the malate–aspartate cycle in the removal of glycolytic NADH from the cytosol. *Symp. Soc. Expt. Biol.*, **27**, 241

18. Scarpa, A. (1979). Transport across mitochondrial membranes. In P.C. Tosteson (ed.), *Transport across Single Biological Membranes*, Ch. 7, pp. 263–355. (New York: Springer-Verlag)

19. Fiskum, G. and Lehninger, A.L. (1980). The mechanisms and regulation of mitochondrial Ca^{2+} transport. *Fed. Proc.*, **39**, 2432

20. Rasmussen, H., Clayberger, C. and Gustin, M.C. (1979). The messenger function of calcium in cell activation. *Symp. Soc. Expt. Biol.*, **33**, 161

21. Jacobus, W.E., Tiozzo, R., Lugli, G., Lehninger, A.L. and Carafoli, E. (1975). Aspects of energy-linked calcium accumulation by rat heart mitochondria. *J. Biol. Chem.*, **250**, 7803

22. Frick, G.P. and Lowenstein, J.M. (1976). Studies of 5'-nucleotidase in the perfused rat heart. *J. Biol. Chem.*, **251**, 6372

23. Murray, A.W. (1971). The biological significance of purine salvage. *Annu. Rev. Biochem.*, **40**, 811

24. Liu, M.S. and Feinberg, H. (1971). Incorporation of [8-^{14}C]adenosine and [8-^{14}C]inosine into adenine nucleotides of perfused rabbit heart. *Am. J. Physiol.*, **220**, 1242

25. Blaustein, M.P. (1974). The interrelationship between sodium and calcium fluxes across cell membranes. *Rev. Physiol. Biochem. Pharmacol.*, **70**, 33

26. Post, R.L., Merritt, C.R., Kinsolving, C.R. and Albright, C.D. (1960). Membrane adenosine triphosphatase as a participant in the active transport of sodium and potassium in the human erythrocyte. *J. Biol. Chem.*, **235**, 1796

27. Krenitsky, T.A. (1969). Tissue distribution of purine and phosphoribosyl transferases in the Rhesus monkey. *Biochim. Biophys. Acta.*, **179**, 506

2
Membrane functions

M. J. PRINGLE

The use of hypothermic conditions for either storage or continuous perfusion of isolated organs has for some years been regarded as a prerequisite for their continuing viability. The rationale for such approaches has remained, however, largely empirical, and is based on the principle that if metabolism is responsible for tissue deterioration, and metabolic processes are temperature-dependent, then a reduction in temperature should lead to extended survival of isolated organs. The very fact that the application of hypothermic techniques has met with some success has proved to be a mixed blessing. On the one hand it has generated much research effort devoted to optimizing both the composition of perfusing media and the operating temperature. On the other hand it has tended to obscure a detailed appraisal of the effects of temperature *per se* on cell function.

It is perhaps not fully appreciated that temperature modulates not only biological processes occurring within tissue cells, but also the structure and function of the cell membranes. Thus, although low temperatures often lead to prolonged survival of isolated tissue, survival is of limited duration and, for example, the loss of mitochondrial function which accompanies hypothermic storage of kidneys, can be attributed, among other factors, to alterations in the mitochondrial membranes. It is, of course, relatively easy to explain the gross cell damage which arises from sub-zero temperatures although even in these circumstances the mechanism of action of cryo-preservatives used for sub-zero protection appears to be more complex than simply the prevention of ice formation. Less severe hypothermia carries with it implications which should be of no less importance to the organ preservationist, and it is the purpose of this chapter to provide a brief outline of the role of temperature in modulating the structure and function of cell membranes. Although much of the experimental data described here derives from a variety of biophysical techniques, it would be beyond the scope of the present chapter to explain either the underlying theory or the experimental methodology.

The first part of this chapter will be devoted to structural considerations, i.e. membrane composition and organization, while the remainder will deal with the interrelationship between structure and function, and the way in which both aspects are modified by changes in temperature.

MEMBRANE STRUCTURE AND ORGANIZATION

Membrane composition

The basic components of all cell membranes are lipids, proteins, and cholesterol. Although an oversimplification, it can be generally assumed that structure resides with the lipid moiety, while proteins provide the functional elements. It will be shown later that cholesterol modulates cell function primarily by its interaction with membrane lipids. Most membrane lipids are derived either from glycerol-3-phosphate or sphingosine (see below):

$$CH = CH \ (CH_2)_{12}CH_3$$

$CH_2 — OH^*$	$CH — OH$
$CH — OH^*$	$CH — NH_2^*$
$CH_2 — OPO_3^{\ominus}{}^{**}$	$CH_2 — OH^{**}$
glycerol-3-phosphate	sphingosine

To those positions marked *, long-chain fatty acids are attached by ester linkages in the case of phospholipids and by an amide linkage in the case of the sphingolipids. To complete the molecules, head-group substituents such as choline, serine, ethanolamine, or sugars are attached to the positions marked **. The wide range of lipids encountered in biomembranes is due not only to variations in the head-groups, but also to the large number of naturally occurring fatty acids. These consist of long, even-numbered hydrocarbon chains which can be fully saturated or partially unsaturated. Although phospholipids are the main lipid class found in cell membranes[1], an individual membrane will contain a wide spectrum of different lipids within this class owing to the large number of possible combinations of head-group and fatty acid. It is also important to realize that the total amount of lipid present in a membrane varies from one cell type to another[2].

Membrane organization

The consensus view of membrane structure remains that which was formalized nearly a decade ago by Singer and Nicolson[3] in terms of a 'fluid-mosaic' arrangement of lipids and proteins. The lipids themselves are aligned in the form of a bilayer with the polar head-groups comprising the inner and outer membrane surfaces, while the long fatty acid chains extend into the membrane interior. These acyl chains are packed together in a more or less parallel manner at right angles to the plane of the membrane.

Membrane proteins are inserted into the lipid matrix such that some are partially submerged in the inner or outer half of the bilayer, while others span the entire width of the membrane. In general terms the shape and disposition of a membrane protein is determined by its biological function.

Thus, ion-carrier proteins are relatively small entities which are able to diffuse from one side of the membrane to the other, while ion-channel proteins can be relatively large, stable structures containing a polar core through which ions can pass, or alternatively they may consist of aggregates of subunits arranged to form a central channel[4]. There is now good evidence that a large number of membrane proteins including cyto-chrome-C oxidase[5], rhodopsin[6], and the acetylcholine receptor[7], span the bilayer and protrude asymmetrically above the two membrane surfaces.

Implicit in the Singer–Nicolson model is the idea of movement within the plane of the membrane, and it will be shown later that lipid composition and temperature are fundamental determinants in the degree of motion which membrane proteins are able to undergo. In order to function as an enzyme, ion-channel, or biological 'trigger' (hormone and neurotrans-mitter receptors), integral proteins must be capable of reversible structural changes. These may involve lateral translation or rotational diffusion of the entire protein molecule, or subtle movements of small segments of the tertiary structure. While some protein conformational changes, for example in excitable membranes, may arise from a direct effect of the electrical field across the membrane (movement of charged groups or dipole realignment), there is now a considerable body of evidence which links protein mobility within the membrane to the fluid nature of the lipid bilayer.

Lipid fluidity

Much of our knowledge of the behaviour of membrane lipids derives from the use of simple model systems. Thus, when a pure phospholipid is dispersed in aqueous buffer it spontaneously forms multilamellar structures known as liposomes[8]. These consist of concentric spheres of lipid arranged in bilayers where each sphere is separated by an aqueous compart-ment. Sonication reduces them to single-shelled liposomes, 200–500 Å in diameter[9]. Such models have proved invaluable in studying structural properties of cell membranes as well as the intra- and extracellular transport of small molecules and ions.

The lipid acyl chains in the bilayer undergo continuous thermal motion, and a variety of so-called spectroscopic probe techniques such as electron spin resonance[10,11], nuclear magnetic resonance[12,13], and fluorescence polarization[14,15], enable one to quantitate this motion and to calculate the degree of order in which the lipid acyl chains are packed together. Most of these methods rely on the use of small 'reporter' molecules (or groups attached to membrane components), where the spectroscopic properties of the molecular 'probes' are dependent upon their microenvironment (fluidity or microviscosity). Taken together, these studies indicate that the interior of a lipid bilayer is in a highly fluid or disordered state. However, the degree of fluidity decreases as one probes outwards, towards the membrane surfaces. Thus, the regions close to the polar head-groups are in a *relatively* ordered state. It has also been established that the degree of order of a lipid membrane depends upon the lipid class, the length of the hydrocarbon chains, and the number of double bonds in the chains. Since these effects are intimately related to the temperature-dependent properties of the lipids, they will be discussed in more detail in the following section. Nevertheless, it should be emphasized that the function of membrane proteins is in many cases critically dependent upon the fluid nature of the lipid environment surrounding them.

TEMPERATURE-DEPENDENT PROPERTIES

Thermotropic behaviour

A key to the understanding of lipids in membranes lies in their so-called thermotropic behaviour. When liposomes (uni- or multilamellar) are prepared from a single type of lipid there is a characteristic temperature at which an abrupt change occurs in the physical state of the lipid. This is known as a phase transition temperature[16]. Most pure lipids exhibit several phase transitions but in the context of biomembranes and cell behaviour, I shall discuss only the main transition temperature, T_c (strictly speaking, the temperature range).

Below T_c, the lipids are arranged in a rigid, hexagonally-packed, crystalline lattice with the hydrocarbon chains in the fully extended (all-*trans*) conformation. This phase is known as the gel state. At the transition temperature, heat is absorbed, there is a sudden increase in thermal motion, and a number of 'kinks' (gauche conformers) appear in the hydrocarbon chains. Above T_c, then, the lipid chains are in a fluid, disordered state. Since the overall structure of the lipid membrane is maintained, this state is known as the liquid crystalline phase. Phase transitions are frequently discussed in terms of their co-operativity, i.e. the efficiency with which heat is dissipated throughout the bilayer. In bilayers consisting of a single type of lipid, thermal energy is very efficiently transmitted from one lipid chain to another. Hence, the main transition is highly co-operative and occurs over a very narrow temperature range. One can measure transition temperatures by many of the spectroscopic probe techniques referred to previously. Alternatively, one can employ differential scanning calorimetry to actually measure the heat absorbed by the liposome dispersion as a function of temperature[17,18]. In the diacylphosphatidylcholine series of lipids, it has been shown that T_c increases with the chain length of the fatty acids and is markedly lowered with increasing unsaturation. Thus, dipalmitoylphosphatidylcholine (a major component of membrane lipids, with $C_{16:0}$ chains) undergoes the main transition at *ca.* 41 °C, a few degrees above the physiological temperature of 37 °C. On the other hand, distearoylphosphatidylcholine ($C_{18:0}$) is in the gel phase below 54 °C, while its mono-unsaturated analogue dioleoylphosphatidylcholine

($C_{18:1}$) remains fluid down to $-22\,°C^{16}$. In bilayers consisting of simple mixtures of lipids, as the temperature is lowered the lipids may (if there is considerable chain mis-matching) crystallize separately[17,19,20] at their respective T_cs. This results in what is called lateral phase separation, where at temperatures between the component T_cs, there exist regions of liquid crystalline lipid and regions of gel-state lipid.

Most natural cell membranes contain a heterogeneous mixture of lipids comprising a variety of fatty acid chains and polar head-groups. Since the respective T_cs encompass a wide temperature range, the thermotropic behaviour of most cell membranes is characterized by very broad, weakly co-operative transitions and lateral phase separations. Furthermore, the presence of cholesterol and membrane proteins has a profound effect on the thermal properties of membranes at low temperature.

Cholesterol

Cholesterol, when it is present, is randomly distributed throughout each half of the membrane bilayer. Model studies with cholesterol-containing liposomes have established that above the lipid T_c, i.e. when the lipid is in the liquid crystalline state, cholesterol reduces fluidity by restricting the thermal motion of the fatty acid hydrocarbon chains[21]. On the other hand, below T_c cholesterol prevents the transition from occurring so that the lipid remains in a fluid state[22,23]. It would seem that cholesterol serves to maintain the cell membrane in a state of optimal fluidity for the normal functioning of integral proteins. It should, however, be appreciated that the sensitivity of a particular membrane to low-temperature crystallization will depend upon the fatty acid composition of the lipids and also upon the amount of cholesterol present. Both of these parameters show a widespread natural variation[2]. Thus, normal erythrocytes do not undergo a phase transition which can be detected calorimetrically, whereas cholesterol-depleted erythrocytes display a very broad transition at low temperature[24].

Cell growth

A great deal of the information concerning the relationship between membrane fluidity and thermotropism on the one hand, and cell growth and viability on the other, stems from bacterial cell culture studies where the membrane lipid composition can often be experimentally controlled by manipulating the fatty acids in the growth media[25,26]. In such cases it has been shown that growth rate is dependent upon the lipid fatty acid composition, and that growth itself can be severely inhibited or abolished if the temperature is below the membrane phase transition, i.e. when the lipids are in the gel state.

Lipid–protein interactions

The effects of intrinsic proteins on the lipid matrix of a cell membrane are complex. In some respects proteins mimic the effect of cholesterol on temperature-dependent properties. For example, the addition of myelin apoprotein to bilayers of dimyristoylphosphatidylcholine broadens the phase transition and, at a high enough concentration, completely abolishes it[27]. This reduction in transition co-operativity can be understood in terms of packing faults introduced into the bilayer by the presence of a relatively large molecule[28]. If the protein concentration is not too high and the temperature is lowered to induce lipid crystallization, membrane proteins will be squeezed out of the crystal lattice because of the packing faults, and a phase separation will occur. This is analogous to the effect of low temperature on a mixed lipid membrane, and it results in a dramatic change in the lateral distribution of membrane components. Whereas in the normal cell membrane the components are randomly distributed, a phase separation will give rise to discrete regions of crystalline, gel state lipid, and clusters of protein aggregates. This phenomenon has been clearly illustrated in electron microscopic studies of lipid vesicles containing the enzyme $Ca^{2+}ATPase$[29].

When we consider the effect of low temperature on protein function we must therefore take into account not only purely kinetic effects, i.e. a reduction in the rate of biochemical processes, but also the possibility of protein aggregation arising from lateral phase separations. Mention has already been made of the role of cholesterol in maintaining membrane fluidity, and recent evidence has shown that cholesterol-depleted thymocytes exhibit both dysfunction and protein aggregation even at 37 °C[30,31].

Measurements of protein rotational diffusion in a biomembrane are a relatively recent innovation[32] but examples have been found where there is a good correlation between the activity of certain membrane-bound enzymes and their ability to undergo rotational motion[33]. However, one cannot make any generalization concerning the functional significance of either rotational or lateral diffusion of membrane proteins. Thus rhodopsin in retinal rod outer segment membranes exhibits extremely rapid motion[34], whereas the integral proteins of the erythrocyte membrane are severely restricted[35], presumably by interactions with the cytoskeletal network[36].

Enzyme activity

It is customary to describe the temperature-dependent activity of enzymes in terms of Arrhenius plots which normally yield linear relationships, provided that the activation energy for the catalytic reaction is constant throughout the temperature range studied. In the case of membrane-bound enzymes this is not always so, and one often finds that at low temperatures the enzyme activity is *less* than would be predicted by extrapolating from high temperatures[37,38]. This is highly indicative of a change occurring in the membrane structure at a particular temperature. For example, the

Arrhenius plot of Ca^{2+}ATPase activity in sarcoplasmic reticulum shows a discontinuity at about 17 °C. However, it is not clear whether this is due to a phase change in the membrane lipids[39], or a conformational change in the protein structure[33].

CONCLUSION

The components of cell membranes are normally randomly distributed in the plane of the membrane, and they exist in dynamic equilibrium with each other. Lowering the temperature of the system can upset this equilibrium by reducing membrane fluidity and by inducing lateral phase separations between different lipids and between lipids and proteins. This may have specific consequences in terms of the functional elements. For example, cardiac activity is controlled by membrane-bound enzymes and it is known that a heart-beat cannot be sustained below 15 °C in non-hibernating animals[40]. Since homeoviscous adaptation to hypothermia involves an increased uptake of unsaturated fatty acids into membrane lipids, it may prove plausible to extend the viability of isolated organs held at low temperatures, by experimentally fluidizing the cell membranes. Anaesthetic agents are known to have this property[41] and current theories suggest that they may act either in this manner or by lowering lipid phase transition temperatures[42]. Such agents, or other similar compounds may prove useful as fluidizing aids in organ preservation.

References

1. Ansell, G. B. and Hawthorne, J. N. (1964). *Phospholipids, Chemistry, Metabolism and Function*. (Amsterdam: Elsevier)
2. Quinn, P. J. (1976). *The Molecular Biology of Cell Membranes*. (London: Macmillan)
3. Singer, S. J. and Nicolson, G. L. (1972). The fluid mosaic model of the structure of cell membranes. *Science*, **175**, 720
4. Singer, S. J. (1977). The fluid mosaic model of membrane structure. In Abrahamsson, S. and Pascher, I. (eds) *Structure of Biological Membranes*, pp. 443–461. (New York: Plenum Press)
5. Henderson, R., Capaldi, R. A. and Leigh, J. S. (1977). Arrangement of cytochrome oxidase molecules in two-dimensional vesicle crystals. *J. Mol. Biol.*, **112**, 631
6. Rosenkranz, J. (1977). New aspects of the ultrastructure of frog rod outer segments. *Int. Rev. Cytol.*, **50**, 25
7. Ross, M. J., Klymkowsky, M. W., Agard, D. A. and Stroud, R. M. (1977). Structural studies of a membrane-bound acetylcholine receptor from *Torpedo californica*. *J. Mol. Biol.*, **116**, 635
8. Bangham, A. D., Standish, M. M. and Watkins, J. C. (1965). Diffusion of univalent ions across the lamellae of swollen phospholipids. *J. Mol. Biol.*, **13**, 238
9. Huang, C. (1969). Studies on phosphatidylcholine vesicles. Formation and physical characteristics. *Biochemistry*, **8**, 344
10. Hubbell, W. L. and McConnell, H. M. (1971). Molecular motion in spin-labeled phospholipids and membranes. *J. Am. Chem. Soc.*, **93**, 314
11. Jost, P., Waggoner, A. S. and Griffith, O. H. (1971). Spin labelling and membrane structure. In Rothfield, L. I. (ed.), *Structure and Function of Biological Membranes*, pp. 83–144. (New York and London: Academic Press)

12. Horowitz, A. F., Horstey, W. J. and Klein, M. P. (1972). Magnetic resonance studies on membrane and model membrane systems: proton magnetic relaxation rates in sonicated lecithin dispersions. *Proc. Natl. Acad. Sci. USA,* **69**, 590

13. Seelig, J. and Niederberger, W. (1974). Deuterium-labeled lipids as structural probes in liquid crystalline bilayers. A deuterium magnetic resonance study. *J. Am. Chem. Soc.,* **96**, 2069

14. Shinitzky, M., Dianoux, A. C., Gitler, C. and Weber, G. (1971). Microviscosity and order in the hydrocarbon region of micelles and membranes determined with fluorescent probes. I Synthetic micelles. *Biochemistry,* **10**, 2106

15. Cogan, U., Shinitzky, M., Weber, G. and Nishida, T. (1973). Microviscosity and order in the hydrocarbon region of phospholipid and phospholipid-cholesterol dispersions determined with fluorescent probes. *Biochemistry,* **12**, 521

16. Chapman, D. (1975). Phase transitions and fluidity characteristics of lipids and cell membranes. *Q. Rev. Biophys.,* **8**, 185

17. Ladbrooke, B. D. and Chapman, D. (1969). Thermal analysis of lipids, proteins and biological membranes. *Chem. Phys. Lipids,* **3**, 304

18. Hinz, H. J. and Sturtevant, J. M. (1972). Calorimetric investigation of the influence of cholesterol on the transition properties of bilayers formed from synthetic L-α-lecithins in aqueous suspension. *J. Biol. Chem.,* **247**, 3697

19. Oldfield, E. and Chapman, D. (1972). Dynamics of lipids in membranes: heterogeneity and the role of cholesterol. *FEBS Lett.,* **23**, 285

20. Chapman, D., Urbina, J. and Keough, K. M. (1974). Biomembrane phase transitions. Studies of lipid–water systems using differential scanning calorimetry. *J. Biol. Chem.,* **249**, 2512

21. Phillips, M. C. and Finer, E. G. (1974). The stoichiometry and dynamics of lecithin–cholesterol clusters in bilayer membranes. *Biochim. Biophys. Acta,* **356**, 199

22. Ladbrooke, B. D., Williams, R. M. and Chapman, D. (1968). Studies on lecithin–cholesterol-water interactions by differential scanning calorimetry and X-ray diffraction. *Biochim. Biophys. Acta,* **150**, 333

23. Schreier-Muccillo, S., Marsh, D., Dugas, H., Schneider, H. and Smith, I. C. P. (1973). A spin probe study of the influence of cholesterol on the motion and orientation of phospholipids in oriented multi-bilayers and vesicles. *Chem. Phys. Lipids,* **10**, 11

24. Ladbrooke, B. D., Jenkinson, T. J., Kamat, V. B. and Chapman, D. (1968). Physical studies of myelin. 1. Thermal analysis. *Biochim. Biophys. Acta,* **164**, 101

25. Chapman, D. and Urbina, J. (1971). Phase transition and bilayer structure of *Mycoplasma laidlawii*. *FEBS Lett.,* **12**, 169

26. Fox, F. C. and Tsukagoshi, T. (1972). The influence of lipid phase transitions on membrane function and assembly. In Fox, C. F. (ed.), *Membrane Research,* p. 145. (London and New York: Academic Press)

27. Curatolo, W., Verma, S. P., Sakura, J. D., Small, D. M., Shipley, G. G. and Wallach, D. F. H. (1978). Structural effects of myelin proteolipid apoprotein on phospholipids: a Raman spectroscopic study. *Biochemistry,* **17**, 1802

28. Chapman, D., Cornell, B. A. and Quinn, P. J. (1977). Phase transitions, protein aggregation and a new method for modulating membrane fluidity. In Semenza, G. and Carafoli, E. (eds) *Biochemistry of Membrane Transport.* FEBS-Symposium No. 42, pp. 72–85. (Berlin: Springer)

29. Hoffmann, W., Sarzala, G. M., Gomez-Fernandez, J. C., Goni, F. M., Restall, C. J., Chapman, D., Heppeler, G. and Kreutz, W. (1980). Protein rotational diffusion and lipid structure of reconstituted systems of Ca^{2+} activated adenosine triphosphate. *J. Mol. Biol.,* **141**, 119

30. Bottomley, J. M., Kramers, M. T. C. and Chapman, D. (1980). Cholesterol depletion from biomembranes of murine lymphocytes and human tonsil lymphocytes. *FEBS Lett.,* **119**, 261

31. Kramers, M. T. C., Patrick, J., Bottomley, J. M., Quinn, P. J. and Chapman, D. (1980). Studies of liposome interactions with rat thymocytes. *Eur. J. Biochem.,* **110**, 579

32. Cherry, R. J. (1979). Rotational and lateral diffusion of membrane proteins. *Biochim. Biophys. Acta,* **559**, 289

33. Hoffmann, W., Sarzala, M. G. and Chapman, D. (1979). Rotational motion and evidence for oligomeric structures of sarcoplasmic reticulum Ca^{2+}-activated ATPase. *Proc. Natl. Acad. Sci. USA,* **76,** 3860

34. Poo, M. M. and Cone, R. A. (1974). Lateral diffusion of rhodopsin in the photoreceptor membrane. *Nature (Lond.),* **247,** 438

35. Fowler, V. and Branton, D. (1977). Lateral mobility of human erythrocyte integral membrane proteins. *Nature (Lond.),* **268,** 23

36. Elgsaeter, A. and Branton, D. (1974). Intramembrane particle aggregation in erythrocyte ghosts. I. The effects of protein removal. *J. Cell Biol.,* **63,** 1018

37. Kimelberg, H. K. and Papahadjopoulos, D. (1972). Phospholipid requirements for (Na^+-K^+)-ATPase activity, head-group specificity and fatty acid fluidity. *Biochim. Biophys. Acta,* **282,** 277

38. Feo, F., Canuto, R. A., Garcea, R., Avogadro, A., Villa, M. and Celasco, M. (1976). Lipid phase transition and breaks in the Arrhenius plots of membrane-bound enzymes in mitochondria from normal rat liver and hepatoma AH-130. *FEBS Lett.,* **72,** 262

39. Inesi, G., Millman, M. and Eletr, S. (1973). Temperature-induced transitions of function and structure in sarcoplasmic reticulum membranes. *J. Mol. Biol.,* **81,** 483

40. Hensel, H., Bruck, K. and Raths, P. (1973). In Precht, H., Christopherson, J., Hensel, H. and Larcher, W. (eds) *Temperature and Life,* p. 505. (Berlin: Springer)

41. Miller, K. W. and Pang, K-Y. Y. (1976). General anaesthetics can selectively perturb bilayer membranes. *Nature (Lond.),* **263,** 253

42. Trudell, J. R., Payan, D. G., Chin, J. H. and Cohen, E. N. (1975). The antagonistic effect of an inhalation anesthetic and high pressure on the phase diagram of mixed dipalmitoyl–dimyristoyl phosphatidylcholine bilayers. *Proc. Natl. Acad. Sci., USA,* **72,** 210

3
Biological significance and therapeutic potential of prostacyclin*

S. MONCADA and J. R. VANE

Prostacyclin and thromboxane A_2 (TXA$_2$) are both derived from arachidonic acid, a fatty acid present in the phospholipids of cell membranes. TXA$_2$ is an unstable ($t_{\frac{1}{2}}$ 30 s at 37 °C), powerful vaso-constrictor agent generated by platelets[1]. Prostacyclin is also unstable ($t_{\frac{1}{2}}$ 3 min at 37 °C) but induces vasodilatation and inhibits platelet aggregation. Prostacyclin and thromboxane A_2 represent, therefore, the opposite poles of a homeostatic mechanism for regulation of platelet aggregability *in vivo*. Manipulation of this control mechanism will affect thrombus and haemo-static plug formation.

The generation of TXA$_2$ in platelets is inhibited by aspirin and other aspirin-like drugs[2] and this is why, prior to the discovery of prostacyclin, aspirin was widely canvassed as an antithrombotic drug. However, it is now clear that these drugs also inhibit prostacyclin formation in the vessel wall and therefore might have the opposite effect.

We have also suggested that drugs which effectively inhibit TXA$_2$ formation will have a superior antithrombotic effect to aspirin. Several of these drugs are now being synthesized and could be ready for testing in humans within the next few years (for extensive review of this point see ref. 3).

Prostacyclin inhibits platelet aggregation by stimulating adenylate cyclase, leading to an increase in cAMP levels in the platelets[4,5]. In this respect prostacyclin is much more potent than either PGE$_1$ or PGD$_2$[5]. In contrast, prostaglandin endoperoxides and TXA$_2$ reduce a raised cAMP activity in platelets[6]. Because of these opposite effects we and others have suggested that a balance between TXA$_2$ and prostacyclin formation regulates platelet cAMP *in vivo* and therefore platelet aggregability. Unlike other prostaglandins such as PGE$_2$ and PGF$_{2\alpha}$, prostacyclin is not inactivated on passage through the pulmonary circulation[7]. Indeed, the lungs constantly release small amounts of prostacyclin into the passing blood perhaps from the huge mass of endothelial cells present[8,9]. The

* This chapter was previously published in *Advanced Medicine 17*, and is reproduced by permission of the authors and the publishers, Pitman Medical Limited, Tunbridge Wells, U.K.

concentration of prostacyclin is higher in arterial than in venous blood for there is about 50% overall inactivation in one circulation through peripheral tissues[7]. This difference, originally obtained in experimental animals, has now been confirmed in humans[10].

Platelets, therefore, may be constantly stimulated by circulating prostacyclin and consequently they may have higher cAMP levels and be less aggregable than has ever been detected by *in vitro* measurements which are only made after a 10–30 min delay during which the blood is processed. In this period, prostacyclin and its effects will decay. Thus, prostacyclin protects the vessel wall against deposition of platelet aggregates and its discovery provides at least a partial explanation of the long-recognized fact that contact with healthy vascular endothelium is not a stimulus for platelet clumping.

Damage to a vessel is followed by platelet adhesion. The degree of injury is an important determinant and there is general agreement that, for the development of thrombosis, severe damage or physical detachment of the endothelium must occur. These observations are in accordance with the distribution of prostacyclin synthetase, for it is abundant in the intima and progressively decreases in concentration from the intima to the adventitia[11]. Moreover, the pro-aggregating elements increase from the sub-endothelium to the adventitia. These two opposing tendencies render the endothelial lining antiaggregatory and the outer layers of the vessel wall much more thrombogenic.

Prostacyclin inhibits aggregation (platelet–platelet interaction) at much lower concentrations than those needed to inhibit adhesion (platelet–collagen interaction) suggesting that prostacyclin allows platelets to stick to damaged vascular tissue and interact with it, while at the same time preventing or limiting thrombus formation[12]. This process of platelet–vessel wall interaction might be important for vessel repair and regeneration.

Lipid peroxides are potent inhibitors of prostacyclin synthetase[13] and selective inhibition of prostacyclin formation by these substances could lead to increased platelet aggregation which in turn could play a role in the development of atherosclerosis. Indeed, lipid peroxidation takes place in plasma as a non-enzymic reaction and it is known to occur in certain pathological conditions[14,15]. Hence, lipid peroxides present in these conditions could be shifting the balance of the system in favour of TXA_2 and may predispose to thrombus formation. In this context it is interesting that there is a strong reduction in prostacyclin formation by the heart or vessel walls of rabbits made atherosclerotic[16]. Similarly, human atherosclerotic tissue does not produce prostacyclin, whereas tissue obtained from a nearby normal vessel does[17].

The role of lipid peroxides in the development of atherosclerosis has been debated for almost 30 years since Glavind and collaborators described the presence of lipid peroxides in human atherosclerotic aortae[15]. They found the peroxide content in diseased arteries to be directly proportional to the severity of the atherosclerosis. Others suggested that Glavind's findings were artefactual, the presence of lipid peroxides being due to their formation during the preparative procedure[18], but others have given support to Glavind's work favouring the suggestion that lipid peroxides are present in atherosclerotic plaques[19]. Whether or not these peroxides act by inhibiting prostacyclin formation and as a consequence reduce the wall's defence mechanism is not clear, but the theory is of interest, especially since other substances related to atherosclerosis such as the cholesterol carriers, low-density lipoproteins (LDL), have also been shown to inhibit prostacyclin formation in endothelial cell cultures[20].

In the few years since the discovery of the PGI_2/TXA_2 balance there are already descriptions of clinical conditions in which the balance might be disturbed. Increased production of TXA_2 *in vitro* by platelets has been found in patients with arterial thrombosis or recurrent venous thrombosis[21]. These conditions are associated with a shortened platelet survival time. In addition, increased sensitivity to aggregating agents and increased release of TXA_2-like activity has been described in rabbits made atherosclerotic by diet[22], and in patients who have survived myocardial infarction[23]. Increased levels of TXB_2 (the stable degradation product of TXA_2) have also been observed in patients with angina during attacks[24]. Moreover, platelets from rats made diabetic release more TXA_2 and their vessel walls produce less prostacyclin[25,26]; these effects are reversed by chronic insulin treatment[25]. Prostacyclin production by blood vessels from patients with diabetes is depressed[27] and circulating levels of 6-oxo-$PGF_{1\alpha}$ are reduced in diabetic patients with proliferative retinopathy[28]. Other diseases associated with changes in prostacyclin production include uraemia, where the haemostatic defect occurring in uraemic patients may be attributable to increased prostacyclin production[29]. On the other hand, a lack of prostacyclin production has been suggested in patients with thrombotic thrombocytopenic purpura[30]. Both diseases are linked by the accumulation during uraemia, or the lack of production during thrombotic thrombocytopaenic purpura, of an ill-defined 'plasma factor' which stimulates prostacyclin synthesis[31]. Finally, increased prostacyclin production has been described in blood vessels of the spontaneously hypertensive rat[32].

As yet, a clear relationship between different diseases and the PGI_2/TXA_2 balance is not established. However, it seems that conditions which favour the development of thrombosis are associated with an increase in TXA_2 and a decrease in prostacyclin formation, whereas an increased prostacyclin formation plus decreased TXA_2 is present in some conditions associated with an increased bleeding tendency.

Prostacyclin or chemical analogues may find a use as a 'hormone replacement' therapy in conditions in which excessive platelet aggregation takes place in the circulation, such as acute myocardial infarction or 'crescendo angina'; it might also be useful in deep vein thrombosis, different types of shock, disseminated intravascular coagulation and organ transplantation. Moreover, we have suggested its use in extracorporeal circulation systems[33], in which the main problems are platelet loss with the formation of micro-aggregates. In cardiopulmonary bypass, micro-aggregates returning to the patient are thought to be responsible for the cerebral and renal impairment sometimes observed[34]. In addition, there are side-effects associated with the chronic use of heparin, especially the development of osteoporosis[35].

Several antiplatelet drugs have been tested in extracorporeal circulations, some with moderate success. PGE_1 has been reported to be beneficial during cardiopulmonary bypass[36]. However, prostaglandins of the E type induce diarrhoea, an effect not shared by prostacyclin[37,38]. Therefore, prostacyclin is not only more potent but more specific in achieving platelet protection. Prostacyclin has now been beneficially used in several systems of extracorporeal circulation in experimental animals and man, including renal dialysis[39], cardiopulmonary bypass[40] and charcoal haemo-perfusion[41,42]. In one of these systems (renal dialysis), prostacyclin can replace heparin altogether[39]. In charcoal haemoperfusion, heparin is also necessary since charcoal particles seem to activate directly the clotting cascade[41].

Following reports that PGE_1 has been used successfully in the treatment of peripheral vascular disease[43], prostacyclin has been shown to have a similar effect, producing a long-lasting increase in muscle blood flow, dis-appearance of ischaemic pain and healing of trophic ulcers after an intra-arterial infusion to the affected limb for 3 days[44]. In a subsequent trial in 30 patients, symptoms were alleviated in 40% for up to 2 months after treatment, while a further 40% exhibited clinical improvement for up to 15 months[45].

Antithrombotic drugs which act on platelets have largely been cyclo-oxygenase inhibitors, the foremost example being aspirin. A newer approach would be represented by the thromboxane synthetase inhibitors, which might have a superior antithrombotic effect as discussed above. However, the arachidonic acid pathway of platelet aggregation is only one of at least three possible types of aggregation, the other two being the thrombin and the ADP pathways which are almost unaffected by aspirin-like drugs. The three pathways of aggregation, however, are all affected by substances which increase cAMP in the platelets either by stimulating the enzyme (adenylate cyclase) which induces this increase (PGE_1, PGD_2 or prostacyclin) or by inhibiting the enzyme which degrades cyclic AMP, dipyridamole being an example of this group.

So far, prostacyclin is the most potent and comprehensive inhibitor of all forms of aggregation. This fact, together with the endogenous nature of prostacyclin, clearly suggests that the future of antithrombotic therapy lies in the development of compounds with a 'prostacyclin' type of action, long-acting, orally active and perhaps free of the cardiovascular effects of prostacyclin.

References

1. Hamberg, M. and Samuelsson, B. (1974). Novel transformations of arachidonic acid in human platelets. *Proc. Natl. Acad. Sci., USA,* **71,** 3400
2. Vane, J. R. (1971). Inhibition of prostaglandin synthesis as a mechanism of action for aspirin-like drugs. *Nature New Biol.,* **231,** 232

3. Moncada, S. and Vane, J.R. (1979). Pharmacology and endogenous roles of prostaglandin endoperoxides, thromboxane A_2 and prostacyclin. *Pharm. Rev.,* **30,** 293

4. Tateson, J.E., Moncada, S. and Vane, J.R. (1977). Effects of prostacyclin (PGX) on cyclic AMP concentrations in human platelets. *Prostaglandins,* **13,** 389

5. Gorman, R.R., Bunting, S. and Miller, O.V. (1977). Modulation of human platelet adenylate cyclase by prostacyclin (PGX). *Prostaglandins,* **13,** 377

6. Miller, O.V. and Gorman, R.R. (1976). Modulation of platelet cyclic nucleotide content by PGE_1 and the prostaglandin endoperoxide PGG_2. *J. Cyclic Nucl. Res.,* **2,** 79

7. Dusting, G.J., Moncada, S. and Vane, J.R. (1977). Disappearance of prostacyclin in the circulation of the dog. *Br. J. Pharmacol.,* **62,** 414P

8. Gryglewski, R.J., Korbut, R. and Ocetkiewicz, A.C. (1978). Generation of prostacyclin by lungs in vivo and its release into the arterial circulation. *Nature (Lond.),* **273,** 765

9. Moncada, S., Korbut, R., Bunting, S. and Vane, J.R. (1978). Prostacyclin is a circulating hormone. *Nature (Lond.),* **273,** 767

10. Hensby, C.N., Barnes, P.J., Dollery, C.T. and Dargie, H. (1979). Production of 6-oxo-$PGF_{1\alpha}$ by human lung in vivo. *Lancet,* **2,** 1162

11. Moncada, S., Herman, A.G., Higgs, E.A. and Vane, J.R. (1977). Differential formation of prostacyclin (PGX or PGI_2) by layers of the arterial wall. An explanation for the anti-thrombotic properties of vascular endothelium. *Thromb. Res.,* **11,** 323

12. Higgs, E.A., Moncada, S., Vane, J.R., Caen, J.P., Michel, H. and Tobelem, G. (1978). Effect of prostacyclin (PGI_2) on platelet adhesion to rabbit arterial subendothelium. *Prostaglandins,* **16,** 17

13. Moncada, S., Gryglewski, R.J., Bunting, S. and Vane, J.R. (1976). A lipid peroxide inhibits the enzyme in blood vessel microsomes that generates from prostaglandin endoperoxides the substance (prostaglandin X) which prevents platelet aggregation. *Prostaglandins,* **12,** 715

14. Slater, T.F. (1972). *Free Radical Mechanisms in Tissue Injury.* (London: Pion Ltd)

15. Glavind, J., Hartmann, S., Clemmesen, J., Jessen, K.E. and Dam, H. (1952). Studies on the role of lipoperoxides in human pathology. II. The presence of peroxidised lipids in the atherosclerotic aorta. *Acta. Pathol. Microbiol. Scand.,* **30,** 1

16. Dembinska-Kiec, A., Gryglewska, T., Zmuda, A. and Gryglewski, R.J. (1977). The generation of prostacyclin by arteries and by the coronary vascular bed is reduced in experimental atherosclerosis in rabbit. *Prostaglandins,* **14,** 1025

17. Angelo, V.D., Villa, S., Mysliwiec, M., Donati, M.B. and De Gaetano, G. (1978). Defective fibrinolytic and prostacyclin-like activity in human atheromatous plaques. *Thromb. Diath. Haemorrh.,* **39,** 535

18. Woodford, F.P., Bottcher, C.J.F., Oette, K. and Ahrens, E.H. Jr. (1965). The artifactual nature of lipid peroxides detected in extracts of human aorta. *J. Atheroscler. Res.,* **5,** 311

19. Iwakami, M. (1965). Peroxides as a factor of atherosclerosis. *Nagoya J. Med. Sci.,* **28,** 50

20. Nordoy, A., Svensson, B., Wiebe, D. and Hoak, J.C. (1978). Lipoproteins and the inhibitory effect of human endothelial cells on platelet function. *Circ. Res.,* **43,** 527

21. Lagarde, M. and Dechavanne, M. (1977). Increase of platelet prostaglandin cyclic endoperoxides in thrombosis. *Lancet,* **1,** 88

22. Shimamoto, T., Kobayashi, M., Takahashi, T., Takashima, Y., Sakamoto, M. and Morooka, S. (1978). An observation of thromboxane A_2 in arterial blood after cholesterol feeding in rabbits. *Jpn. Heart J.,* **19,** 748

23. Szczeklik, A., Gryglewski, R.J., Musial, J., Grodzinska, L., Serwonska, M. and Marcinkiewicz, E. (1978). Thromboxane generation and platelet aggregation in survivals of myocardial infarction. *Thromb. Diath. Haemorrh.,* **40,** 66

24. Lewy, R.I., Smith, J.B., Silver, M.J., Saia, J., Walinsky, P. and Wiener, L. (1979). Detection of thromboxane B_2 in peripheral blood of patients with Prinzmental's angina. *Prostaglandins Med.,* **2,** 243

25. Harrison, H.E., Reece, A.H. and Johnson, M. (1978). Decreased vascular prostacyclin in experimental diabetes. *Life Sci.,* **23,** 351

26. Johnson, M., Reece, A.H. and Harrison, H.E. (1978). Decreased vascular prostacyclin in experimental diabetes. *7th Int. Cong. Pharmacology, Paris, Abstracts,* p. 342. (Oxford: Pergamon Press)

27. Johnson, M., Harrison, H. E., Raftery, A. T. and Elder, J. B. (1979). Vascular prostacyclin may be reduced in diabetes in man. *Lancet,* **1**, 325
28. Dollery, C. T., Friedman, L. A., Hensby, C. N., Kohner, E., Lewis, P. J., Porta, M. and Webster, J. (1979). Circulating prostacyclin may be reduced in diabetes. *Lancet,* **2**, 1365
29. Remuzzi, G., Cavenaghi, A. E., Mecca, G., Donati, M. B. and De Gaetano, G. (1977). Prostacyclin (PGI$_2$) and bleeding time in uremic patients. *Thromb. Res.,* **11**, 919
30. Remuzzi, G., Misiani, R., Marchesi, D., Livio, M., Mecca, G., De Gaetano, G. and Donati, M. B. (1978). Haemolytic-uraemic syndrome: deficiency of plasma factor(s) regulating prostacyclin activity. *Lancet,* **2**, 871
31. MacIntyre, D. E., Pearson, J. J. and Gordon, J. L. (1978). Localisation and stimulation of prostacyclin production in vascular cells. *Nature (Lond.),* **271**, 549
32. Pace-Asciak, C. R., Carrara, M. C., Rangaraj, G. and Nicolaou, K. G. (1978). Enhanced formation of PGI$_2$, a potent hypotensive substance, by aortic rings and homogenates of the spontaneously hypertensive rat. *Prostaglandins,* **15**, 1005
33. Moncada, S. and Vane, J. R. (1979). Arachidonic acid metabolites and the interactions between platelets and blood vessel walls. *N. Engl. J. Med.,* **300**, 1142
34. Branthwaite, M. A. (1972). Neurological damage related to open heart surgery. *Thorax,* **27**, 748
35. Griffith, G. C., Nichols, G., Asher, J. D. and Flanagan, B. (1965). Heparin osteoporosis. *J. Am. Med. Assoc.,* **193**, 91
36. Balanowski, P. J. P., Bauer, J., Machiedo, G. and Neville, W. E. (1977). Prostaglandin influence on pulmonary intravascular leukocytic aggregation during cardiopulmonary bypass. *J. Thorac. Cardiovasc. Surg.,* **73**, 221
37. Ubatuba, F. B., Moncada, S. and Vane, J. R. (1979). The effect of prostacyclin (PGI$_2$) on platelet behaviour, thrombus formation in vivo and bleeding time. *Thromb. Diath. Haemorrh.,* **41**, 425
38. Robert, A., Hanchar, A. J., Lancaster, C. and Nezamis, J. E. (1979). Prostaglandin inhibits enteropooling and diarrhea. In Vane, J. R. and Bergstrom, S. (eds.), *Prostacyclin,* pp. 147–158. (New York: Raven Press)
39. Woods, H. F., Ash, G., Weston, M. J., Bunting, S., Moncada, S. and Vane, J. R. (1978). Prostacyclin can replace heparin in haemodialysis in dogs. *Lancet,* **2**, 1075
40. Coppe, D., Wonders, T., Snider, M. and Salzman, E. W. (1979). Preservation of platelet number and function during extracorporeal membrane oxygenation (ECMO) by regional infusion of prostacyclin. In Vane, J. R. and Bergstrom, S. (eds.), *Prostacyclin,* pp. 371–383. (New York: Raven Press)
41. Bunting, S., Moncada, S., Vane, J. R., Woods, H. F. and Weston, M. J. (1979). Prostacyclin improves hemocompatibility during charcoal hemoperfusion. In Vane, J. R. and Bergstrom, S. (eds.), *Prostacyclin,* pp. 361–369. (New York: Raven Press)
42. Gimson, A. E. S., Hughes, R. D., Mellon, P. J., Woods, H. F., Langley, P. G., Canalese, J., Williams, R. and Weston, M. J. (1980). Prostacyclin to prevent platelet activation during charcoal haemoperfusion in fulminant hepatic failure. *Lancet,* **1**, 173
43. Carlson, L. A. and Olsson, A. G. (1976). Intravenous prostaglandin E$_1$ in severe peripheral vascular disease. *Lancet,* **2**, 810
44. Szczeklik, A., Nizankowski, R., Skawinski, S., Szczeklik, J., Gluszko, P. and Gryglewski, R. J. (1979). Successful therapy of advanced arteriosclerosis obliterans with prostacyclin. *Lancet,* **1**, 1111
45. Szczeklik, A., Gryglewski, R. J., Nizankowski, R., Skawinski, S., Gluszko, P. and Korbut, R. (1980). Prostacyclin therapy in peripheral artery disease. *Thromb. Res.,* **19**, 191

4
A free radical approach to tissue injury

H. H. THAW, J. O. FORSBERG, R. F. DEL MAESTRO, B. GERDIN,
F. N. McKENZIE and K.-E. ARFORS

Problems associated with hypoxic tissue damage emerge as central constraints in cardiovascular, neurosurgical and transplantation surgery. Achievements in these fields have been predominantly the results of advances in surgical techniques, medical and intensive-care methods.

Tissue hypoxia, regardless of the initiating cause, produces a spectrum of undesired effects. The crucial problem is how to prevent the effects of tissue hypoxia that always accompany impaired organ perfusion.

The causes of ischaemic injury are multifactorial: the severity and duration of ischaemia, nutritional, hormonal and metabolic status, the presence of coincidental disease, age, and sex, all play indeterminate roles. A functional vascular delivery system and the integrity of cellular components are both necessary for utilization of substrates required for energy production, such as oxygen and glucose. A decrease in the availability of either of these substrates may be extremely debilitating to energy production. One of the predominant effects of ischaemia and inadequate energy production is the disruption of the energy-dependent cell membrane pumps responsible for maintaining transcellular ionic gradients. Thus, the breakdown of energy-rich nucleotides is of great importance when considering the maintenance of membrane integrity.

Some recent experimental findings suggest that hypoxia, as such, might not be the only cause of 'hypoxic' tissue damage. Incomplete cerebral ischaemia as compared with complete ischaemia produced a higher frequency of irreversible brain damage during corresponding time periods in both cats and monkeys[1]. Kalimo and co-workers also demonstrated that brain tissue which was exposed to 30 min of total ischaemia showed only moderate ultrastructural changes before recirculation[2]. Siesjö and co-workers showed that the use of extremely low concentrations of oxygen during brain ischaemia resulted in less mitochondrial damage during reflow than when oxygen was present in higher concentrations during the ischaemia[3]. Hearse et al. demonstrated that significant myocardial damage can appear in the recirculation phase following ischaemia[4]. Buckberg reported that a major component of the damage of myocardial ischaemia occurs during the early phases of reoxygenation, where he found a marked inability to utilize delivered oxygen, even with coronary blood flow and oxygen content at normal levels[5]. Following myocardial ischaemia, Hearse and associates observed that the release of creatinine kinase (CK) correlated with the oxygen content of the perfusate[6].

The microvascular changes occurring during reperfusion after ischaemia are complex. In kidney, brain and heart, the no-reflow phenomenon, or more accurately, the flow-then-no-flow phenomenon appears to play a prominent role in propagating injury[7-9].

Transient changes in oxygen delivery may lead to complex cellular alterations. It is obvious that the delivery of abundant oxygen to tissue in the face of ischaemic changes does not assure that the cells can utilize this oxygen to repair ischaemic damage or reconstitute depleted energy stores. The background presented has led us to the belief that the lack of oxygen as such, within a reasonable time scope, may not be the only cause of 'hypoxic' cell damage. Lack of oxygen may create a condition within the cell where molecular oxygen that is supplied by reperfusion is reduced to toxic free radicals, i.e. that it is the reperfusion rather than the hypoxia that is deleterious.

OXYGEN FREE RADICALS

Mitochondria generate ATP, performing this function by their ability to reduce oxygen to H_2O. This controlled reduction requires the addition of four electrons, and the cytochrome oxidase complex of the mitochondria accomplishes this in one step. In doing so, it bypasses the formation of a group of toxic free radical intermediates which include the superoxide anion radical (O_2^-), hydrogen peroxide (H_2O_2), and hydroxyl radical ($\cdot OH$). A small fraction of oxygen, however, escapes the controlled pathway and is reduced in this uncontrolled manner (Figure 4.1). This 'uncontrolled' reduction of oxygen is called the 'univalent pathway' because the electrons are added one by one, and the free radical intermediates are formed. The effect of uncontrolled free radical production on the cell may be the initiation of lipid peroxidation, with the

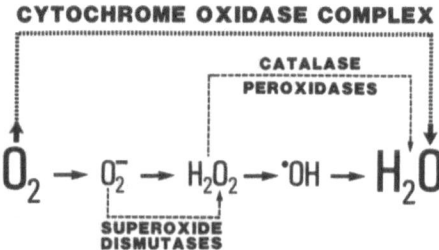

Figure 4.1 The univalent pathway for oxygen reduction gives rise to the superoxide radical (O_2^-), hydrogen peroxide (H_2O_2), and the hydroxyl radical ($\cdot OH$). Enzymatic defence mechanisms bypass and prevent the accumulation of these reactive intermediates of 'uncontrolled' oxygen reduction

subsequent release of fatty acids (i.e. arachidonic acid). Since these are important components of mitochondrial and cell membranes, the peroxidative processes can lead to deleterious consequences for cell vitality.

Mitochondria, and other cell components, normally maintain efficient control systems (scavengers) which protect themselves and the cells from the destructive effects of free radicals. Superoxide dismutases (SOD), which convert O_2^- to H_2O_2, and catalase (CAT) and glutathione peroxidase (GSH-Px) which reduce H_2O_2 to H_2O are the major enzymatic control systems. In addition a spectrum of endogenous cellular antioxidants exists comprising vitamin E; glutathione; thiol amino acids; ascorbic acid; thiolic, phenolic, and catecholic amino acids; selenium; corticosteroids; to name only a few. The presence of these enzyme and scavenger systems in both mitochondrial and cytosolic compartments suggests that at least a part of normal oxygen reduction is via the univalent pathway and results in a flux of O_2^-.

EXPERIMENTAL STUDIES

The investigations carried out in our laboratory have been concerned with the possible mechanism(s) by which oxygen-derived free radicals and active oxygen species may result in tissue injury[10]. The model systems used for these investigations may provide some insight into the possibility for the involvement of free radicals in reperfusion injury (these are shown in Table 4.1). Under aerobic conditions hypoxanthine and xanthine are metabolized to urate by the enzyme xanthine oxidase. This enzyme has been extensively studied and is capable of producing free radicals[11].

Table 4.1 Model systems

Microvascular system	Cell components	Interstitial space macromecules
Hamster cheek pouch	Glial cells	Hyaluronic acid

We have utilized a hypoxanthine-xanthine oxidase (Hx–XO) system which produces both O_2^- and H_2O_2, and secondarily $\cdot OH$[12] to generate a flux of O_2-derived free radicals in our biological models.

Hyaluronic acid, a biopolymer, was degraded by our free radical generating system. The free radical induced degradation was inhibited by ethanol (10 mmol/l), mannitol (10 mmol/l), or Me_2SO (50 μmol/l). This suggests that the $\cdot OH$ was responsible (selective scavenging principle), and since the combination of both SOD (10 μg/ml) and CAT (10 μg/ml) could also prevent the breakdown, both O_2^- and H_2O_2 appear to be involved in the process.

Human glial cells *in culture* were irreversibly injured following a 1 min exposure to the Hx–XO system. Acute changes in cell behaviour and morphology were seen somewhat akin to those induced by exposure of the

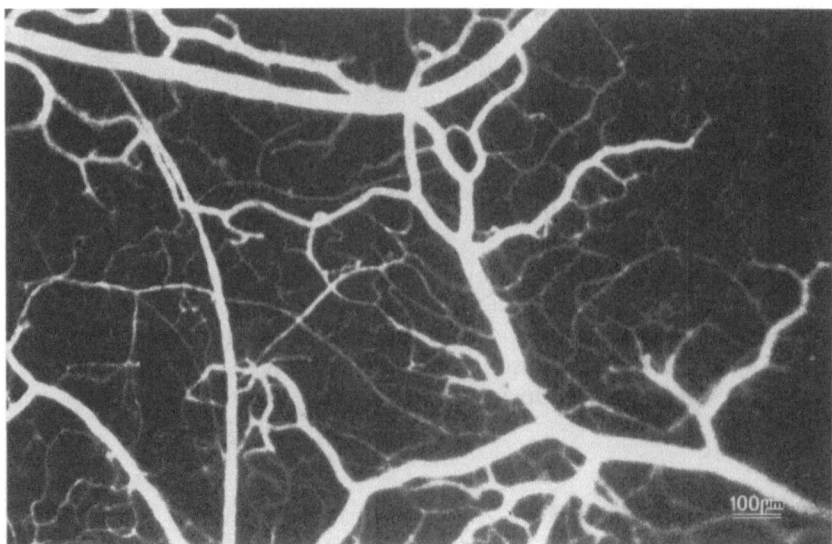

Figure 4.2 A light micrograph of cheek pouch microcirculation taken in fluorescent light immediately prior to topical application of free radical generating system

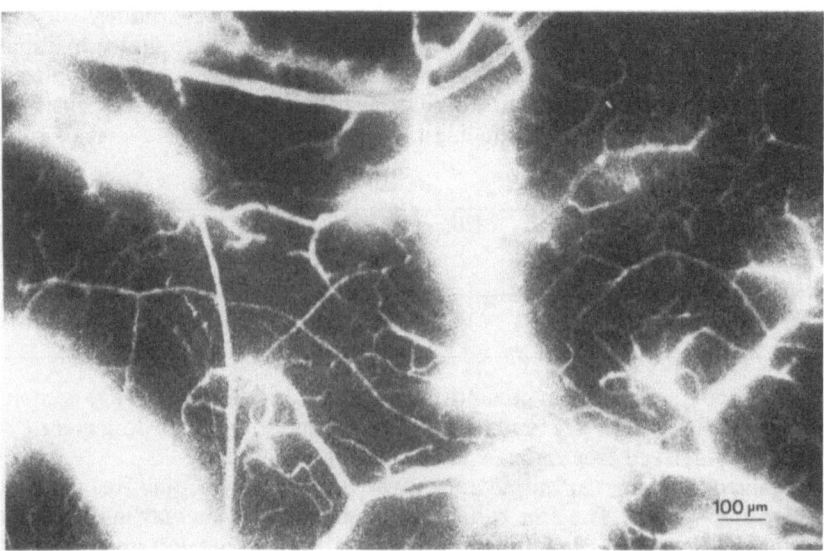

Figure 4.3 Same region as seen in Figure 4.2, 15 min following 1 min of free radical generation. FITC-dextran 150 is seen leaking from post-capillary venules, appearing as intense areas of fluorescence

similar cells to 20 000 rad of X-irradiation. Pretreatment of the cells with DMSO (5 μmol/l), or dexamethasone (0.5 μmol/l) preserved cellular integrity and inhibited these changes. The damage to which the cells

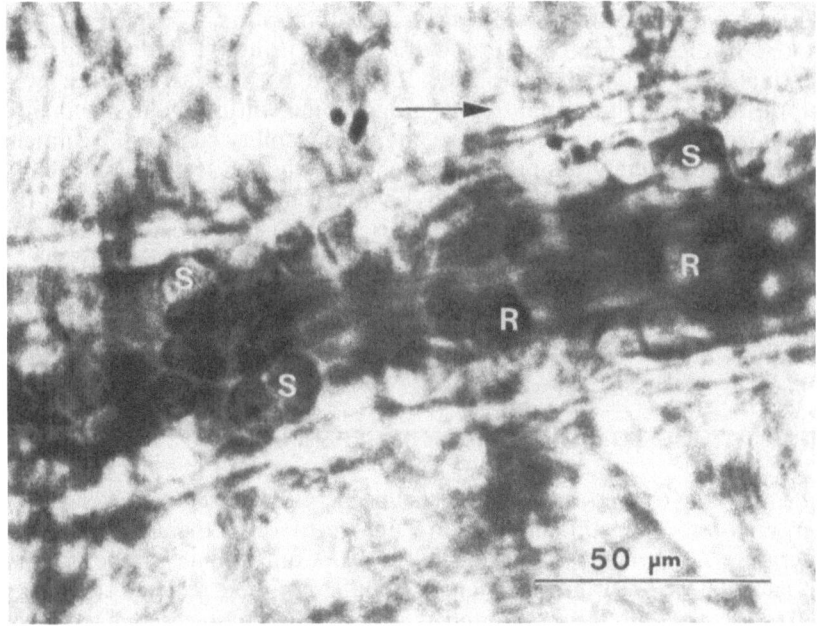

Figure 4.4 A light micrograph of a venule in the cheek pouch microcirculation. Granulocyte sticking (S) and rolling (R) were demonstrated following free radical generation

succumb appears to be mediated through changes in membrane stability, induced by a potent oxidizing species (probably $\cdot$OH).

Continuous observation of the microvasculature of the hamster cheek pouch under fluorescent microscopy is made possible using fluorescein-labelled dextran MW 150000 (FITC-dextran 150) which is injected intravenously (Figure 4.2). Exposing the microcirculatory system to a 1 min flux of oxygen free radicals by topical application of the Hx–XO system resulted in extravasation of the FITC-dextran 150 (Figure 4.3). The majority of leakage sites were in post-capillary venules and granulocyte adhesion was also prominent at these sites. Some leakage did occur from larger veins ($> 50 \mu m$) as well. The number of leakage sites/cm$_2$ was reduced significantly by adding SOD or CAT ($10 \mu g/ml$), Me$_2$SO ($10 mmol/l$), or L-methionine ($10 mmol/l$) to the cheek pouch reservoir immediately prior to the xanthine oxidase. These results are consistent with the concept that $\cdot$OH is involved in inducing alterations in permeability of the microcirculation of the hamster cheek pouch.

An O_2^--dependent lipid hydroperoxide that is generated on the cheek pouch of the hamster by the Hx–XO system caused a dramatic modulation of granulocyte–endothelial interactions (Figure 4.4). Granulocyte velocity decreased, and this was accompanied by an increase in the frequency of rolling granulocytes and granulocyte adhesion. SOD ($50 \mu g/ml$) completely inhibited these changes, while CAT ($50 \mu g/ml$) and L-methionine were without effect. These results support the observations by McCord of an

O_2^--dependent plasma factor that is chemotactic both *in vitro* and *in vivo*[13].

In a reperfusion model dealing with cat intestine, Granger and co-workers studied permeability in low flow states using [^{125}I]albumin[14]. The intestinal flow was reduced to 20% for 1 h, and this was followed by a restoration period of normal flow. Antihistamine, antibradykinin and anti-prostaglandin agents were unable to alter permeability changes. Treatment with SOD completely inhibited the change in microvascular permeability seen, indicating that O_2^- was directly involved in the pathogenesis of the mucosal lesions produced by intestinal ischaemia. In a recent study using the Langendorff heart preparation, Guarnieri *et al.* demonstrated a correlation between the amount of tissue damage occurring during the reperfusion phase and the decrease in both SOD and GSH–Px during ischaemia[15].

IMPLICATIONS TO ISCHAEMIA AND REPERFUSION

A decrease in oxygen availability results in the immediate utilization of energy stores. The mitochondria are unable to fulfil their basic role of generating ATP, and lactic acidosis results. Components of the energy-producing electron transport chain accumulate in their reduced states and in the presence of trace amounts of oxygen (incomplete ischaemia or hypoxia) may lead to spontaneous oxidations and hence uncontrolled free radical formation. It is doubtful that this occurs under conditions of complete ischaemia (anoxia), and this may contribute towards the explanation of why incomplete ischaemia is less well tolerated than complete ischaemia. The subsequent increased free radical flux may result in peroxidative injury to biomembranes, degradation of macromolecules and alterations in permeability[10].

The catabolism of high-energy adenine nucleotides (ATP) is known to increase in tissues during hypoxia, and these then readily diffuse from the tissues. Berne reported that the amount of hypoxanthine released by perfused cat hearts was inversely proportional to the oxygen tension of the perfusate[16]. During conditions of ischaemia and hypoxia, high tissue levels of hypoxanthine are formed[17], in the reperfusion phase these levels are rapidly returned to normal by metabolism to xanthine and urate. Xanthine oxidase catalyses the oxidation of hypoxanthine first to xanthine then to uric acid, using oxygen as a substrate. Evidence exists that the enzyme actually exists *in vivo* in a non-O_2^--producing form. However, *in vitro* exposure of this enzyme to proteolytic enzymes or hypoxia may result in a rapid conversion to a form capable of producing superoxide (McCord, J. M., personal communication). Xanthine oxidase was the first known biological source of superoxide, reported by McCord and Fridovich[11], and this enzyme has been well studied. Unfortunately, technology has not advanced to the point where the direct *in vivo* measurement of free radical production is possible. The use of allopurinol, an inhibitor of xanthine oxidase, which provides protection against myocardial ischaemia, arrest and haemorrhagic shock, furnishes some circumstantial evidence supporting the possible involvement of active oxygen species[18-20]. Whether the mechanisms underlying the protective effects of xanthine oxidase inhibition on anoxia, hypoxia and ischaemia are related to free radical production or to preservation of high-energy phosphates, remains to be elucidated by further investigations.

Finally, an inflammatory component associated with ischaemic lesions may be initiated or perhaps speeded up by oxygen free radical production. The release of chemoattractant substances from the injured tissue, an O_2^--dependent chemotactic factor, or the production of both O_2^- and H_2O_2 by invading inflammatory cells may further extend damage to the already injured tissues.

CONCLUSION

Free radical aspects of tissue injury have attracted much attention and are

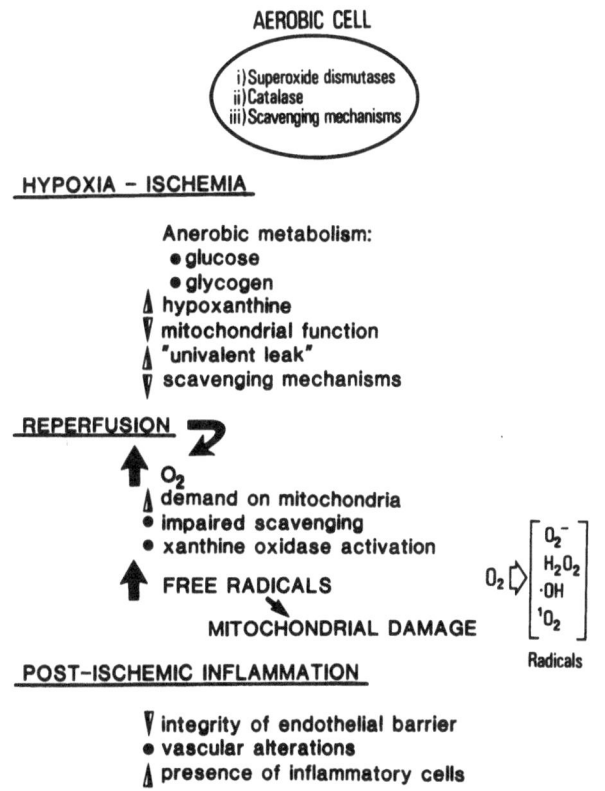

Figure 4.5 Evolutionary development of primitive anaerobic cells into aerobic cells has been associated with the development of free radical scavenging mechanisms. During hypoxia, aerobic cells convert to anaerobic metabolism. The reperfusion of anoxic or hypoxic cells with oxygen may result in a sudden increase of free radical production that could increase cellular damage. Inflammation may also be an important secondary component contributing to the damage initiated by hypoxia

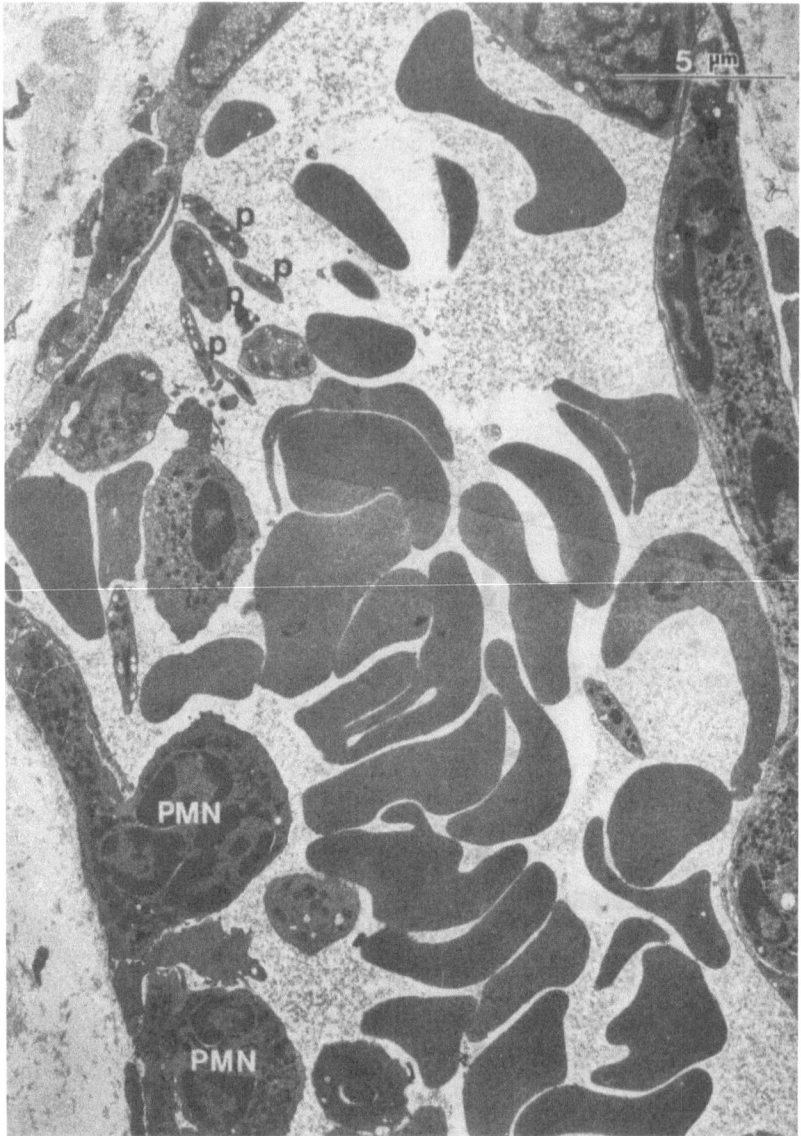

Figure 4.6 A transmission electron micrograph of a section of the cheek pouch micro-circulation in the early minutes following free radical generation. Inflammatory cells (PMN) and platelets (p) can be seen along the endothelial border

the subject of many excellent reviews[21-23]. Our discussions have centred around a free radical theory of reperfusion injury (Figure 4.5).

We have shown that glial cells are irreversibly injured, and others have shown that endothelial cells in culture are also damaged[24] by the same free radical generating system we have used. Free radical generation has a striking effect on the microcirculation, both on microvascular permeability (Figure 4.2) and on blood cell–endothelial interactions (Figures 4.4 and 4.6). Endothelial cell alterations occur very early and are often very pronounced after ischaemia and reperfusion.

Thus far, hypothermia and hypothermic perfusion are the outstanding methods for achieving organ survival for reasonable time periods. Control of, and protection against, free radicals might be another approach to increasing the time during which tissue can tolerate hypoxia.

Acknowledgements

This work was supported in part by the Alexander Medical Foundation and the Canadian Medical Research Council. We are grateful to Professor Ulf Brunk, Erik Arro, and the Institute of Pathology, University of Uppsala for their assistance. Special recognition is due to Annie Lindbom for careful preparation and typing of the manuscript, and to Erik Johansson for skilful design of artwork and figures.

References

1. Hossmann, K. A. and Kleihues, P. (1973). Reversibility of ischemic brain damage. *Arch. Neurol.*, **29**, 375
2. Kalimo, H., Garcia, J. H., Kamijyo, Y., Tanaka, J. and Trump, F. (1977). The ultrastructure of 'brain death'. II. Electron microscopy of feline cortex after complete ischaemia. *Virchows Arch. B. Cell Pathol.*, **25**, 207
3. Rehncrona, S., Mela, L. and Siesjö, B. K. (1979). Recovery of brain mitochondrial function in the rat after complete and incomplete cerebral ischaemia. *Stroke,* **10**, 437
4. Hearse, D. J., Humphrey, S. M., Naylor, W. G., Slade, A. and Border, D. (1975). Ultrastructural damage associated with reoxygenation of the anoxic myocardium. *J. Molec. Cardiol.,* **7**, 315
5. Buckberg, G. D. (1979). A proposed 'solution' to the cardioplegic controversy. *J. Thorac. Cardiovasc. Surg.,* **77**, 803
6. Hearse, D. J., Stewart, D. A. and Braimbridge, M. V. (1976). Cellular protection during myocardial ischemia. The development and characterization of a procedure for the induction of reversible ischemic arrest. *Circulation,* **54**, 193
7. Summers, W. K. and Jamison, R. L. (1971). The no reflow phenomenon in renal ischemia. *Lab. Invest.,* **25**, 635
8. Majno, G., Ames, III, A., Chiang, J. and Wright, R. L. (1967). No reflow after cerebral ischemia. *Lancet,* **2**, 635
9. Willerson, J. T., Powell, W. J. Jr, Gruiney, T. E., Stark, J. I., Saunders, C. A. and Leaf, A. (1972). Improvement in myocardial function and coronary blood flow in ischemic myocardium after mannitol. *J. Clin. Invest.,* **51**, 2989
10. Del Maestro, R. F., Thaw, H. H., Björk, J., Planker, M. and Arfors, K.-E. (1980). Free radicals as mediators of tissue injury. In Lewis, D. H. and Del Maestro, R. F. (eds) *Acta Physiol. Scand.,* **492** (suppl.), 43
11. McCord, J. M. and Fridovich, I. (1969). Superoxide dismutase, an enzymatic function for erythrocuprein. *J. Biol. Chem.,* **244**, 6049
12. Beauchamp, C. and Fridovich, I. (1970). A mechanism for the production of ethylene from methional. The generation of the hydroxyl radical by xanthine oxidase. *J. Biol. Chem.,* **245**, 4641
13. McCord, J. M., Wong, K., Stokes, S. H., Petrone, W. F. and English, D. (1980). Super-

oxide and inflammation: a mechanism for the anti-inflammatory activity of superoxide dismutase. In Lewis, D. H. and Del Maestro, R. F. (eds) *Acta Physiol. Scand.,* **492** (suppl.), 25

14. Granger, D. N., Rutili, G. and McCord, J. M. (1982). Superoxide radicals in intestinal ischemia. *Gastroenterology* (In press)

15. Guarnieri, C., Flamigni, F. and Carlarera, C. M. (1980). Role of oxygen in the cellular damage induced by re-oxygenation of the hypoxic heart. *J. Mol. Cell Cardiol.,* **12,** 797

16. Berne, R. M. and Rubio, R. (1974). Adenine nucleotide metabolism in the heart. *Circ. Res.,* **35,** 109

17. Saugstad, O. D., Schrader, H. and Aasen, A. O. (1976). Alteration of hypoxanthine level in cerebro-spinal fluid as an indicator of tissue hypoxia. *Brain Res.,* **112,** 188

18. Crowell, J. W., Jones, C. E. and Smith, E. E. (1969). Effect of allopurinol on haemorrhagic shock. *Am. J. Physiol.,* **216,** 744

19. Baker, C. H. (1972). Protection against irreversible haemorrhagic shock by allopurinol. *Proc. Soc. Exp. Biol. Med.,* **141,** 694

20. Parker, J. C. and Smith, E. E. (1972). Effects of xanthine oxidase inhibition in cardiac arrest. *Surgery,* **71,** 339

21. Pharmacia Symposium No. 1: Free Radicals (1980). *Free Radicals in Medicine and Biology, Acta Physiol. Scand.,* **492** (suppl.)

22. Ciba Foundation Symposium 65 (new series) (1979). *Oxygen Free Radicals and Tissue Damage.* (Amsterdam: Excerpta Medica)

23. Pryor, W. A. (1976–80). *Free Radicals in Biology.* (Vols. I-V). (New York: Academic Press)

24. Sacks, T., Moldow, C. F., Craddock, P. R., Bowers, T. K. and Jacob, S. (1978). Oxygen radicals mediate endothelial cell damage by complement-stimulated granulocytes. *J. Clin. Invest.,* 1161

5
Endothelial cell function and organ preservation *ex vivo*

J. D. PEARSON, A. HUTCHINGS and J. L. GORDON

The endothelial cell monolayer that lines blood vessels forms the interface between circulating blood and extravascular tissue, and it controls the egress of soluble blood components and formed elements of the blood. Excessive leakage of small molecules or of blood cells is prevented, whilst the transport of appropriate nutrients is permitted, as is the emigration of specific classes of white cell from the vessel lumen under certain circumstances.

A substantial body of data suggests that compromised endothelial function (or frank endothelial injury) leads to oedema near damaged vessels or ischaemia distal to occluded small vessels, and this is one of the major reasons for unsuccessful organ preservation *ex vivo*[1-3]. It results in increasing tissue weight and vascular resistance when the organ is reperfused. A contributing cause to the occlusion of small vessels is the production of thrombi (or emboli therefrom). Endothelial cells normally form a non-thrombogenic surface, and damage to endothelium can promote thrombus formation or blood clotting as well as the oedema noted above.

Endothelium can be damaged by physical disruption (e.g. cooling and re-warming tissue inappropriately, or osmotic shock) or by more subtle alterations of cellular metabolism – either general (e.g. depletion of energy stores or alteration of plasma membrane permeability) or specific (e.g. inhibition of antithrombotic functions). Additionally it has been recently recognized that rejection of a transplanted organ is frequently due to the consequences of host immunological reactions directed against donor endothelium[4,5].

This review will not deal with the practicalities of organ preservation in relation to endothelial function, but will summarize some of the aspects of endothelial biology that are concerned with the maintenance of vascular integrity and therefore important in organ preservation. Recent reviews describing the functions of endothelium *in vivo* and the characteristics of cultured endothelial cells include those by Thorgeirsson and Robertson[6], Gimbrone[7] and Weksler[8].

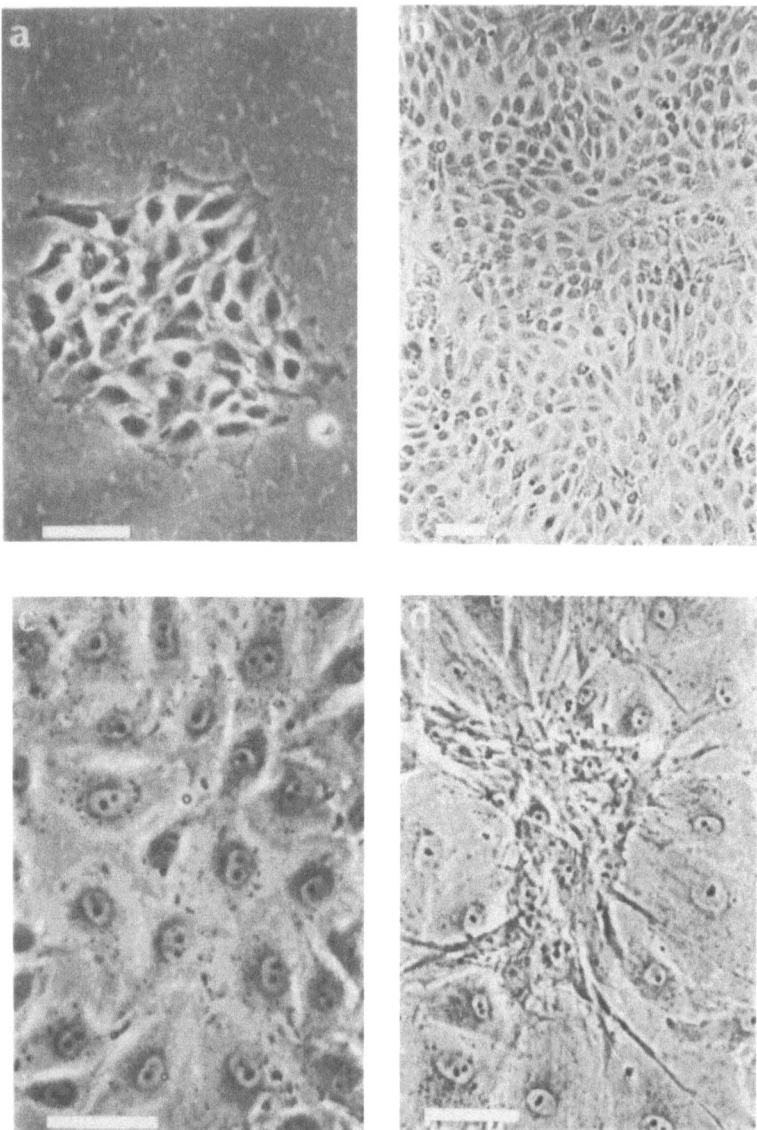

Figure 5.1 Morphology of endothelial cells cultured from newborn pig aorta. Micrographs of living cells; the bar in each case represents $40\,\mu\text{m}$. (a) An island of cells shortly after isolation and attachment to the culture dish. (b) A confluent monolayer of cells in primary culture. (c) A confluent monolayer of subcultured cells, at higher magnification. (d) The appearance of endothelial cells contaminated with smooth muscle cells. The monolayer of endothelium is overgrown by multilayered patches of overlapping cells

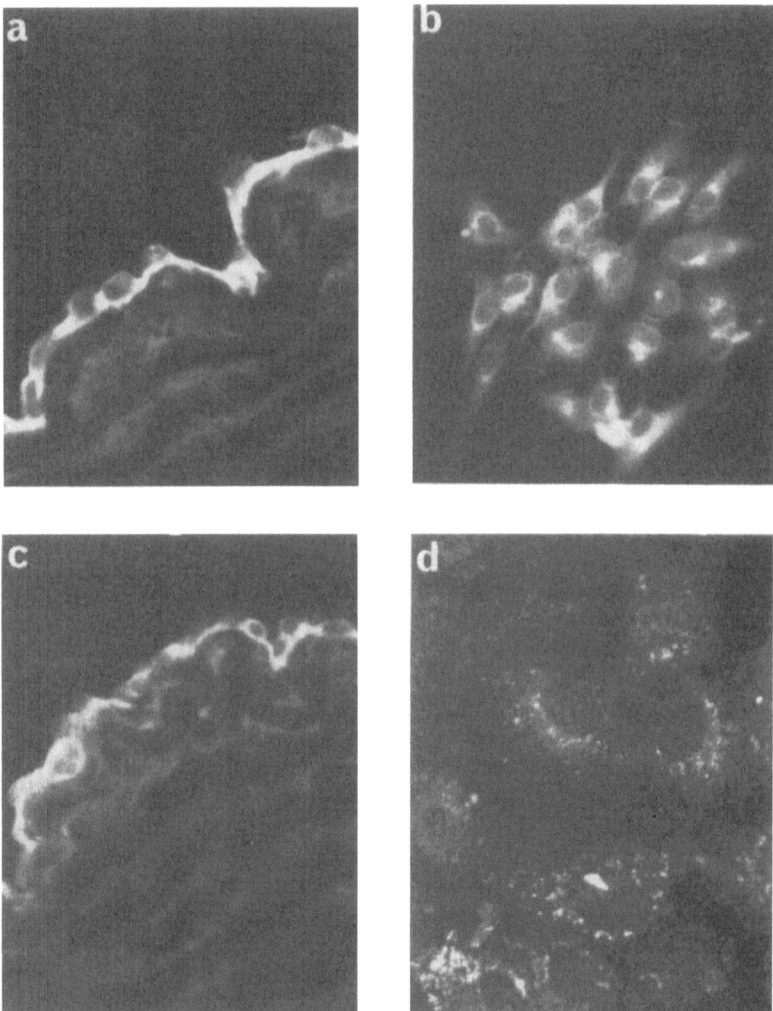

Figure 5.2 Localization of specific products by immunofluorescence in endothelial cells cultured from newborn pig aorta. The bar in each case represents $20\,\mu$m. (a) and (b) transverse section of aorta and primary culture of endothelial cells respectively. Each was fixed, incubated with goat antiserum to porcine angiotensin-converting enzyme and stained with fluorescein isothiocyanate conjugated to anti-goat IgG. Note that staining in (a) is restricted to the endothelial monolayer; subjacent smooth muscle cells are unstained (the faintly visible fluorescence in the media is autofluorescence due to elastin). Cultured smooth muscle cells or endothelial cells incubated with non-immune serum did not stain. (c) and (d) transverse section of aorta and subcultured endothelial cells respectively. Each was fixed, incubated with rabbit antiserum to porcine Factor VIII and stained with fluorescein isothiocyanate conjugated to anti-rabbit IgG. Staining in (c) is restricted to the endothelium; (d) shows the characteristic punctate cytoplasmic staining. Cultured smooth muscle cells or endothelial cells incubated with non-immune serum did not stain. We wish to thank Dr Una Ryan for anti-converting enzyme, and Drs Dominique Meyer and Eric Preston for anti-Factor VIII

CULTURED ENDOTHELIUM

Endothelial cells have now been cultured successfully from medium-sized to large arteries or veins from many species, and in nearly every case the technique used has been based on that introduced in 1972 by Jaffe[9], i.e. brief exposure of the cells to a dilute solution of bacterial collagenase at 37°C filling the lumen of the vessel. Endothelial cells are then obtained in small sheets by flushing the vessel with growth medium, and these adhere to culture flasks, spread out, and multiply to form a confluent monolayer of characteristic morphology (Figure 5.1). By using cells from various species, several of the general distinguishing biochemical features of endothelium have now been delineated. Unfortunately, little has been published on fundamental aspects of endothelial energy metabolism, such as the proportion of ATP derived from aerobic versus anaerobic respiration, or the susceptibility of endothelium to injury caused by acidosis or hypoxia, and a greater knowledge of these would be of value in organ preservation. Endothelium in culture requires a greater concentration of serum (~20%) for satisfactory growth than do many other cell types, perhaps reflecting the fact that its position *in vivo* exposes it (unlike all other cells apart from the formed elements of the blood) to 100% plasma.

The plasma membrane of endothelium *in vivo* and in culture is unique in possessing angiotensin-converting enzyme on its surface[10] (see Figure 5.2). This ectoenzyme, which converts angiotensin I to angiotensin II and also inactivates bradykinin, is apparently one example of metabolic functions, many of them specific to endothelium, that are involved in the inactivation of circulating vasoactive agents. *In vivo*, the uptake and metabolism of several prostaglandins and amines have been attributed to endothelium[11,12], although it has proved difficult to confirm some of these properties using cultured cells[13]. We have shown that cultured porcine endothelial cells have an active transport process for adenosine (a powerful vasodilator) which is rapidly incorporated into adenine nucleotides after its intracellular uptake[14]. Furthermore, endothelium possesses a system of ectoenzymes that degrades circulating ATP, ADP and AMP to adenosine[15], which suggests that the regulation of adenosine levels in the coronary vasculature during reactive hyperaemia could be controlled by the endothelium.

ENDOTHELIAL CELLS AND THE HAEMOSTATIC PROCESS

Under normal conditions endothelium *in vivo* and *in vitro* forms a non-thrombogenic surface. Many endothelial metabolic functions are now recognized as being involved in the body's active response to an altered haemostatic state, and four major topics of current research interest in this area are outlined below.

Prostanoids

Soon after the discovery that vascular tissue can release a labile prosta-

46

glandin that potently inhibits platelet aggregation, this compound was characterized and named prostacyclin (or PGI_2). Prostacyclin, which is synthesized and secreted by vascular tissue or cultured endothelial cells[16-18], will also disperse preformed platelet clumps; it exerts its effect by binding to specific receptors at the platelet surface and raising cytoplasmic cAMP levels in the platelet by stimulating adenylate cyclase[19]. Although prostacyclin powerfully inhibits platelet–platelet aggregation, it is much less able to prevent platelet adherence to cultured endothelium or to exposed subendothelium *in vivo*[20-22]. The degree of adhesion of activated platelets to cultured endothelial cells is, however, lower than to other cell types even when endothelial prostacyclin synthesis is blocked, implying that other endothelial properties, as yet not well characterized, though perhaps involving surface glycosaminoglycan composition are involved.

The secretion of prostacyclin by endothelium *in vivo* or *in vitro* is stimulated by several vasoactive agents (e.g. bradykinin) and by thrombin – although this response may be restricted to certain species or sites of endothelium[18,23,24]. The interactions between thrombin and endothelial cells are considered in more detail below, but it should be remembered that as well as being the penultimate element of the coagulation cascade, thrombin is a potent platelet activator. Consequently, thrombin can stimulate endothelium by its direct effect, as well as indirectly via platelet activation. Firstly, prostaglandin endoperoxides released by aggregating platelets can be taken up by adjacent endothelial cells and converted to prostacyclin[25,26]. Secondly, the polypeptide growth factor released from the alpha granules of stimulated platelets is a powerful stimulator of prostacyclin release[27]. This is important because it provides a potential feedback mechanism for limiting thrombus formation.

Thrombin

Thrombin is avidly bound by endothelial cells *in vitro*, and it is cleared from the circulation by the same process *in vivo*[28]. It binds to a small number of high-affinity sites (not present on smooth muscle cells or fibroblasts) and also to a larger population of lower affinity sites[29]. Following binding, thrombin can stimulate the secretion of prostacyclin and the release of purine nucleotides from cultured endothelium[30]; neither of these processes is, however, inhibited when the high-affinity thrombin-binding sites are blocked[31,32]. Thus the biological function of these sites is not apparently to stimulate secretion; rather, they may be involved in the binding and inactivation of circulating thrombin.

The anticoagulant effect of heparin is a consequence of its ability to inactivate thrombin, and this inactivation is catalysed by antithrombin III, a protein present on the surface of endothelial cells[33,34]. Heparan and dermatan sulphates are synthesized by endothelium[35,36], and these glycosaminoglycans have been shown to have anticoagulant activity *in vitro*[37]; it therefore seems likely that they act in conjunction with antithrombin III to inactivate thrombin at the endothelial surface. Activation of platelets could affect this natural anticoagulant property of endothelium; one of the proteins released from platelet alpha granules (along with the polypeptide growth factor) is platelet factor (PF) 4. Until recently no intrinsic biological function had been ascribed to PF4, although it was known to exhibit anti-heparin activity *in vitro,* but Busch *et al.* have now demonstrated that PF4 binds with high affinity to the surface of endothelium, probably to heparan sulphate or other glycosaminoglycans[38]. PF4 can be displaced into the circulation by heparin, to which it binds with higher affinity, and its biological role may therefore be to modulate the ability of endothelial cells to inactivate thrombin.

Plasminogen activator

It has been known for many years that vascular tissue (particularly endo-thelial cells) can release enzymic activity that in the presence of plasmino-gen degrades fibrin, thus initiating the dissolution of a stabilized haemostatic plug or blood clot[39,40]. Release of this plasminogen activator *in vivo* is stimulated by several vasoactive agents including noradrenaline and bradykinin[41] and immunological studies support the concept that this circulating activity is derived from vascular cells[42]. Studies with isolated and cultured endothelial cells confirmed that they synthesize and secrete plasminogen activator[43], but more recent work indicates that the control of plasminogen activator expression is complex; endothelium also synthesizes an inhibitor of plasminogen activator, and serum components and the growth state of the cells can both affect plasminogen activator levels[43,44].

Pro-coagulant activities

Endothelial cells exhibit at least two procoagulant properties. In common with many other cell types, they contain 'tissue factor' or thromboplastin, which promotes clotting by the extrinsic pathway via Factor VII. This is probably lipoprotein in nature, and is exposed when tissue is damaged[45]. Endothelial cells also synthesize and secrete molecules with Factor VIII activities. Purified Factor VIII is a combination of molecules with three properties; (1) VIII antigen (VIII_{AG}) identified by heterologous antibody precipitation; (2) Von Willebrand factor (VIII_{VW}), deficient in patients with von Willebrand's disease (these patients have prolonged bleeding times and defective platelet adhesion to exposed basement membrane, apparently because VIII_{VW} is an essential cofactor for this reaction); (3) coagulant factor (VIII_C), absent in patients with haemophilia A.

Initial immunofluorescent studies localized VIII_{AG} to vascular intima; Jaffe *et al.*[9,46] then demonstrated that cultured endothelium synthesizes VIII_{AG} and VIII_{VW}. This has been confirmed by other workers (see Figure 5.2) but more recent studies have suggested that the cultured cells may secrete VIII_{AG} that is not identical to the circulating antigen[47]. VIII_C activity has not been detected in cultures of endothelium, but VIII_C is sensitive to proteolytic inactivation, and proteolytic activities (such as plasminogen activator) at the surface of endothelial cells *in vitro* are sufficient to destroy VIII$_C$, so it still remains possible that endothelium *in vivo* synthesizes and secretes all the components of Factor VIII[47,48].

ENDOTHELIAL INTERACTIONS WITH LEUKOCYTES

Endothelial cells interact specifically with each of the three classes of blood leukocyte; lymphocytes, monocytes and granulocytes. Recirculating lymphocytes normally cross endothelium in large numbers within lymph nodes at sites where the endothelial cells (in most species) have a characteristically 'plump' appearance in what are termed high endothelial venules (HEV). Although it has long been supposed that some special feature of HEV regulates lymphocyte adhesion and emigration, few clues to the mechanism involved have yet emerged. A promising technique to study this was first used by Woodruff, who demonstrated that isolated re-circulating lymphocytes adhere specifically to HEV in sections of lymphoid tissue[49]. In addition to their interaction with HEV, however, large numbers of lymphocytes traverse the endothelium of blood vessels other than those in lymph nodes, at sites of chronic inflammatory injury in response to antigen[50,51], or in a rejecting transplanted organ.

Monocyte emigration from blood vessels, a necessary stage in the development of tissue macrophages, also involves interactions with endo-thelial cells, but this process has been little studied. The adhesion and emigration of granulocytes has been the subject of more intensive investigation, perhaps because of the dramatic local increase in this process that occurs at sites of acute inflammation.

In the following subsections, we shall first consider the nature of the interaction between granulocytes and endothelium, then briefly discuss the interaction of endothelial cells with lymphocytes with emphasis on the events that can occur in a transplanted organ.

Granulocytes

There have been recent reviews of this subject from several research groups including our own, and the reader can refer to these for details[52-54]; we will here only briefly present our views on the interactions between granulocytes and endothelium, views which are based primarily on results we obtained using an *in vitro* model in which autologous peripheral blood granulocytes suspended in defined media were in continuous motion over monolayers of cultured endothelium.

Granulocytes *in vivo* have a blood transit time of $< 24\,$h, and they are in dynamic equilibrium between a freely circulating and a marginated pool. The cells of the latter are adherent to endothelial cells, mainly in small blood vessels, on which they crawl and between which they emigrate, to reach the tissues spaces. Granulocytes (unlike lymphocytes) do not return to the bloodstream from the extravascular tissue. At acute inflammatory sites there is a rapid and massive enhancement of this granulocyte traffic, presumably directed by chemotactic agents.

In vitro studies have shown that granulocytes adhere preferentially to endothelial cells rather than to any other cell type, implying that there is recognition of some specific feature of the endothelial cell surface. Adhesion requires divalent cations and viable granulocytes, and it can be modified by agents that affect the endothelial cell surface, although the surface components involved in this specific interaction have not yet been systematically investigated[55,56]. This interaction is highly dependent on shear forces; over a range of low rates of flow, adhesion is inversely related to flow, whilst at flow rates greater than those usually experienced in small blood vessels very few granulocytes will adhere to endothelium *in vitro*[55]. Migration of granulocytes between endothelial cells to reach the substratum beneath the monolayer occurs *in vitro* in the absence of added stimuli such as chemokinetic or chemotactic agents[57], suggesting that specific features of the endothelium may contribute to granulocyte emigration *in vivo*; this could be amplified and directed by inflammatory stimuli altering local blood flow and/or producing a transendothelial gradient of chemotactic factor(s).

Lymphocytes

Experiments with endothelium and lymphocytes *in vitro* are currently leading to a better understanding of several aspects of the involvement of endothelial cells in normal lymphocyte traffic (as noted above) and in the production of an immune response. In a rejecting graft, particularly during acute or hyperacute rejection, vascular damage rapidly leads to ischaemia and necrosis of the donor tissue. In hyperacute rejection this is often due to humorally mediated destruction of donor endothelium by pre-existing circulating antibodies, and serological tests have recently revealed that these antibodies recognize a group of antigens restricted to endothelium alone, or to endothelial cells plus granulocytes and/or monocytes[58-60]. Acute rejection involves a complex series of events, including the initial adherence of lymphocytes (and other leukocytes) to small vessel endothelium followed over 2–5 days by leukocyte migration beneath the endothelium, hypertrophy and damage to endothelial cells, and multiplication of lymphocytes beneath the endothelium[4,61]. Co-culture studies *in vitro* have shown that endothelial cells can directly stimulate lymphocyte proliferation and that this is almost certainly due to the expression of Ia-like (HLA-Dr) antigens by endothelium[62,63] – these antigens otherwise being restricted mainly to leukocytes.

In experiments on lymphocyte adherence to cultured endothelium (similar to those with granulocytes) de Bono has shown that endothelium is a preferred cellular substratum for lymphocyte adhesion, and that altering endothelial surface properties affects this interaction[64]. Homologous or autologous lymphocytes adhered but did not migrate well and adhesion was only temporary[64]. Lymphocytes sensitized by mixed lymphocyte culture or grafting adhered to donor endothelium *in vitro* in increased numbers, migrated through the monolayer, and were cytotoxic in the presence of complement[65], exactly as might be expected from observations made *in vivo*.

In summary, it seems that the interaction between granulocytes and endothelium may involve a single recognition phenomenon producing adhesion, and that modulation of granulocyte behaviour by exogenous stimuli leads to increased migration. The interactions between lymphocytes and endothelial cells are apparently more complex. In addition to a recognition phenomenon regulating normal lymphocyte traffic, separate immune determinants are involved in the reactions between endothelial cells and lymphocytes in an allogeneic situation or when lymphocytes emigrate to reach the site of a chronic inflammatory injury.

CONCLUSION

Vascular endothelial cells can no longer be regarded as simple lining elements forming a passive blood-compatible surface. Satisfactory methods for culturing endothelium *in vitro* have been developed only within the last 8 years; in that time, as a direct consequence of being able to study endothelial biology under defined conditions and without the complications of contributing reactions from other cell types, our knowledge of the physiology and biochemistry of the endothelium has progressed rapidly.

It is now clear that endothelial cells actively contribute to the maintenance of vascular homeostasis in many ways; notably by synthesizing and secreting a wide range of pro- and anticoagulant factors, and by expressing surface components that modulate coagulation reactions, platelet activation and interactions with granulocytes and lymphocytes.

Because of the importance of endothelium in regulating the properties of the circulating blood and in maintaining normal vascular permeability, it is evident that measures designed to protect endothelial integrity are an important factor in organ preservation. In order to optimize such measures we need to know more about the biology of endothelial cells and their responses to damaging stimuli and to environmental change. It is to this end that much of the research in several laboratories, including our own, is currently being directed.

References

1. Pegg, D. E. (1971). Vascular resistance of the isolated rabbit kidney. *Cryobiology*, **8**, 431
2. Belzer, F. O., Hoffman, R., Huang, J. and Downes, G. (1972). Endothelial damage in perfused dog kidney and cold sensitivity of vascular Na-K-ATPase. *Cryobiology*, **9**, 457
3. Pegg, D. E. and Green, C. J. (1973). The functional state of kidneys perfused at 37°C with a bloodless fluid. *J. Surg. Res.*, **15**, 218

4. Dvorak, H. F., Mihm, M. C., Dvorak, A., Barnes, B. A., Manseau, E. J. and Galli, S. J. (1979). Rejection of first-set skin allografts in man. The microvasculature is the critical target of the immune response. *J. Exp. Med.*, **150**, 322

5. Paul, L. C., Van Es, L. A., Van Rood, J. J., Van Leeuwen, A., de la Riviere, G. B. and de Graeff, J. (1979). Antibodies directed against antigens on the endothelium of peritubular capillaries in patients with rejecting renal allografts. *Transplantation*, **27**, 175

6. Thorgeirsson, G. and Robertson, A. L. (1978). The vascular endothelium – pathobiologic significance. *Am. J. Pathol.*, **93**, 803

7. Gimbrone, M. A. (1976). Culture of vascular endothelium. In Spaet, T. H. (ed.), *Progress in Hemostasis and Thrombosis*. Vol. III, pp. 1–28. (New York: Grune & Stratton)

8. Weksler, B. B. (1982). Prostaglandins and the endothelial cell. In Herman, A. G., Vanhoutte, P. M., Denolin, H. and Goossens, A. (eds.) *Cardiovascular Pharmacology of the Prostaglandins*. (New York: Raven Press) (In press)

9. Jaffe, E. A., Hoyer, L. W. and Nachman, R. L. (1973). Synthesis of antihemophilic factor antigen by cultured human endothelial cells. *J. Clin. Invest.*, **52**, 2757

10. Ryan, U. S., Ryan, J. W., Whitaker, C. and Chiu, A. (1976). Localization of angiotensin converting enzyme II immunocytochemistry and immunofluorescence. *Tissue Cell*, **8**, 125

11. Bakhle, Y. S. and Vane, J. R. (1974). Pharmacokinetic functions of the pulmonary circulation. *Pharmacol. Rev.*, **54**, 1007

12. Gillis, C. N. and Roth, J. A. (1976). Pulmonary disposition of circulating vasoactive hormones. *Biochem. Pharmacol.*, **25**, 2547

13. Trevethick, M. A., Olverman, H. J., Pearson, J. D., Gordon, J. L., Lyles, G. A. and Callingham, B. A. (1981). Monoamine oxidase activities of porcine vascular endothelial and smooth muscle cells. *Biochem. Pharmacol.*, **30**, 2209

14. Pearson, J. D., Carleton, J. S., Hutchings, A. and Gordon, J. L. (1978). Uptake and metabolism of adenosine by pig aortic endothelial and smooth muscle cells in culture. *Biochem. J.*, **170**, 265

15. Pearson, J. D., Carleton, J. S. and Gordon, J. L. (1980). Metabolism of adenine nucleotides by ectoenzymes of vascular endothelial and smooth muscle cells in culture. *Biochem. J.*, **190**, 421

16. Moncada, S., Gryglewski, R., Bunting, S. and Vane, J. R. (1976). An enzyme isolated from arteries transforms prostaglandin endoperoxides to an unstable substance that inhibits platelet aggregation. *Nature (Lond.)*, **263**, 663

17. Weksler, B. B., Marcus, A. J. and Jaffe, E. A. (1977). Synthesis of prostaglandin I_2 by cultured human and bovine endothelial cells. *Proc. Natl. Acad. Sci., (USA)*, **74**, 3922

18. MacIntyre, D. E., Pearson, J. D. and Gordon, J. L. (1978). Localization and stimulation of prostacyclin production in vascular cells. *Nature (Lond.)*, **271**, 549

19. Best, L. C., Martin, T. J., Russell, R. G. G. and Preston, F. E. (1977). Prostacyclin increases cyclic AMP levels and adenylate cyclase activity in platelets. *Nature (Lond.)*, **267**, 850

20. Czervionke, R. L., Smith, J. B., Fry, G. L., Hoak, J. C. and Haycraft, D. L. (1979). Inhibition of prostacyclin by treatment of endothelium with aspirin. Correlation with platelet adherence. *J. Clin. Invest.*, **63**, 1089

21. Curwen, K. D., Gimbrone, M. A. and Handin, R. I. (1980). *In vitro* studies of thrombo-resistance. The role of prostacyclin in platelet adhesion to cultured normal and virally transformed human vascular endothelial cells. *Lab. Invest.*, **42**, 366

22. Higgs, E. A., Moncada, S., Vane, J. R., Caen, J. P., Michel, M. and Tobelem, G. (1978). Effect of prostacyclin on platelet adhesion to rabbit arterial subendothelium. *Prostaglandins*, **16**, 17

23. Weksler, B. B., Ley, C. W. and Jaffe, E. A. (1978). Stimulation of endothelial prostacyclin production by thrombin, trypsin, and the ionophore A23187. *J. Clin. Invest.*, **62**, 923

24. Hong, S. L. (1980). Effect of bradykinin and thrombin on prostacyclin synthesis in endothelial cells from calf and pig aorta and human umbilical vein. *Thromb. Res.*, **18**, 787

25. Needleman, P., Wyche, A. and Raz, A. (1979). Platelet and blood vessel arachidonate metabolism and interactions. *J. Clin. Invest.*, **63**, 345

26. Marcus, A. J., Weksler, B. B., Jaffe, E. A. and Broekman, M. J. (1980). Synthesis of prostacyclin from platelet-derived endoperoxides by cultured human endothelial cells. *J. Clin. Invest.*, **66**, 979
27. Coughlin, S. R., Moskowitz, M. A., Zetter, B. R., Antoniades, H. N. and Levine, L. (1980). Platelet-dependent stimulation of prostacyclin synthesis by platelet-derived growth factor. *Nature (Lond.)*, **288**, 600
28. Lollar, P. and Owen, W. G. (1980). Clearance of thrombin from circulation in rabbits by high-affinity binding sites on endothelium. *J. Clin. Invest.*, **66**, 1222
29. Awbrey, B. J., Hoak, J. C. and Owen, W. G. (1979). Binding of human thrombin to cultured endothelial cells. *J. Biol. Chem.*, **254**, 4092
30. Pearson, J. D. and Gordon, J. L. (1979). Vascular endothelial and smooth muscle cells in culture selectively release adenine nucleotides. *Nature (Lond.)*, **281**, 384
31. Lollar, P. and Owen, W. G. (1980). Evidence that the effects of thrombin on arachidonate metabolism in cultured human endothelial cells are not mediated by a high affinity receptor. *J. Biochem.*, **255**, 8031
32. Lollar, P. and Owen, W. G. (1981). Active site dependent, thrombin-induced release of adenine nucelotides from cultured human endothelial cells. *Ann. N. Y. Acad. Sci.*, **307**, 51
33. Chan, V. and Chan, K. (1979). Anti-thrombin III in fresh and cultured human endothelial cells: a natural anticoagulant from the vascular endothelium. *Thromb. Res.*, **15**, 209
34. Kowalski, S. and Finlay, T. H. (1979). Heparin and the inactivation of thrombin by antithrombin III. *Thromb. Res.*, **14**, 387
35. Buonassisi, V. (1973). Sulfated mucopolysaccharide synthesis and secretion in endothelial cell cultures. *Exp. Cell Res.*, **76**, 363
36. Busch, C., Ljungman, C., Holdin, C.-M., Waskson, E. and Obrink, B. (1979). Surface properties of cultured endothelial cells. *Haemostasis*, **8**, 142
37. Long, W. F., Williamson, F. B., Kindness, G. and Edward, M. (1980). The anticoagulant activity of dermatan sulphates. *Thromb. Res.*, **18**, 493
38. Busch, C., Dawes, J., Pepper, D. S. and Wasteson, A. (1980). Binding of platelet factor 4 to cultured human umbilical vein endothelial cells. *Thromb. Res.*, **19**, 129
39. Todd, A. S. (1959). The histological localisation of fibrinolysin activator. *J. Pathol. Bacteriol.*, **78**, 281
40. Pugatch, E. M. J. and Poole, J. C. F. (1969). Studies on the fibrinolytic activity of an extract from vascular endothelium. *Q. J. Exp. Physiol.*, **54**, 80
41. Izaki, S. and Kitaguchi, H. (1977). Calcium dependent and independent release of plasminogen activator from the vessel wall. *Thromb. Res.*, **10**, 765
42. Rijken, D. C., Wijngaards, G. and Welbergen, J. (1980). Relationship between tissue plasminogen activator and the activators in blood and vascular wall. *Thromb. Res.*, **18**, 815
43. Loskutoff, D. J. and Edgington, T. S. (1977). Synthesis of a fibrinolytic activator and inhibitor by endothelial cells. *Proc. Natl. Acad. Sci., (USA)*, **74**, 3903
44. Levin, E. G. and Loskutoff, D. J. (1980). Serum-mediated suppression of cell-associated plasminogen activator activity in cultured endothelial cells. *Cell*, **22**, 701
45. Maynard, J. R., Dreyer, B. E., Stemerman, M. B. and Pitlick, F. A. (1977). Tissue factor coagulant activity of cultured human endothelial and smooth muscle cells and fibroblasts. *Blood*, **50**, 387
46. Jaffe, E. A., Hoyer, L. E. and Nachman, R. L. (1974). Synthesis of von Willebrand factor by cultured human endothelial cells. *Proc. Natl. Acad. Sci., (USA)*, **71**, 1906
47. Shearn, S. A. M., Peake, I. R., Giddings, J. C., Humphrys, J. and Bloom, A. L. (1977). The characterisation and synthesis of antigens related to factor VIII in vascular endothelium. *Thromb. Res.*, **11**, 43
48. Stead, N. W. and McKee, P. A. (1979). The effect of cultured endothelial cells on factor VIII procoagulant activity. *Blood*, **54**, 560
49. Woodruff, J. J. and Kuttner, B. J. (1980). Adherence of lymphocytes to the high endothelium of lymph nodes in vitro. *CIBA Found. Symp.*, **71**, 243

50. Graham, R. C. and Shannon, S. L. (1972). Peroxidase arthritis II lymphoid cell–endothelial interactions during a developing immunologic inflammatory response. *Am. J. Pathol.,* **69,** 7

51. Smith, J. B., McIntosh, G. M. and Morris, B. (1970). The migration of cells through chronically inflamed tissues. *J. Pathol.,* **100,** 21

52. Wilkinson, P. C. and Lackie, J. M. (1979). The adhesion, migration and chemotaxis of leucocytes in inflammation. *Curr. Top. Pathol.,* **68,** 47

53. MacGregor, R. R. (1980). Granulocyte adherence. In Weissman, G. (ed.), *Cell Biology of Inflammation,* pp. 267–298. (Amsterdam: Elsevier)

54. Pearson, J. D. and Gordon, J. L. (1981). Granulocyte interactions with endothelium. In Gordon, J. L. and Dingle, J. T. (eds.) *Cellular Interactions,* pp. 107–118. (Amsterdam: Elsevier)

55. Beesley, J. E., Pearson, J. D., Carleton, J. S., Hutchings, A. and Gordon, J. L. (1978). Interactions of leukocytes with vascular cells in culture. *J. Cell Sci.,* **33,** 85

56. Lackie, J. M. and Smith, R. P. C. (1980). Interactions of neutrophil granulocytes and endothelium. In Curtis, A. S. G. and Pitts, J. D. (eds.) *Cell Adhesion and Motility,* pp. 235–272. (Cambridge: Cambridge University Press)

57. Beesley, J. D., Pearson, J. D., Hutchings, A., Carleton, J. S. and Gordon, J. L. (1979). Granulocyte migration through endothelium in culture. *J. Cell Sci.,* **38,** 237

58. Thompson, J. S., Overlin, V., Severson, C. D., Parsons, T. J., Herbick, J., Strauss, R. G., Burns, C. P. and Claas, F. H. J. (1980). Demonstration of granulocyte, monocyte, and endothelial cell antigens by double fluorochromatic microcytotoxicity testing. *Transpl. Proc.,* **12** (suppl. 1), 26

59. Stasny, P. (1980). Endothelial-monocyte antigens. *Transpl. Proc.,* **12** (suppl. 1), 32

60. Cerilli, J. and Brasile, L. (1980). Endothelial cell alloantigens. *Transpl. Proc.,* **12** (suppl. 1), 37

61. Porter, K. A., Calne, R. Y. and Zukoski, C. F. (1964). Vascular and other changes in 200 canine renal homotransplants treated with immunosuppressive drugs. *Lab. Invest.,* **13,** 809

62. Hirschberg, H., Moen, T. and Thorsby, E. (1979). Specific destruction of human endothelial cell monolayers by anti-DRW antisera. *Transplantation,* **28,** 116

63. Burger, D. R., Ford, D., Hamblin, A. and Dumonde, D. (1981). Endothelial cell presentation of antigen to human T cells. *Hum. Immunol.,* **2** (In press)

64. De Bono, D. (1976). Endothelium–lymphocyte interactions *in vitro.* I. Adherence of non-allergised lymphocytes. *Cell Immunol.,* **26,** 78

65. De Bono, D. (1979). Endothelium–lymphocyte interactions *in vitro.* II. Adherence of allergised lymphocytes. *Cell Immunol.,* **44,** 64

6
The principles of organ storage procedures

D. E. PEGG

A period of ischaemia is inevitable in any organ transplantation procedure; the duration may be brief, perhaps 20 min when a living donor is used, but it is always total, and more usually it lasts a number of hours, sometimes days. The function, then, of preservation methods, is to prevent ischaemic damage. Ischaemia should be carefully differentiated from anoxia and hypoxia, the total or partial lack of oxygen; anoxia is merely one of the many consequences of lack of a blood supply. The effects of ischaemia are best discussed after first considering the normal functions of the blood circulation. What follows is elementary and familiar, but it provides the essential foundation for an analysis of preservation methods.

SOME ESSENTIAL FUNCTIONS OF THE CIRCULATION

The circulation provides an internal heat-exchange system that maintains the temperature of the organs with which we are concerned, within very close limits. Ischaemia in an excised organ therefore produces cooling. The circulation is also responsible for maintaining a remarkably constant composition of the extracellular fluid: the osmolality remains close to 300 mosmol/kg and cells will tolerate a variation of only ~10% without harm. The majority of cells are in osmotic equilibrium with the extra-cellular fluid and therefore also have an internal osmolality of about 300 mosmol/kg. External pH is maintained within the range pH 7.31–7.43, although most cells will actually tolerate a much wider range (e.g. pH 6.6–7.8 in a typical tissue culture). Inorganic ions (sodium, potassium, calcium, magnesium, chloride, bicarbonate and phosphate) have all been shown to be essential in both tissue culture and biochemical studies, in more or less the same concentrations that are found in plasma. The circulation provides metabolites of which the most important, in the short term, are the fuels for respiration: glucose is not the only such substrate; in fact fatty acids and ketone bodies are the preferred fuels for many tissues. Respiration is predominantly aerobic in most tissues, red cells and renal medulla being notable exceptions, and their oxygen requirements are considerable, 20 litres of oxygen/h/g kidney dry weight for renal cortex, for instance. The amount of oxygen that can be physically dissolved in tissue fluid is small, about 24 ml/kg, so that the switch-off of aerobic energy production is exceedingly rapid in ischaemia. In the longer term metabolites other than those required for energy production – amino acids, vitamins, glutathione, coenzymes and many other factors are necessary. However, there is little evidence that these compounds are essential in the short time-scale we are considering. The vascular system is also responsible for the removal of the products of cellular metabolism. Taken together, these properties of the circulation enable organs to function in a remarkably constant environment. Granted this constancy, two cellular functions seem essential to survival under normal physiological conditions: the continual trapping of chemical energy and the maintenance of large ionic gradients across the plasma membrane.

It would be inappropriate to review here the details of energy metabolism: this has been discussed at greater length elsewhere[1]. Some of the more important features will, however, be summarized. When glucose or glycogen is the fuel, the rate of the initial reaction sequence, the *glycolytic pathway,* is regulated by the enzyme phosphofructokinase (PFK) which is activated by adenosine diphosphate (ADP) and inorganic phosphate, and is inhibited by moderate levels of adenosine triphosphate (ATP) and by citrate: hence when the Krebs cycle and electron transport chain are actively generating citrate and ATP, glycolysis is retarded. It should also be noted that PFK is inhibited by a low pH. The subsequent cleavage of fructose-1,6-bisphosphate to yield 2 mol of glyceraldehyde-3-phosphate generates 1 mol of reduced coenzyme (NADH) and 1 mol of hydrogen ions. The overall efficiency of glycolysis is exceedingly low, about 3%, and it must be remembered that glycolysis is the only means of producing ATP in the absence of oxygen. Moreover, oxidized coenzyme (NAD+) is required for the cleavage of fructose-1,6-bisphosphate, and in the absence of oxygen this can be produced only by the reduction of pyruvate to lactate: hence, when the Po_2 is low, glycolysis leads to the accumulation of lactate and H+, and since the latter inhibits PFK, the production of energy by anaerobic means is exceedingly limited.

The normal aerobic fate of pyruvate is oxidation in the Krebs cycle; the *pentose phosphate shunt* provides an alternative aerobic means of completely oxidizing glucose. Fatty acids and ketone bodies are also oxidized aerobically via the Krebs cycle, with an overall efficiency similar to that of carbohydrate – 40–50%. Whether produced by glycolysis or aerobic means, trapped energy is stored as the high-energy phosphate compounds ATP and ADP and their concentration provides a convenient index of the energy status of cells and tissues.

The second cellular function that is essential for survival is the regulation of exchanges of ions and water between cells and their environment. Typically, cell membranes are some 50–100 times more permeable to potassium and chloride than to sodium, and yet they maintain a high internal concentration of potassium and a low concentration of sodium. As is well known, this is achieved by the so-called sodium pump: sodium is extruded in exchange for potassium, and each then leaks back. Because potassium permeates so much more rapidly than sodium, the cell contents acquire a negative charge, which opposes the further loss of potassium and leads to an equilibrium state with a stable membrane potential. Anions, which in general are not actively pumped, necessarily distribute in accordance with that charge: much of the internal anion is non-permeating, but chloride diffuses freely, and consequently the internal Cl^- concentration is very low. In effect then, the sodium pump extrudes sodium chloride, and because the cell membrane has no rigidity to withstand an actual pressure gradient, there is an osmotic flow of water out of the cell in the molecular ratio of approximately 180 H_2O to 1 Na^+ or Cl^-. It can be seen therefore that the sodium pump controls cell volume as well as ion distribution. All active pumps require energy, in the form of ATP, so that the membrane function of cells is in turn dependent on their energy metabolism.

Having briefly considered these essential functions of the circulation we can examine the effects of ischaemia.

ISCHAEMIA

When an organ is excised for grafting two physical changes occur immediately: the temperature drops and the vascular system collapses. With solid organs the rate of cooling is slow (<1°C/min initially) unless it is deliberately augmented, and the final temperature is quite high (~22°C). Hypothermia is the single most important factor in preservation, and will be discussed in more detail below. Collapse of the vascular system is only partial: in small arteries and arterioles complete obliteration of the lumen may occur when the internal pressure falls below the so-called *critical closing pressure*, but plasma and blood cells remain in the capillaries and venous system. The loss of a hydrostatic pressure gradient across the capillary walls leads to an osmotic influx of isotonic fluid, while depletion of ATP in the erythrocytes causes a massive increase in their rigidity[2]. The net result is that the vasculature of an ischaemic organ becomes progressively more difficult to reperfuse as the duration of ischaemia is prolonged, the so-called *no-reflow* phenomenon[3]. This is a most important factor in so-called *warm ischaemic injury*.

Most attention has been given to the metabolic consequences of ischaemia. The most critical effect is due to anoxia: glycogen reserves provide an adequate fuel supply for most tissues for short ischaemia times, but cessation of the supply of molecular oxygen arrests the electron transport chain causing accumulation of NADH and H^+, and depletion of ATP. The Krebs cycle is arrested by low NAD^+ levels. The lactate dehydrogenase reaction generates limited amounts of NAD^+ with the accumulation of lactate, but glycolysis is the only means of generating ATP. However, falling pH blocks the activity of PFK, thus limiting the already meagre supplies of ATP provided by glycolysis. Thus, the generation of ATP is inhibited both by lack of substrates (O_2 initially, then glucose) and by the accumulation of lactate and H^+. The rapidity with which high-energy phosphate compounds are lost is dramatic[4].

An important immediate consequence of lack of ATP is cessation of the Na^+ pump: intracellular sodium $(Na^+)_i$ rises and $(K^+)_i$ falls. However, $(Na^+)_i$ rises more than $(K^+)_i$ falls because of the intracellular impermeant anion, and as the membrane potential is reduced Cl^- also enters. The net effect is therefore that NaCl enters the cells, together with the necessary osmotic quota of water, and causes the cells to swell – the so-called *cloudy swelling* of the pathologist.

The function of preservation methods then is to prevent these harmful consequences of ischaemia without introducing new damaging factors.

PRESERVATION

There are basically two possible approaches: the first is to restore conditions, as quickly as possible, towards the normal physiological state, that is, to use normothermic perfusion; the second is to use the general slowing of reaction rates that is produced by cooling, to retard those processes that cause deterioration.

NORMOTHERMIA

It is not difficult to supply the known functions of a circulation by normothermic perfusion, but it has so far proved impossible to do so without introducing new and serious problems. The maximum preservation period possible is in the region of 7 h when function is assayed by transplantation[5], the problems being associated with damage to blood vessels and blood cells (see ref. 6 for discussion). The use of fluorocarbon emulsions may improve on this position, but for the present, normothermic perfusion cannot rival hypothermia for preservation purposes.

HYPOTHERMIA

The more important consequences of cooling will now be examined, and it will be shown that not all of them are helpful in avoiding ischaemic damage.

Effect on reaction rates

Reactions occur only between activated molecules. The fraction of molecules in a given system with an energy E is given by the expression $\exp(-E/RT)$ where R is the gas constant and T is absolute temperature. If the logarithm of the rate at which a reaction occurs is plotted against T^{-1}

(an Arrhenius plot), the resulting line will have a slope of $-E/R$, which therefore indicates the temperature-dependence of that reaction. An alternative way of representing temperature dependence is the Q_{10}, which can be shown to be related to E, the activation energy, by the equation

$$E = \frac{RT^2 \log_e Q_{10}}{10}$$

Q_{10} values of 2 and 3 correspond respectively to activation energies of 13 and 21 kcal/mol respectively. By reducing the rate at which substrates are metabolized, cooling makes cells less dependent on their supply. It should be pointed out, however, that not all reaction rates are affected to the same extent, or even in the same manner, by cooling: the effects of cooling on an integrated metabolizing system are complex, and it is at least theoretically possible that interconnected pathways may be dislocated, with harmful consequences. An illustration of the complex effects of cooling is provided in the next section.

Effect on energy metabolism

We know that the supply of oxygen is the most critical metabolic factor in ischaemia. In the 1950s Fuhrman established the temperature-dependence of oxygen consumption for a wide range of tissues[7]; the Q_{10} values were all between 2 and 2.5 down to 10 °C and rather larger at lower temperatures. Thus cooling by 25–35 °C produced a reduction in oxygen requirements of between 6 and 30 times. The ratio is given by the expression:

$$Q_{10} \exp \left(\frac{t_1 - t_2}{10} \right)$$

There is relatively little quantitative information available on the effect of temperature on the requirements for other metabolites: it is clear, however, that the preference for different substrates and the relative contributions of glycolysis and aerobic oxidation may change with temperature. Huang et al.[8], studying well-oxygenated renal cortex slices, found that whereas glucose, amino acids, ketone bodies and fatty acids were all consumed at 38 °C, only short-chain fatty acids and ketone bodies were metabolized at 10 °C. In hypothermically perfused canine kidneys, Pettersson et al.[9] found very little glucose uptake at 6 °C, most of that being metabolized to lactate, whereas the eight-carbon fatty acid caprylic acid was completely oxidized. Slaatelid's findings agree with this[10]. The Po_2 in these experiments was probably in the region of 150–250 mmHg. In rabbit kidneys we also concluded that glycolysis was the principal source of energy at 10 °C when the Po_2 was 150 mmHg, but that oxidation of caprylic acid was the main fuel when the Po_2 was raised to 650 mmHg[4]. Data published by Fischer's group in fact show that the amount of caprylate oxidized is highly dependent on the P_{O_2} of the perfusate, increasing almost 20-fold as the P_{O_2} is raised from 11 to 250 mmHg[11].

These experimental results show that the effects of cooling on metabolism are indeed complex and poorly understood at the present time. The simple notion that cooling produces a uniform retardation of all processes is not tenable.

Effects on active ion transport

The sodium pump and other active pumps are turned off by cooling: thus the *effect* is similar to that produced by anoxia although the *mechanism* is different: there may be ample supplies of ATP present, but at a low temperature the pump itself is unable to utilize ATP. At the temperatures commonly used for preservation ($>10\,°C$) there is essentially no (Na^+-K^+)-ATPase activity in most, if not all tissues[1]. Thus hypothermia has no very useful effect on this consequence of ischaemia, although the passive diffusion of ions and water is slowed somewhat. It may be mentioned here that the fact that cooling causes cells to swell, but prevents the no-reflow phenomenon, makes it unlikely that endothelial cell swelling plays any part in that phenomenon[12].

Thermal shock

This is an ill-understood phenomenon whereby some cells are damaged by rapid cooling even in the absence of freezing. It has long been known to occur in some micro-organisms, spermatozoa and modified erythrocytes. It may be caused by mechanical stress on cell membranes, induced by differential thermal contraction[13]. Its relevance to organ preservation is that Jacobsen and his colleagues have recently shown a deleterious effect of rapid cooling in rabbit kidneys (see Chapter 23). A cooling rate of 7.2 °C/min was necessary to produce this effect: its mechanism is not yet fully understood, but the observation warns us that ultra-rapid cooling should be avoided.

Conclusions

The main beneficial effect of cooling is in the slowing of chemical reactions and hence the reduced demand for oxygen and other metabolites. The detailed effects on metabolism are complex, however, not necessarily entirely beneficial, and certainly require closer study. Cooling has no useful effect on cell swelling or the redistribution of ions, and ultra-rapid cooling may be injurious.

APPLICATIONS OF HYPOTHERMIA

Low temperature has been used in three fundamentally different ways to achieve the preservation of ischaemic organs. The assumptions upon which each approach is based will be examined, and their advantages and disadvantages discussed. (It is realized that not all protagonists of each method will agree with my analysis, or indeed with each other, but it is hoped that this somewhat didactic presentation will help to stimulate discussion!)

Continuous perfusion at ~10 °C

It is assumed that a moderate degree of hypothermia will reduce metabolic needs, but that continuous perfusion will still be needed to support the remaining metabolism, and remove the products of that metabolism. The remaining metabolism is assumed to be sufficient for fluid and ionic movements to be controlled by active, biochemical processes. Thus the perfusate is of plasma-like composition and osmolality, it is well oxygenated, contains fatty acids and glucose, and is perfused at a pressure sufficient to achieve complete and even tissue perfusion[14]. The assumption that metabolism continues at 10 °C is clearly justified by the studies already referred to. The most important metabolite to supply is oxygen: in the absence of exogenous fuels endogenous lipids are burned[15], but it does seem prudent to avoid this by supplying short-chain fatty acids and glucose. In view of the evidence that significant glycolysis occurs even at oxygen tensions as high as 150–250 mmHg, it may be useful to consider higher oxygen tensions. If significant glycolysis does occur, or there has been significant prior warm ischaemia, perfusion has the advantage that it washes out lactate and $H+$ and thereby removes the potential block on PFK. Perfusion has two other advantages when there has been significant warm ischaemia prior to preservation: it permits the collapsed, partially blocked microcirculation to be gradually cleared at a safe temperature, over several hours if necessary[12], and if the appropriate substrates are provided (oxygen, respiratory fuel, and hypoxanthine or adenine), it permits resynthesis of depleted adenine nucleotide during preservation[4]. It seems unlikely that the method can prevent transmembrane ion and water movements, however, because of the temperature sensitivity of the pump, and indeed some protagonists of continuous perfusion have increased both the $K+$ concentration[16] and the osmolality[17] of the perfusate to overcome the problem. In practice continuous perfusion has been shown to permit the longest periods of preservation[16] and it is the most effective method for kidneys with significant warm ischaemic injury[18]. The disadvantages of the method are its complexity, its cost, and the fact that it is possible to cause vascular damage by inexpert or inappropriate perfusion methods[19].

Initial perfusion and storage at ~0 °C

This approach assumes that, with the use of somewhat lower temperatures, it is unnecessary to support metabolism: control of ion and water distribution between the intracellular and extracellular compartments is achieved by physical, not biochemical, means. Since the driving force for sodium loading and potassium depletion is the different ion balance in extracellular fluid, and since the driving force for net fluid entry is the impermeant intracellular anion, both changes can be prevented by altering the composition of the extracellular fluid; this can be achieved by brief perfusion of the excised organ with an appropriately formulated solution. Following the original studies of Keeler et al.[20], Collins was the first to establish a practical method: his solution contained 115 mmol/l K^+, 30 mmol/l Mg^{2+}, 30 mmol/l SO_4^{2-}, 58 mmol/l phosphate and 140 mmol/l glucose; it was potassium- and magnesium-rich and contained slowly permeating anions and neutral solutes[21]. Similar solutions were subsequently utilized by Sacks[22] and Ross and Marshall[23], and the general approach has proved highly effective for 24 or even 48 h preservation of kidneys and some other organs, providing there was no significant warm ischaemic injury. The practical value of the special ionic balance is open to question however and there is even some evidence that high levels of K^+[12] and of Mg^{2+} (see Chapter 26) can be harmful in some situations. The importance of impermeant solutes is firmly established, however[24-26]. It is interesting that in fact none of the solutions used so far has really closely mimicked intracellular fluid, and although the intracellular impermeant anion probably amounts to no more than 20 mosmol/kg concentrations of glucose, sucrose and mannitol in the 100–200 mosmol/kg range have generally been used. Robinson in fact showed[27] that 20 mosmol/kg of a relatively low molecular weight polymer (~6000 daltons) was able to maintain a normal water content in non-metabolizing renal cortex, and we confirmed this in whole rabbit kidneys[28]. It would be interesting to see whether a solution of ionic balance closer to the true intracellular fluid, and containing 20 mosmol/kg of such a polymer would improve results with this method of preservation.

The limitations of this approach are two: substrates for metabolism are not provided and a collapsed, blocked microcirculation may remain so until the organ is transplanted, with resulting severe damage. Both deficiencies assume particular importance when there has been significant prior warm ischaemia. The technique can be modified to take some account of these problems: biochemical substrates can be included in the solution, not only glucose, but also hypoxanthine or adenine, and inhibitors of 5'-nucleotide activity[29]; Fischer's technique of retrograde oxygen persufflation may make sufficient supplies of molecular oxygen available without the complications and risks of continuous perfusion[30]. Removal of inspissated red cells can be facilitated by the inclusion of low molecular weight dextran[31], or other suitable solutes to draw more fluid into the vascular system. It remains likely, however, that continuous perfusion will remain the optimal method for preserving and even improving the quality of organs with significant warm ischaemic injury.

Cryopreservation at $< 0\,°C$

This approach attempts to hold organs at much lower temperatures in a state of truly suspended animation, where storage can be indefinite. It assumes that methods that have been developed for a very wide range of single-cell systems, such as red cells, lymphocytes and tissue culture cells, can be successfully applied to whole organs. Such methods rely on the use of cryoprotective agents and the control of cooling rate and warming rate; by careful optimization it is possible to obtain greater than 80% survival of a large number of cell types[32]. There are, however, theoretical obstacles to such a convenient extrapolation, obstacles that ought not to be completely ignored by experimenters! They may be listed as follows:

(1) *Geometry.* Cell suspensions can be packaged in convenient shapes that permit accurate control of cooling and warming rates: solid organs are 'pre-packed' in very inconvenient shapes, with a low surface area:volume ratio, making heat exchange a major problem at all but very slow rates.

(2) *Mixed cell types.* Cells differ in their requirements for preservation, and effective techniques for erythrocytes, lymphocytes and fertilized ova, for instance, are quite different. In an organ there are many cell types, and any effective method has to secure the survival of them all.

(3) *Packing density.* The highly successful techniques for single cells are almost exclusively used with low packed-cell volumes, certainly $< 10\%$. It is now known that, with many combinations of cryo-protectant, cooling rate and warming rate, survival is severely impaired when the system consists of $> 50\%$ cells. The mechanisms are not yet completely clear, but the phenomenon may well apply to solid organs[33].

(4) *General architecture.* In a cell suspension only the cells matter: events in the extracellular space are of no direct consequence, and extracellular ice is innocuous. In an organ, the extracellular architecture of basement membranes and other extracellular materials is vital to function, and their disruption, and the disturbance of the normal cell-to-cell relations may be just as damaging as injury to the cells themselves.

(5) *Vascular system.* Organs require an intact vascular system in order that they may function: 100% recovery of parenchyma will be of no value unless the microcirculation is undamaged. It appears that although endothelial cells will survive cryopreservation, their attachments to the basement membrane may be disrupted, leading to occlusion after re-establishing the circulation.

These difficulties are formidable; not necessarily insuperable. It must, however, be stated unequivocally that neither theoretical considerations, nor the results of direct experimentation to date, justify the expectation that cryopreservation will provide indefinite storage in the immediate future.

PRACTICAL METHODS

For practical purposes the choice for all organs now being transplanted lies between continuous hypothermic perfusion and preliminary perfusion followed by refrigeration at $\lessgtr 0\,°C$. The general conclusion must be that continuous perfusion is superior where there has been either significant prior warm ischaemia or where very long preservation is needed. When, as is usually the case today, these requirements do not apply, the simpler method is to be preferred. The present situation for the four most commonly transplanted organs may be summarized thus.

(1) *Kidney.* When there has been no significant warm ischaemia and preservation is needed for less than 48 h, then initial perfusion with Collins'[21] or Ross and Marshall's solution[23] followed by storage at 0–4 °C is effective. If these conditions are not satisfied, then continuous perfusion with plasma protein fraction seems to be the best choice[18].

(2) *Liver.* It is essential that there be no prior warm ischaemia: initial perfusion with either Collins' solution[34] or plasma protein fraction with an elevated K^+ concentration[35] followed by refrigeration at 0–4 °C will provide up to 10 h storage.

(3) *Heart.* Up to 24 h preservation is possible after initial perfusion with a hyperosmolar, potassium-rich solution[36]: the optimal composition is unclear; the concentration of Ca^{2+} is probably critical for longer preservation times, but more work is needed to clarify this[37]. Again, it is essential to avoid warm ischaemia.

(4) *Pancreas.* When there has been no significant warm ischaemia, up to 24 h preservation has been demonstrated using a range of washout solutions with elevated K^+ content and osmolality. We have evidence that a high Mg^{2+} concentration may be deleterious with this organ (see Chapter 26). Others have shown that the introduction of a colloid may permit prolongation to 48 h[38]. Continuous perfusion has not been shown to permit longer or more effective preservation.

References

1. Pegg, D.E. (1981). The biology of cell survival in vitro. In Karow, A.M. Jr. and Pegg, D.E. (eds) *Organ Preservation for Transplantation.* 2nd edn, pp. 31–52. (New York: Marcel Dekker)
2. Weed, R.I., La Celle, P.L. and Merrill, E.W. (1969). Metabolic dependence of red cell deformability. *J. Clin. Invest.,* **48**, 795
3. Sheehan, H.L. and Davis, J.C. (1959). Renal ischaemia after failed reflow. *J. Path. Bacteriol.,* **78**, 105
4. Pegg, D.E., Wusteman, M.C. and Foreman, J. (1981). The metabolism of normal and ischemically injured rabbit kidneys during perfusion for 48 hours at 10 °C. *Transplantation,* **32**, 437
5. Cassie, G., Couch, N., Dammin, G. and Murray, J.C. (1959). Normothermic perfusion and reimplantation of the excised dog kidney. *Surg. Gynec. Obstet.,* **109**, 721
6. Pegg, D.E. (1971). Vascular resistance of the isolated rabbit kidney. *Cryobiology,* **8**, 431

7. Fuhrman, F. A. (1956). Oxygen consumption of mammalian tissues at reduced temperatures. In *The Physiology of Induced Hypothermia*. Pub. 451 (Nat. Acad. Sci.-Nat. Res. Council: Washington), pp. 50–51

8. Huang, J. S., Downes, G. L., Childress, G. L., Felts, J. M. and Belzer, F. O. (1974). Oxidation of ^{14}C-labelled substrates by dog kidney cortex at 10 and 38 °C. *Cryobiology*, **11**, 387

9. Pettersson, S., Claes, G. and Scherstén, T. (1974). Fatty acid and glucose utilization during continuous hypothermic perfusion of dog kidney. *Eur. Surg. Res.*, **6**, 79

10. Slattelid, O., Flatmark, A. and Skrede, S. (1976). The importance of perfusate control of free fatty acids for dog kidney preservation. *Scand. J. Clin. Lab. Invest.*, **36**, 239

11. Fischer, J. H., Armbruster, D., Grebe, W., Czerniak, A. and Isselhard, W. (1980). Effects of differences in substrate supply on the energy metabolism of hypothermically perfused canine kidneys. *Cryobiology*, **17**, 135

12. Pegg, D. E. (1978). An approach to hypothermic renal preservation. *Cryobiology*, **15**, 1

13. Lovelock, J. E. (1955). Haemolysis by thermal shock. *Br. J. Haematol.*, **1**, 117

14. Belzer, F. O., Ashby, B. S. and Dunphy, J. E. (1967). 24-hour and 72-hour preservation of canine kidneys. *Lancet*, **2**, 536

15. Huang, J. S., Downes, G. L. and Belzer, F. O. (1971). Utilization of fatty acids in perfused hypothermic dog kidneys. *J. Lipid Res.*, **12**, 622

16. Johnson, R. W. G., Cohen, G. L. and Ballardie, F. D. (1979). The limitations of continuous perfusion with plasma protein fraction. In Pegg, D. E. and Jacobsen, I. A. (eds.) *Organ Preservation II*, pp. 18–30. (Edinburgh: Churchill Livingstone)

17. Pegg, D. E., Jacobsen, I. A. and Walter, C. A. (1977). Hypothermic perfusion of rabbit kidneys with solutions containing gelatin polypeptides. *Transplantation*, **24**, 29

18. Johnson, R. W. G. (1972). The effect of ischaemic injury on kidneys preserved for 24 hours before transplantation. *Br. J. Surg.*, **59**, 765

19. Cerra, F. B., Raza, S., Andres, G. A. and Siegal, J. H. (1977). The endothelial damage of pulsatile renal preservation and its relationship to perfusion pressure and colloid osmotic pressure. *Surgery*, **81**, 534

20. Keeler, R., Swinney, J., Taylor, R. M. R. and Uldall, M. B. (1966). The problem of renal preservation. *Br. J. Urol.*, **38**, 653

21. Collins, G. M., Bravo-Shugarman, M. and Terasaki, P. I. (1969). Kidney preservation for transportation. Initial perfusion and 30-hours ice storage. *Lancet*, **2**, 1219

22. Sacks, S. A., Petritsch, P. H. and Kaufman, J. J. (1973). Canine kidney preservation using a new perfusate. *Lancet*, **2**, 1024

23. Ross, H., Marshall, V. C. and Escott, M. L. (1976). 72-hour canine kidney preservation without continuous perfusion. *Transplantation*, **21**, 498

24. Collins, G. M., Hartley, L. C. J. and Clunie, G. J. A. (1972). Kidney preservation for transportation. Experimental analysis of optimum perfusate composition. *Br. J. Surg.*, **59**, 187

25. Downes, G., Hoffman, R., Huang, J. S. and Belzer, F. O. (1973). Mechanism of action of washout solutions for kidney preservation. *Transplantation*, **16**, 46

26. Green, C. J. and Pegg, D. E. (1979). Mechanism of action of 'intra-cellular' renal preservation solutions. *World J. Surg.*, **3**, 115

27. Robinson, J. R. (1971). Control of water content of non-metabolizing kidney slices by sodium chloride and polyethylene glycol (PEG 6000). *J. Physiol.*, **213**, 227

28. Pegg, D. E. (1977). The water and cation content of non-metabolizing perfused rabbit kidneys. *Cryobiology*, **14**, 160

29. Buhl, M. R., Kemp, E. and Kemp, G. (1979). Purine nucleotide and nucleoside administration to kidneys: The effect on tolerance to ischaemia. In Pegg, D. E. and Jacobsen, I. A. (eds.) *Organ Preservation II*, pp. 247–252. (Edinburgh: Churchill Livingstone)

30. Fischer, J. H., Czerniak, A., Hauer, U. and Isselhard, W. (1978). A new simple method for optimal storage of ischaemically damaged kidneys. *Transplantation*, **25**, 43

31. Wusteman, M. C., Jacobsen, I. A. and Pegg, D. E. (1978). A new solution for initial perfusion of transplant kidneys. *Scand. J. Urol. Nephrol.*, **12**, 281

32. Pegg, D. E. (1976). Long-term preservation of cells and tissues: a review. *J. Clin. Pathol.*, **29**, 271

33. Pegg, D.E. (1981). The effect of cell concentration on the recovery of human erythrocytes after freezing and thawing in the presence of glycerol. *Cryobiology,* **18,** 221
34. Benichou, J., Halgrimson, C.G., Weill III, R., Koep, L.J. and Starzl, T.E. (1977). Canine and human liver preservation for 6–18 hours by cold perfusion. *Transplantation,* **24,** 407
35. Calne, R.Y. (1981). Liver. In Karow, A.M., Jr. and Pegg, D.E. (eds.) *Organ Preservation for Transplantation.* 2nd edn, pp. 617–624. (New York: Marcel Dekker)
36. Watson, D.C. (1977). Consistent survival after prolonged donor heart preservation. *Transplant Proc.,* **9,** 297
37. Armitage, W.J. and Pegg, D.E. (1978). The influence of gelatin polypeptides, potassium, calcium and osmolality on the hypothermic perfusion of rabbit hearts. *Cryobiology,* **15,** 537
38. Toledo-Pereyra, L.H., Chee, M., Condie, R.M., Najarian, J.S. and Lillehei, R.C. (1979). Forty-eight hours hypothermic storage of whole canine pancreas allografts. Improved preservation with a colloid hyperosmolar solution. *Cryobiology,* **16,** 221

PART II
EFFECTS OF ISCHAEMIA
AND ANOXIA

7
Recovery of renal function in the rat after warm ischaemia: functional and morphological changes

V. MARSHALL, P. JABLONSKI, B. HOWDEN, E. LESLIE, D. RAE and J. TANGE

Where cardiac arrest is used as the criterion of death and organ removal for transplantation, significant renal damage occurs prior to removal, and is a major factor in subsequent preservation. Pre-treatment regimens may reduce ischaemic damage but little is known concerning the events leading to recovery, the extent of recovery or the factors that influence recovery from warm ischaemic damage. This preliminary study was planned to determine functional and morphological changes occurring in the rat kidney after warm ischaemia.

METHODS

Male Sprague–Dawley rats (250–350 g) were anaesthetized and heparinized. The right renal artery was then occluded by a soft silver clip (Weck) for ischaemic periods of 30 sec, 30, 45 or 60 min. Contralateral nephrectomy was performed after the clip was removed.

Serum creatinine and urea were determined 2, 4, 7 and 14 days after ischaemia. Urine volume, osmolality, Na, K and creatinine were also determined. Early and late function after ischaemia were also assessed by perfusion of the damaged kidney in a standardized *in vitro* normothermic perfusion circuit described previously[1], 5 min and 14 days after ischaemia. Ischaemic kidneys were examined histologically after fixation in buffered formalin at 1, 2, 4 and 14 days.

RESULTS

All animals survived 30 sec warm ischaemia, whereas 75–80% survived

30–45 min, and 67% survived 60 min. Deaths occurred from 2 to 7 days after ischaemic damage. Two days after any period of warm ischaemia, serum creatinine and urea were elevated, and the concentration was related to the duration of warm ischaemia (creatinine, means ± SEM: controls 44 ± 4; 30 sec 70 ± 12; 30 min 68 ± 6; 45 min 222 ± 87; 60 min 368 ± 80 μmol/l. Urea, means ± SEM: controls 5.5 ± 0.2; 30 sec 7.2 ± 0.5; 30 min 7.8 ± 0.6; 45 min 20.9 ± 7.4; 60 min 37.8 ± 6.6 mmol/l). After 4 days serum creatinine returned towards normal levels in those animals where the ischaemic period was less than 60 min (e.g. 45 min 67 ± 13 μmol/l vs 60 min 268 ± 111 μmol/l) and after 14 days serum creatinine was normal in all groups. Serum urea appeared to be a more sensitive index of damage and was still elevated 14 days after 45 or 60 min warm ischaemia (30 min 5.0 ± 0.8; 45 min 7.7 ± 0.7 and 60 min 9.5 ± 0.7 mmol/l).

Four days after ischaemic damage the animals secreted large volumes of dilute urine (30 sec 7.6 ± 1.3; 30 min 12.9 ± 1.6; 45 min 16.8 ± 2.0; 60 min 29.3 ± 4.9 ml/24 h). Urine volume and osmolality were related to the duration of ischaemia. After 14 days the volumes were smaller (30 sec 9.1 ± 0.8; 30 min 12.1 ± 1.7; 45 min 11.6 ± 2.9; 60 min 18.1 ± 2.4 ml/24 h) and urine osmolality was only marginally lower than that of controls (30 sec 1660 ± 140; 30 min 1520 ± 120; 45 min 1280 ± 90; 60 min 1340 ± 150 mosmol/kg). Total sodium and potassium excretion were similar to control 4 days after ischaemia.

Isolated perfusion of kidneys 5 min after ischaemic damage demonstrated a marked diminution in glomerular filtration rate (GFR: control 0.68 ± 0.04; 30 min 0.36 ± 0.05; 60 min 0.17 ± 0.04 ml/min); urinary/plasma inulin ratio (U/P inulin: control 21.9 ± 2.3; 30 min 7.4 ± 0.8; 60 min 2.3 ± 0.2); total Na reabsorption: (T_{Na} control 97.6 ± 5.9; 30 min 51.6 ± 5.9; 60 min 14.8 ± 3.7 μmol/min) and percentage Na reabsorption (control 96.8 ± 0.04; 30 min 88.8 ± 1.4; 60 min 55.6 ± 6.1%). Urinary flow rate (control 36 ± 4; 30 min 56 ± 9; 60 min 70 ± 15 μg/min) and Na excretion (control 3.2 ± 0.5; 30 min 6.2 ± 1.1; 60 min 9.5 ± 2.1 μmol/min) were increased. The magnitude of these changes was related to the duration of the ischaemia. After 14 days the GFR (0.20 ± 0.05 ml/min) and T_{Na} (28.9 ± 7.4 μmol/min) were still diminished, U/P inulin and percentage Na reabsorption had returned to normal and urinary flow rate (14 ± 3 μg/min) and sodium excretion (0.7 ± 0.2 μmol/min) were below those of the control group. All kidneys were hypertrophied (2–2.5 times control weight) so renal functional parameters expressed per g weight would have been even further depressed.

Warm ischaemia of 30 min or longer resulted in necrosis of the proximal convoluted tubule. Glomeruli appeared normal. The acute effect could be seen at 1 day but was most evident at 2 days when the severity of the lesion was graded histologically, as follows: (1) mitoses and necrosis of individual cells (Figure 7.1); (2) necrosis of all cells in adjacent proximal convoluted tubules, with survival of surrounding tubules (Figure 7.2); (3) necrosis of the distal third of the proximal convoluted tubule – a band of necrosis extending across the inner cortex (Figure 7.3); (4) necrosis affecting the whole of the proximal convoluted tubule (Figure 7.4).

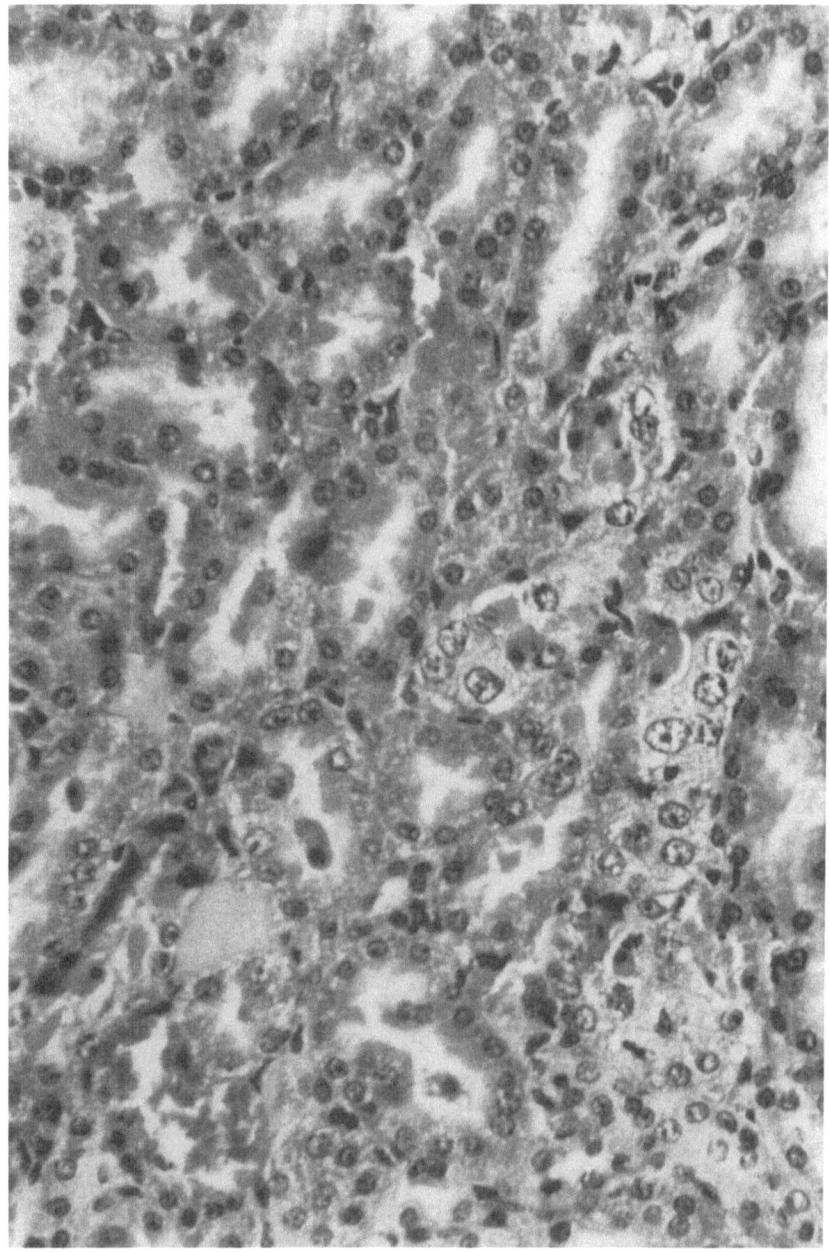

Figure 7.1 Photomicrograph of rat proximal convoluted tubules showing isolated necrotic cells and mitotic figures. Grade 1 necrosis. H&E × 324

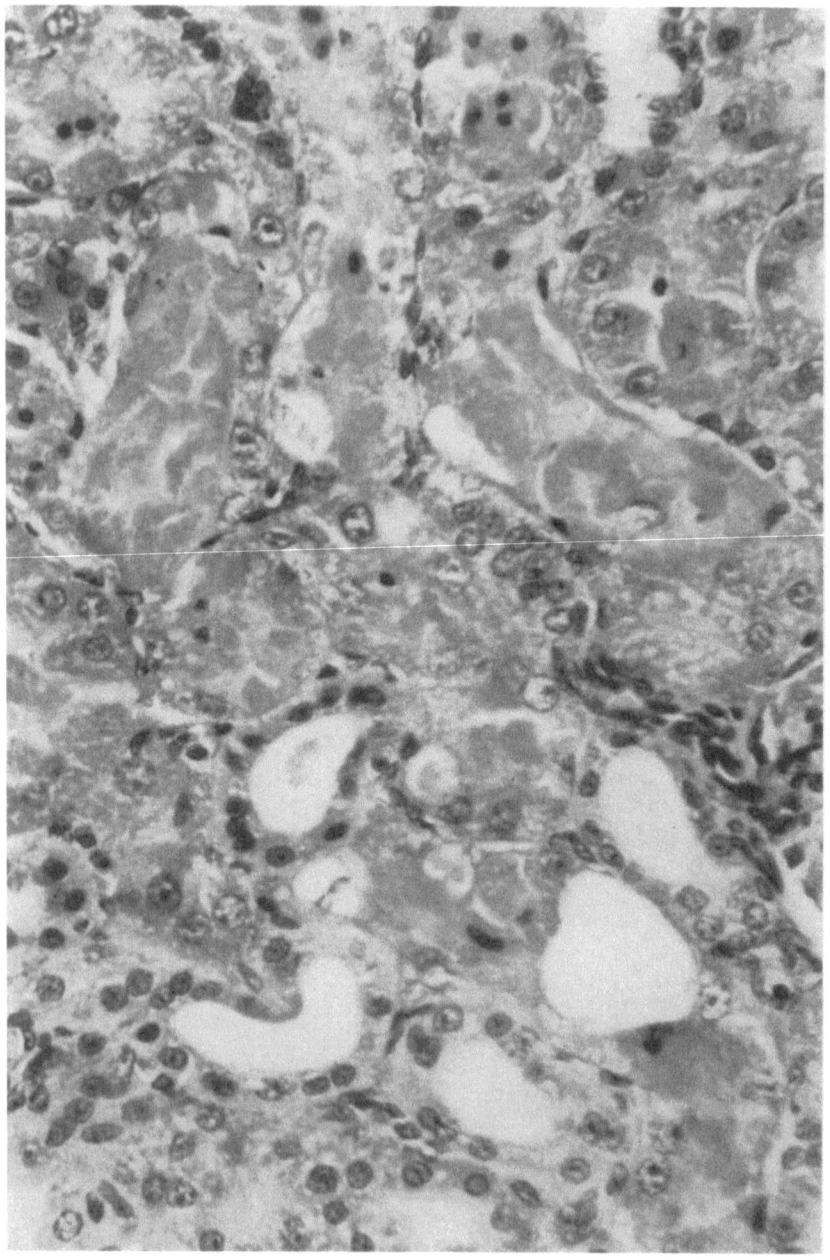

Figure 7.2 Necrosis of all cells in groups of proximal convoluted tubules. Grade 2 necrosis.
H&E × 324

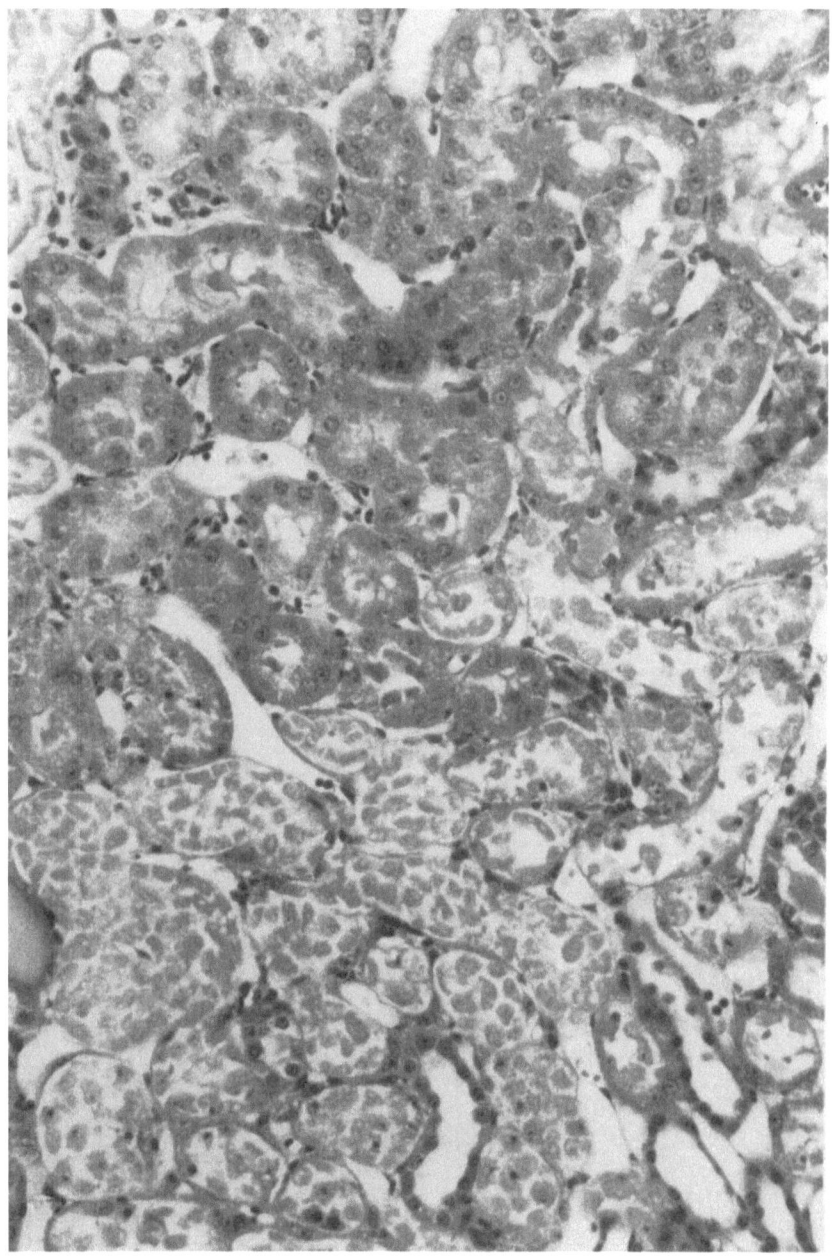

Figure 7.3 Necrosis of the distal third of the proximal convoluted tubules. Grade 3 necrosis. H&E × 216

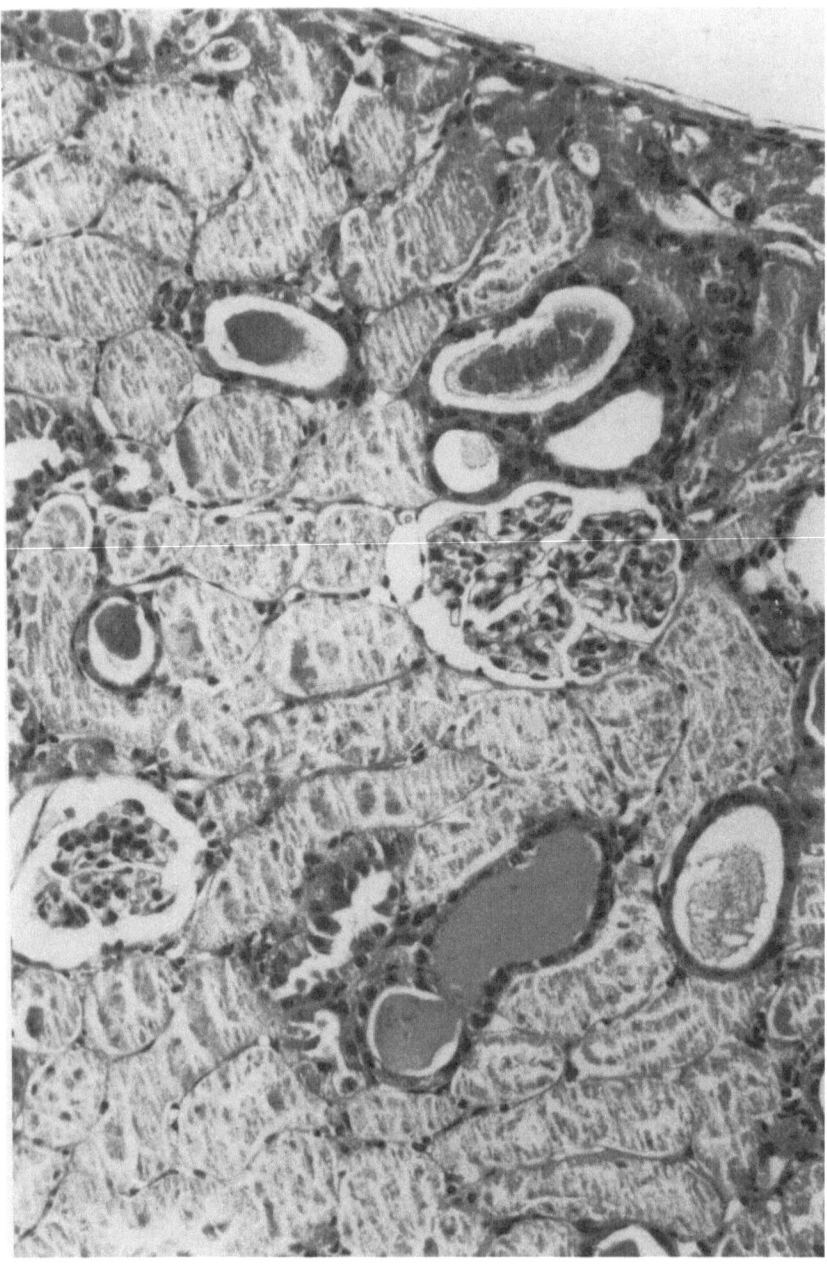

Figure 7.4 Necrosis involving the whole of the proximal convoluted tubule. Grade 4 necrosis. H&E × 216

The severity of necrosis was related to the period of ischaemia. Grade 4 necrosis was not found after 30 min ischaemia whereas this degree of necrosis was found in 35% of kidneys after 45 min and in 60% after 60 min ischaemia. Grade 3 necrosis was found in 40% after 30 min, 50% after 45 min and 36% after 60 min ischaemia. After 30 min warm ischaemia 55% of kidneys had grade 2 lesions whereas this degree of necrosis was present in only 5% after 60 min and in 15% after 45 min. Regeneration of tubular epithelium was present at 2 days and re-epithelialization was virtually complete after 14 days. There was always some residual cortical damage. This consisted of groups of tubules with contracted lumens and lined by epithelium with basophilic cytoplasm. There was an increase in surrounding interstitial tissue and some tubular basement membranes were thickened. These tubulo-interstitial changes were graded as mild: 0–10% residual damage; moderate: 10–20% damage; severe: > 20% damage; and the severity of the long-term effect was also related to the duration of ischaemia. Severe damage was noted in 67% of kidneys after 60 min ischaemia and in 36% after 45 min. Moderate damage occurred in 33% of kidneys after 60 min and in 27% after 45 min. Only mild damage was evident after 30 min ischaemia. Mild and moderate damage was restricted to the deeper cortex, but with severe damage residual changes were found in the proximal convoluted tubule throughout the whole cortex and there was extensive calcium deposition in tubule lumens.

DISCUSSION

These results indicate that survival, renal function and morphology after different periods of warm ischaemia are directly related to the duration of ischaemia. However, it is apparent that the use of only one of these para-meters as a measure of the efficacy of any treatment regimen may provide an inadequate assessment. Animals survive with remarkably poor renal function and severe morphological changes; even then serum creatinine and urea can approach control values. Assessment of both functional and morphological changes produced by renal ischaemia is necessary if results of different experiments are to be compared. It cannot be assumed that the severity of tubular necrosis or the extent of interstitial nephritis following a given period of ischaemia is constant for each study[2].

The isolated perfused kidney has provided additional information about the effects of renal tubular ischaemia. Early in recovery isolated kidney perfusion is unreliable because of leakage of inulin across damaged tubules[3,4]. This is no longer present at 14 days[2] and the fall in GFR still demonstrable at this time with high constant perfusion rates indicates the interplay of other factors besides the fall of renal blood flow observed *in vivo*[2].

Acknowledgement

This work was supported in part by a grant from the National Health and Medical Research Council.

References

1. Jablonski, P., Howden, B., Marshall, V. and Scott, D. F. (1980). Evaluation of citrate flushing solution using the isolated perfused rat kidney. *Transplantation,* **30,** 239
2. Finn, W. F. and Chevalier, R. L. (1979). Recovery from postischemic acute renal failure in the rat. *Kidney Int.,* **16,** 113
3. Donohoe, J. F., Venkatachalam, M. A., Bernard, D. B. and Levinsky, N. G. (1978). Tubular leakage and obstruction after renal ischaemia: structural–functional correlations. *Kidney Int.,* **13,** 208
4. Olbricht, C., Mason, J., Takabatake, T., Hohlbrugger, G. and Thurau, K. (1977). The early phase of experimental acute renal failure. II: Tubular leakage and the reliability of glomerular markers. *Pflügers Arch.,* **372,** 251

8
The dynamics of regional blood flow after ischaemic trauma of the rat kidney

L. FRÖDIN, L. KARLBERG, Ö. KÄLLSKOG, B. J. NORLÉN and M. WOLGAST

The vascular resistance increases in kidneys subjected to ischaemic trauma, be it warm ischaemia[1], cold ischaemia[2], or cold continuous perfusion[3]. By reperfusion after different periods of hypothermic storage using a cold colloidal perfusate it was shown that this increased resistance was more pronounced in the deeper parts of the renal cortex and subsequently in the renal medulla[2]. This same pattern of regional perfusion was found in recipients immediately after transplantation[4]. The functional characteristics as studied by micropuncture techniques in transplanted kidneys also support the conclusion that the renal medulla is of primary interest for the understanding of the pathophysiology of acute renal failure after ischaemic trauma[5]. The observation of medullary vascular congestion in humans[6] and other species[7,8] supports this statement.

The present investigation was designed to evaluate total, cortical and medullary blood flow after renal artery clamping for 45 min. Blood flow conditions were examined 10 min after recirculation and 1, 7 and 28 days thereafter.

METHODS

Fifty male Sprague–Dawley rats weighing 255–350 g were used for the experiments. After heparinization (100 IU), acute renal failure was induced by clamping the left renal artery for 45 min. The right kidney was used as a control. Blood flow was measured with a catheter placed in the aortic root. Ligatures were placed around the pedicles of both kidneys.

The experiments were conducted by injecting about 2×10^5 [113]Sn-labelled 10 μm microspheres and about 20 μCi of [^{86}Rb]chloride through the carotid artery catheter. Before the injection, the reference blood sample was withdrawn at 0.75 ml/min. Exactly 30 sec after one-half of the total dose had been injected, sampling was stopped and both renal pedicles were ligated. The kidneys were then rapidly removed for subsequent microdissection.

Specimens from the cortex and the medulla were obtained. The medulla was subdivided into the outer stripe of the outer zone, the inner stripe of the outer zone and the inner zone. The specimens and the rest of the kidney were then weighed and the ^{86}Rb and the [113]Sn activities were measured in a gamma spectrophotometer shielded with a 3 mm thick brass cylinder to reduce beta-radiation.

The blood flow in ml/min/mg in the samples and the whole kidney was calculated as:

$$F = \frac{(M_{\text{tissue}}) \, (0.75)}{(M_{\text{blood}}) \, (\text{tissue weight})}$$

where F is the blood flow, 0.75 the blood sampling rate in ml/min, M_{tissue} the activity in the specimen and M_{blood} the activity found in the reference blood sample. The microsphere method[9] was used for total and cortical flow estimations and the ^{86}Rb extraction method[10] for estimations of the renal medullary blood flow.

RESULTS

The kidneys were pale and swollen when inspected 10 min and 24 h after recirculation. After 28 days the kidneys had a normal colour but were smaller than normal. Scars and crypts were scattered over the surface. The cut surfaces were typical with a dark zone in the inner stripe of the outer zone of the medulla 10 min after recirculation. This dark zone had mostly disappeared after 24 h but persistent oedema could be seen 7 days after the insult. No changes could be seen in the contralateral kidneys. Total renal blood flow was 3.8 ml/min/g 10 min after recirculation and 4.0 ml/min/g 24 h after the ischaemia. A remarkable reduction was found after 1 week when the total renal blood flow was only 1.2 ml/min/g but increased to 3.4 ml/min/g after 28 days. The same pattern was found for the cortex, but in the medulla the conditions were quite different. Ten minutes after recirculation the blood flow in the inner stripe of the outer zone was only 0.2 ml/min/g. After 7 days (when the total renal blood flow was markedly reduced) the blood flow in this zone was 0.3 ml/min/g. Taking into account the reduction of total renal blood flow this value is high and after 28 days the flow to the inner stripe was 1.4 ml/min/g which is a normal value.

Comparisons were made to normal values measured in separate experiments using the same methods[10].

DISCUSSION

The dynamics of blood flow after an ischaemic trauma may explain the diverging results presented by other authors, since blood flow studies have been performed at different times after the induction of acute renal

78

failure[11-13]. The polyuric isosthenuria found immediately after the trauma develops into anuria after 24h due to a progressive medullary dysfunction[14]; thereafter functions slowly improve. The most important functions which successively return to normal are the ability to excrete potassium and to concentrate urine.

Total renal blood flow and cortical flow is depressed to very low levels 1 week after the trauma. This is explained by an altered resistance first in the afferent and then also the efferent, artery. This finding is in accordance with the 'vasomotor nephropathy' suggested by Oken[15]. In our model, high intratubular pressures resulting from a proposed medullary block could possibly act on the glomeruli and result in the same response of the afferent artery, as shown in connection with ureteral obstruction[16]. As a consequence, the flow to peritubular capillaries will diminish, adding ischaemia to the tubular cells.

However, the most striking finding seems to be the greatly depressed reflow to the medulla immediately after reperfusion. The cause of this phenomenon could arise before recirculation, since vascular resistance was found to increase during the bloodless hypothermic state as recorded in experiments measuring regional perfusion after different periods of hypothermic storage by reperfusion with cold perfusate[2]. This is most probably due to cellular dysfunction developing during the ischaemic period when metabolic activity is low and membrane functions are disturbed, creating oedema during reperfusion.

After reperfusion, casts and debris in the tubular lumen[17] and blood cells in the vasculature[14] have been shown to add to the blockage in the deep part of the kidney. The accumulation of blood corpuscles is more prone to occur since albumin leaks through the membranes, thus concentrating blood in the vessels[14].

Several factors could be involved. The medulla differs from the cortex not only anatomically, containing the thin vasa recta and the loops of Henle, but also many other factors are different in this area. One interesting point is the difference in metabolic activity with the ability in the renal medulla to continue with anaerobic metabolism when oxygen supply has ceased. This activity will alter the regional pH[18]. The local formation of free radicals is possible. The disintegration of cell membranes and subsequent osmotic and oncotic forces would result in cellular oedema. In addition the removal of liquid through lymph channels is likely to be minimal in this part of the kidney.

The formation of vasoactive substances differs in the deep parts of the cortex and the medulla compared to other parts of the kidney[19]. The problem is even more complicated on account of rheological factors, viscosity changes, endothelial disorders, altered muscular functions and the possible actions of unknown metabolites formed in the ischaemic kidney both during the ischaemic period and in the recovery phase.

From the clinical viewpoint our findings could explain some well-known facts. The clinical effects of mannitol and furosemide are apparent if they are used in connection with reperfusion when the medullary block is incomplete and water could still be removed from the medulla. This theory can also explain the positive role of hyperosmolar perfusates in preservation procedures.

Furthermore, knowledge of the extreme depression of cortical and total renal blood flow in the recovery phase should teach us to interpret with extreme caution the findings on angiograms, renograms, gamma camera scintigrams and computed sequence tomograms. The possibility of the kidney regaining function could be good in spite of very low flows.

Preservation research associated with renal transplantation has always faced two basically different problems. One is the acute renal failure resulting in a 'no onset of function' but with a relatively good prognosis. The other problem is the non-viable kidney which never starts to function or where the end-result is very poor. It has hitherto been difficult to sort out these kidneys. It is of great interest whether the first-mentioned disorder progresses into the other, or if some other definite change in the kidney is responsible. From our studies it is possible to explain the non-viable kidney as the end-result of acute renal failure; if too many nephrons in the recovery phase become ischaemic to the critical point were the cells lose their ability to survive in spite of some recovery of blood flow. Another possibility is that at a critical point, reflow becomes totally impossible. Which ever of these speculations will prove to be true it seems logical, with our experimental data as a background, to try to intervene in the development of the observed medullary block in order to prevent the ischaemic damage in kidney transplants and in other situations which include ischaemic trauma to the kidney.

References

1. Frödin, L. (1975). Renal transplantation in the rat. II. In vitro perfusion of rat kidneys before transplantation. *Scand. J. Clin. Lab. Invest.*, **35**, 455
2. Harvig, B., Källskog, Ö. and Norlén, B. J. (1980). Effects of cold ischemia on the preserved rat kidney: intrarenal distribution of perfusate. *Cryobiology*, **17**, 478
3. Andrén, T., Frödin, L. and Harvig, B. (1982). Continuous perfusion and transplantation of rat kidneys. (In preparation)
4. Norlén, B. J., Engberg, A., Källskog, Ö. and Wolgast, M. (1978). Intrarenal hemo-dynamics in the transplanted rat kidney. *Kidney Int.*, **14**, 1
5. Norlén, B. J., Engberg, A., Källskog, Ö. and Wolgast, M. (1978). Nephron function of the transplanted rat kidney. *Kidney Int.*, **14**, 10
6. Thiel, G., de Rougemont, D., Thorhorst, J., Kaufmann, A., Peters-Haefeli, L. and Brunner, F. P. (1980). Importance of tubular obstruction and its prevention in ischemic acute renal failure in the rat. *Renal Pathophysiology*, p. 223 (New York: Raven Press)
7. Frega, N. S., Di Bona, D. R., Gaertler, B. and Leaf, A. (1976). Ischemic renal injury. *Kidney Int.*, **10**, 17
8. Diethelm, A. G. and Wilson, S. J. (1971). Obstruction to the renal microcirculation after temporary ischemia. *J. Surg. Res.*, **11**, 265
9. Källskog, Ö., Lindbom, L. O., Ulfendahl, H. R. and Wolgast, M. (1975). Regional and single glomerular blood flow in the rat kidney prepared for micropuncture. A methodological study. *Acta Physiol. Scand.*, **94**, 145
10. Karlberg, L., Källskog, Ö., Öjteg, G. and Wolgast, M. (1981). Renal medullary blood flow studied with the 86-Rb extraction method. Methodological considerations. *Acta Univ. Upsaliensis*, **381**, 1

11. Hollenberg, N. K., Epstein, M., Rosen, S. M., Basch, R. J., Oken, D. E. and Merril, J. P. (1968). Acute oliguric renal failure in man: Evidence for preferential renal cortical ischaemia. *Medicine,* **47,** 455

12. Churchill, S., Zarlengo, M. D., Carvalho, J. S., Gottlieb, M. N. and Oken, D. E. (1977). Normal renocortical flow in experimental acute renal failure. *Kidney Int.,* **11,** 246

13. Karlberg, L., Norlén, B. J., Öjteg, G. and Wolgast, M. (1981). Impaired medullary circulation in postischemic acute renal failure. *Acta Univ. Upsaliensis,* **381,** 1

14. Karlberg, L., Källskog, Ö., Nygren, K. and Wolgast, M. (1982). Erythrocyte and albumin distribution in the kidney following warm ischemia. A study in rats. *Scand. J. Urol. Nephrol.* (In press)

15. Oken, D. E. (1971). Nosologic considerations in the nomenclature of acute renal failure. *Nephron,* **8,** 550

16. Arendshorst, W. J., Finn, W. F. and Gottschalk, C. W. (1974). Nephron stop-flow pressure response to obstruction of 24 hours in the rat kidney. *J. Clin. Invest.,* **53,** 1497

17. Steinhausen, M., Thederan, H. and Nolinski, D. (1978). Further evidence of tubular blockage after acute ischemic renal failure in tupaia belangeri and rats. *Virchows Arch. A. Pathol. Histol.,* **381,** 13

18. Needleman, P., Passonean, J. V. and Lowry, O. H. (1968). Distribution of glucose and related metabolites in rat kidneys. *Am. J. Physiol.,* **215,** 655

19. Dunn, M. J. and Hood, V. L. (1977). Prostaglandins and the kidney. *Am. J. Physiol.,* **233,** F169

9
Renal function impairment in swelling with and without anoxia

J. JAMART and L. LAMBOTTE

As improvement in organ preservation has been obtained with hyperosmolar solutions, it has been deduced that inhibition of cellular swelling was beneficial, and that cellular swelling was one of the major pathways leading to cellular death. Disruption of cellular architecture and spatial separation of key enzymes are the suspected mechanisms. If this is the case, swelling in absence of anoxia should produce the same defects as anoxia. We have therefore attempted to produce similar swelling by flushing kidneys with hypotonic solutions or by submitting them to normothermic anoxia. The effects on glomerular function tested immediately or after 24 h were markedly different according to the origin of the oedema.

METHODS

Twenty-four mongrel dogs of an average weight of 20 kg were used. Anaesthesia was induced and maintained with sodium pentobarbital and the animal was ventilated via an intratracheal tube. A catheter introduced into the jugular vein allowed slow infusion of 1 litre of 0.9% NaCl solution during operation. A priming dose of $25 \mu Ci$ of 3H-labelled inulin was given intravenously and a second infusion containing $50 \mu Ci$ of tritiated inulin mixed in 500 ml 5% glucose solution was started at the time of anaesthesia and maintained at an infusion rate of 1 ml/min using a constant-flow pump. Blood samples were taken after 1 and 2 h to assess that equilibrium state was effectively reached. A midline laparotomy was performed. A careful dissection of aorta, vena cava and renal vessels was made and both kidneys completely freed from retroperitoneal tissue. Thereafter catheters were introduced into both ureters. Urine was collected by gravity during 30 min while three blood samples were taken from the femoral artery at 0, 15 and 30 min for determination of inulin. Renal blood flow (RBF) was measured using an electromagnetic flowmeter. These values were used as control values for each kidney, before the experimental procedure described below.

Twelve dogs were used for comparing hypotonic and isotonic flushing. After determination of control values a catheter was introduced into the aorta via the right iliac artery, with its tip pushed below the origin of the left renal artery. A ligature was tied around the catheter 2 cm below its tip and the aorta was clamped above the origin of the right renal artery. A similar catheter was then introduced via the iliac vein into the vena cava. Both kidneys were then flushed with an isotonic saline solution (NaCl 0.9%; 308 mosmol/l) at 37 °C and with a pressure of 125 cmH$_2$O, until the returning liquid was clear. The vessels of one kidney were then clamped while the other kidney was flushed during 5 min with a hypotonic solution (NaCl 0.225%; 77 mosmol/l). After this period, the vessels were also clamped for 5 min while the contralateral kidney was flushed with isotonic solution. The kidneys were therefore submitted to either an isotonic or a hypotonic solution for 10 min. Biopsies were taken at that time from both renal cortices. Both kidneys were again flushed for 2 min with isotonic solution and then the aortic clamp and catheters were removed. Iso- and hypotonic solutions were given alternately to left and right kidneys in consecutive dogs. Blood samples and 30 min urine samples were taken as described for control values, respectively at 10–40, 55–85 and 100–130 min after revascularization.

In six dogs of this series no catheter was pushed into the vena cava and continuity of the right iliac artery was restored. After performing measurements during 2 h after revascularization the kidneys were fixed to the muscular posterior wall to avoid twisting, and cutaneous ureterostomies were performed. The abdomen was closed while 0.25 mg atropine and 125 mg methylprednisolone were given. Twenty-four hours later both ureters were catheterized as earlier. Two series of blood samples and 30 min urine samples were taken as described above. Thereafter cortical tissue was taken for determination of water content.

Twelve dogs were used for comparing anoxia with isotonic or hypotonic flushing. One kidney was flushed for 2 min with isotonic solution, then its artery and vein were clamped for 60 min. The contralateral kidney was flushed as described above with isotonic or hypotonic solution. Measurements were performed for 2 h after revascularization and 24 h later.

Tritiated inulin in blood and urine samples was measured in a liquid scintillation counter in duplicate. Inulin clearance (Cl$_{IN}$) was computed for 30 min periods using the usual equation. Determination of water content in cortical tissue was estimated after desiccating tissue in an oven at 120 °C for 24 h.

As the presence of a contralateral kidney does not really influence the function of an injured kidney as determined by clearance tests[1], each kidney was considered as independent of the contralateral one. Three groups of kidneys were thus studied: isotonic group (I, $n = 18$); hypotonic group (H, $n = 18$) and anoxic group (A, $n = 12$). Statistical analysis was by the usual methods. All values are expressed as mean ± SEM.

RESULTS

Ischaemic period

Values of water content in the H (5.05 ± 0.12) and A (5.13 ± 0.11) groups, which do not differ significantly between themselves, are higher than in the I group (4.34 ± 0.14) and in a group of unflushed kidneys (3.59 ± 0.10). (H vs I: $p \lhd 0.01$; A vs I, H vs N and A vs N: $p < 0.001$). Water content in the I group is greater than in unflushed kidneys ($p < 0.01$). These results show that oedema induced by 60 min anoxia and by hypotonic flushing is similar as far as water gain is concerned.

Total ischaemia time did not differ significantly between the I (15.5 ± 0.4 min) and H (14.8 ± 0.5 min) groups.

Revascularization period

Twenty-four hours after revascularization, the water content of cortical tissue in the H (3.81 ± 0.15) and A (4.32 ± 0.11) groups was statistically smaller than water content obtained immediately after flushing or after anoxia ($p < 0.001$). The water content after 24 h is greater in the A group than in the H group ($p < 0.05$). Similarly the ratio of water content after 24 h to water content after flushing or after anoxia is greater in the A group (0.84 ± 0.03) than in the H group (0.75 ± 0.03) ($p < 0.05$). Oedema is thus reduced in both groups after 24 h, but more so after hypotonic perfusion than after anoxia.

RBF (Figure 9.1) decreased significantly in all three groups during the

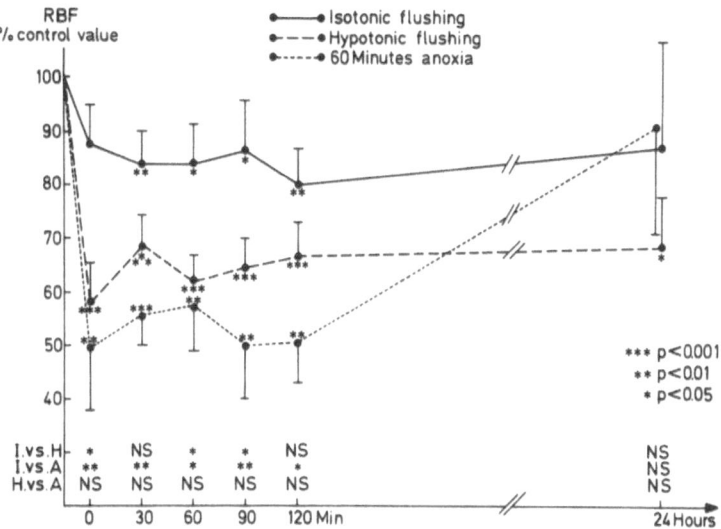

Figure 9.1 Renal blood flow in kidneys flushed with isotonic solution, hypotonic solution or submitted to 60 min of anoxia

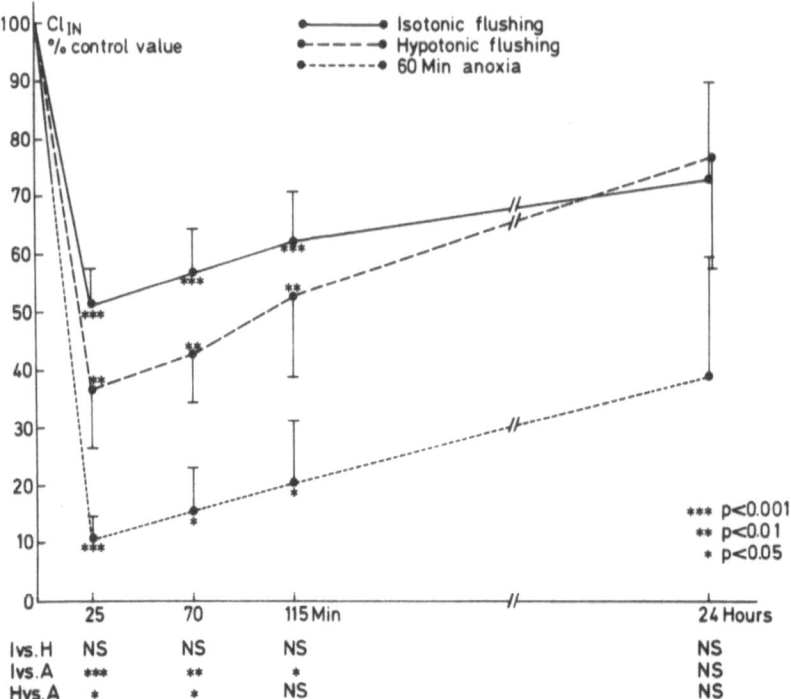

Figure 9.2 Inulin clearance in kidneys flushed with isotonic solution, hypotonic solution or submitted to 60 min of anoxia

first 2 h after revascularization, and after 24 h in group H. RBF is smaller in the H and A groups than in group I. RBF in group H never differed significantly from RBF in group A.

The elapsed time between revascularization and the appearance of the first drop of urine was 0.3 ± 0.3 min in group I and 13.1 ± 2.9 min in group H. One anoxic kidney never produced urine and the mean time for the other kidneys of group A was 30.5 ± 5.7. Comparison shows statistically significant differences between I and H ($p < 0.001$), I and A ($p < 0.001$) and H and A ($p < 0.01$) groups.

During the first 2 h, values of Cl_{IN} (Figure 9.2) were reduced in all three groups. They were lower for group A ($11 \pm 4\%$ of control value 25 min after revascularization and $20 \pm 11\%$ after 2 h) than for groups I (respectively $52 \pm 8\%$ and $70 \pm 11\%$) and H (respectively $42 \pm 17\%$ and $60 \pm 21\%$) groups. The values of Cl_{IN} observed in groups I and H did not differ significantly.

DISCUSSION

Physiopathologic consequences of ischaemia which finally result in cellular death are poorly understood. Two major pathways can lead to depression of mitochondrial function and cellular death. The first is a metabolic effect such as acidosis resulting from the anaerobic production of energy by the glycolytic chain[2], accumulation of wastes like ammonia[3] or of other toxic substances[4], or another mechanism. The second pathway is the mechanical effect of swelling which may separate reactive sites of enzymes bound to membranes, increase membrane permeability or modify organelles (clumping of nuclear chromatin, dilatation of endoplasmic reticulum or condensation of mitochrondria[5]).

Our experiments demonstrate different impairment of renal function in kidneys flushed with an isotonic or hypotonic solution or submitted to anoxia of 60 min. According to some authors, irreversible damage may already be present after 15 min of anoxia[6]. However, it has been reported by many others that kidney preservation is not impaired after such a period of normothermic ischaemia[7-10]. In our experiments similar ischaemia times of about 15 min in both groups I and H allow us to assign the differences in function to the difference in osmolality between the two solutions tested. Differences in glomerular function observed between these two groups are small and do not reach a statistically significant level, even if the duration of anuria is different.

By contrast, kidney function is clearly more impaired after an anoxic period of 60 min than after flushing with a hypotonic solution, even though both produce the same gain in tissue water. This consequence of anoxia may thus be considered due to other mechanisms than cellular swelling, if it is accepted that the water-gain is mainly intracellular, both in anoxia and in hypotonic flushing. The fact that the decrease in blood flow, a consequence of intracellular swelling, is similar in both groups supports this hypothesis.

Thus, our experiments show that non-anoxic oedema is much less damaging than anoxic oedema. If the increase of water content induced by hypotonic solution and by anoxia are manifestations of an identical cellular swelling, it can be deduced that the injury of anoxia is not the simple consequence of spatial disruption of cell architecture and that the metabolic disturbances are more important than the mechanical one in the physiopathologic process leading to cellular death.

These results make one question the mechanism of action of intracellular organ preservation solutions. Since the original work of Collins and associates[11], many authors have shown the beneficial effect of intracellular solutions, which was attributed by Downes and his co-workers[12] to their higher osmolality rather than their ionic composition. More recently Green and Pegg[13] have also claimed that the important factor in the mechanism of action of intracellular solutions is the elevation of osmolality with impermeant neutral solute and replacement of chloride by an impermeant anion. It has thus been generally deduced that the effectiveness of intracellular solutions depends upon the prevention of cellular swelling. In fact, these studies demonstrate only that under hypothermic conditions anoxia is better tolerated in the absence of swelling.

It can thus be concluded that swelling alone or anoxia alone is less deleterious than the combination of both factors. Several hypotheses may be proposed to explain this cumulative injury. Anoxia could prevent restoration of cellular membranes disrupted by swelling, and the lack of energy could make the cell unable to recover its physiological volume. Our results showing that swelling is more persistent in the anoxic group than in the hypotonic group are in agreement with this hypothesis. On the other hand, oedema may become deleterious when prolonged. In this respect, combined losses of potassium and intracellular anions may be considered as a possible consequence of swelling. These losses occur progressively in osmotically swollen liver cells[14].

Mechanisms of action other than prevention of cellular swelling may also be involved. Some authors have shown that Collins' solution gives better results in organ preservation than solutions with a higher osmolality such as Sacks', Ross' hypertonic citrate or Lambotte's KMgS solutions[15,16]. Moreover some preservation solutions with a similar osmolality give different results[13,17,18]. The success of kidney preservation with Euro-Collins' solution (allowing preservation up to $50 h$[19]) shows that $MgSO_4$ is not necessary, and a beneficial effect of one or several of the other components of Collins' solutions, such as glucose or phosphate, cannot be excluded.

References

1. Fischer, J. H., Czerniak, A., Hauer, U. and Isselhard, W. (1978). A new simple method for optimal storage of ischemically damaged kidneys. *Transplantation, 25*, 43
2. Krebs, H. (1971). Report of a meeting: workshop on organ preservation. *Surgery, 69*, 321
3. Abouna, G. M., Lim, F., Cook, J. S., Grubb, W., Craig, S. S., Seibel, H. R. and Hume, D. M. (1972). Three-day canine kidney preservation. *Surgery, 71*, 436
4. Pontegnie-Istace, S. and Lambotte, L. (1977). Liver adenine nucleotide metabolism during hypothermic anoxia and a recovery period in perfusion. *J. Surg. Res., 23*, 339
5. Macknight, A. D. C. and Leaf, A. (1977). Regulation of cellular volume. *Physiol. Rev., 57*, 510
6. Cohn, H. and Moses, M. (1966). The critical interval in cadaver kidney transplantation: function of canine renal autotransplants after variable periods of ischemia. *Surgery, 60*, 750
7. Grana, L., Donnellan, W. L. and Swenson, O. (1971). Low flow hypothermic renal perfusion. *Surg. Gynecol. Obstet., 133*, 401
8. Collins, G. M., Taft, P., Green, R. D., Ruprecht, R. and Halasz, N. A. (1977). Adenine nucleotide levels in preserved and ischemically injured canine kidneys. *World J. Surg., 1*, 237
9. Grundmann, R., Eichmann, J., Keckstein, J., Raab, M., Meusel, E. and Pichlmaier, H. (1977). Relationship between the prolongation of warm ischemia and the maximum available preservation period. *Surgery, 81*, 512
10. Grundmann, R., Bischoff, A., Albrod, A. and Pichlmaier, H. (1979). Canine kidney perfusion after various warm ischaemic periods. In Pegg, D. E. and Jacobsen, I. A. (eds.) *Organ Preservation II*, pp. 33–45. (Edinburgh: Churchill Livingstone)
11. Collins, G. M., Bravo-Shugarman, M. and Terasaki, P. I. (1969). Kidney preservation for transportation. Initial perfusion and 30 hours' ice storage. *Lancet, 2*, 1219
12. Downes, G., Hoffman, R., Huang, J. and Belzer, F. O. (1973). Mechanism of action of washout solutions for kidney preservation. *Transplantation, 16*, 46
13. Green, C. J. and Pegg, D. E. (1979). The effect of variation in electrolyte composition and osmolality of solutions for infusion and hypothermic storage of kidneys. In Pegg, D. E. and Jacobsen, I. A. (eds.) *Organ Preservation II*, pp. 86–100. (Edinburgh: Churchill Livingstone)
14. Lambotte, L. and Wojcik, S. (1979). Ouabain inhibits the recovery of cellular volume in liver perfused with hypo-osmolar solution. *Arch. Int. Phys. Bioch., 87*, 335

15. Opelz, G. and Terasaki, P. I. (1976). Kidney preservation: perfusion versus cold storage – 1975. *Transplant. Proc.,* **8,** 121

16. Fischer, J. H., Miyata, M., Isselhard, W. and Casser, H. R. (1979). Hypotherme lagerung unter aeroben bedingungen. Einfluss unterschiedlicher freispüllösungen auf die function-serhaltung der niere. *Langenbecks Arch. Chir.,* suppl., 307

17. Sterling, W. A., Datnow, B. and Diethelm, A. G. (1976). Sachs I solution and 7% mannitol solution for renal preservation. *J. Surg. Res.,* **20,** 103

18. Green, C. J. and Pegg, D. E. (1979). Mechanism of action of 'intracellular' renal preservation solutions. *World J. Surg.,* **3,** 115

19. Squifflet, J. P., Pirson, Y., Gianello, P., Van Cangh, P. and Alexandre, G. P. J. (1981). Safe preservation of human renal cadaver transplants by Euro-Collins' solution up to 50 hours. *Transplant. Proc.,* **13,** 693

10
Prostacyclin and the ischaemic kidney

A. R. MUNDY, J. M. RESTORICK and M. BEWICK

We have recently shown[1] that pretreatment with prostacyclin will protect a kidney against the adverse effects of warm ischaemia induced by clamping the renal artery, as judged by postoperative renal function. Prostacyclin is the most potent inhibitor of platelet aggregation yet discovered[2] and a potent vasodilator with profound effects on renal circulation[1]. It was therefore suggested that this protective effect of prostacyclin might be due to prevention of platelet aggregation within the microvasculature during the period of ischaemia. Thus, on removing the vascular clamp, reperfusion of the kidney would not be impaired by intravascular obstructive platelet aggregates or thrombi. The present experiments were designed to find the maximum period of warm ischaemia (WI) the kidney could tolerate with return of normal function after prostacyclin pre-treatment.

METHODS

Forty mongrel dogs with a mean weight of $19.9 \, kg \pm 2.1$ (SD) were anaesthetized with thiopentone sodium ($25 \, mg/kg$) and maintained with oxygen–nitrous oxide–halothane by spontaneous respiration. Unilateral nephrectomy was performed with cross-clamping of the contralateral renal artery with an atraumatic vascular clamp for 30, 45, 60 or 75 min. There were 10 dogs in each of these four groups. Within each group five dogs received an infusion of prostacyclin $300 \, ng/min$ in glycine buffer (pH 10.5)[1,2] into the renal artery for 5 min before and 5 min after the cross-clamping; the other five dogs received the glycine buffer alone. Postoperatively the serum creatinine was measured daily for 7 days, then on alternate days for 2 more weeks. Urine was collected on alternate days and examined for haematuria. At 21 days the glomerular filtration rate (GFR) was measured using [^{51}Cr]EDTA. The dogs were then sacrificed and the kidneys removed for histological examination.

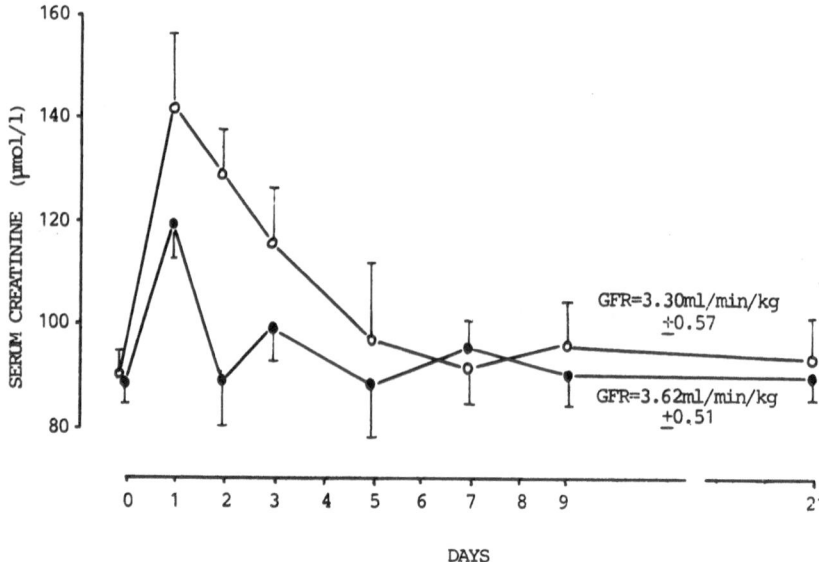

Figure 10.1 Daily postoperative serum creatinine levels and GFR at 21 days in dogs subjected to unilateral nephrectomy and cross-clamping of the contralateral renal artery for 30 min. ●——●, five dogs pretreated with prostacyclin in glycine buffer; ○——○, five dogs pretreated with glycine buffer alone. All values are the mean of five experiments ±1 SD

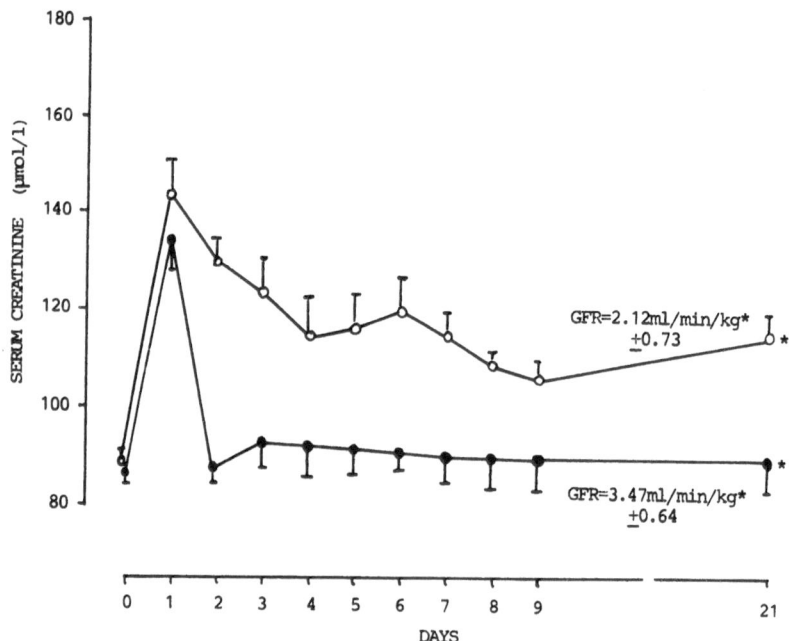

Figure 10.2 Effects of 45 min WI. For key see legend to Figure 10.1.
* Indicates a significant difference between paired results ($p < 0.05$)

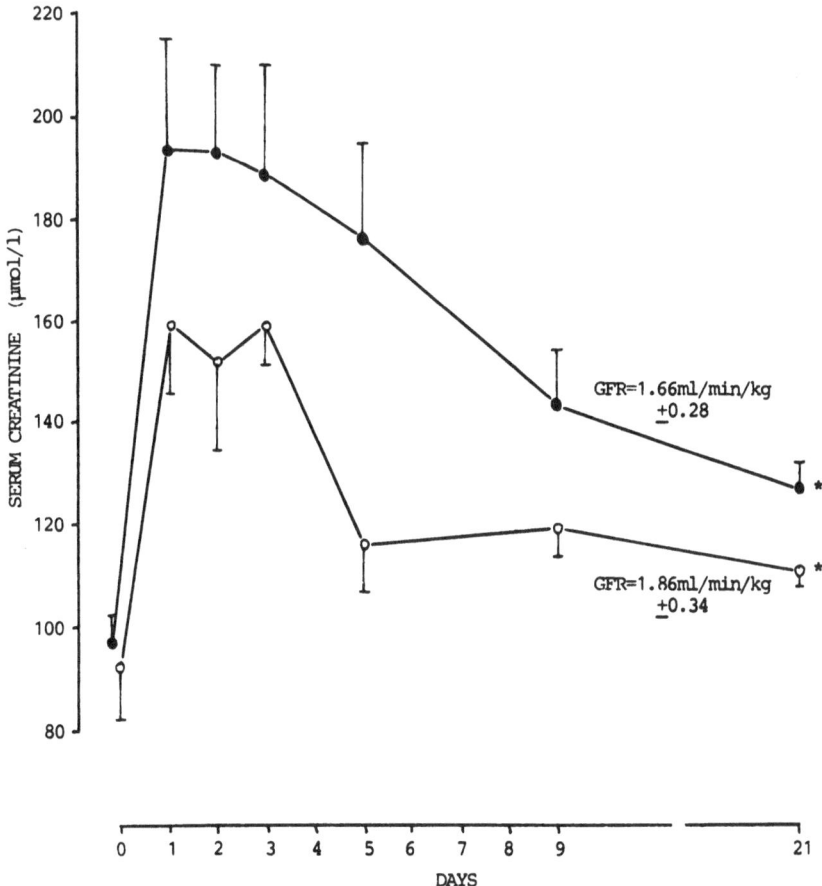

Figure 10.3 Effects of 60 min WI. For key see legend to Figure 10.1.
* Indicates a significant difference between paired results ($p < 0.05$)

RESULTS

The daily serum creatinine levels and the GFR at 21 days in each group of dogs are shown in Figures 10.1–10.4. After 30 min WI renal function was ultimately normal in all dogs, but returned to normal earlier in prostacyclin-treated dogs. After 45 min WI renal function returned to normal in prostacyclin-treated dogs but not in untreated dogs. After 60 and 75 min WI the situation was reversed with untreated dogs showing better functional recovery. Furthermore, although less quantifiable, haematuria persisted for longer in treated dogs in these groups and interstitial haemorrhage (in addition to the characteristic features of ischaemic damage) was more marked on light microscopy.

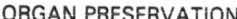

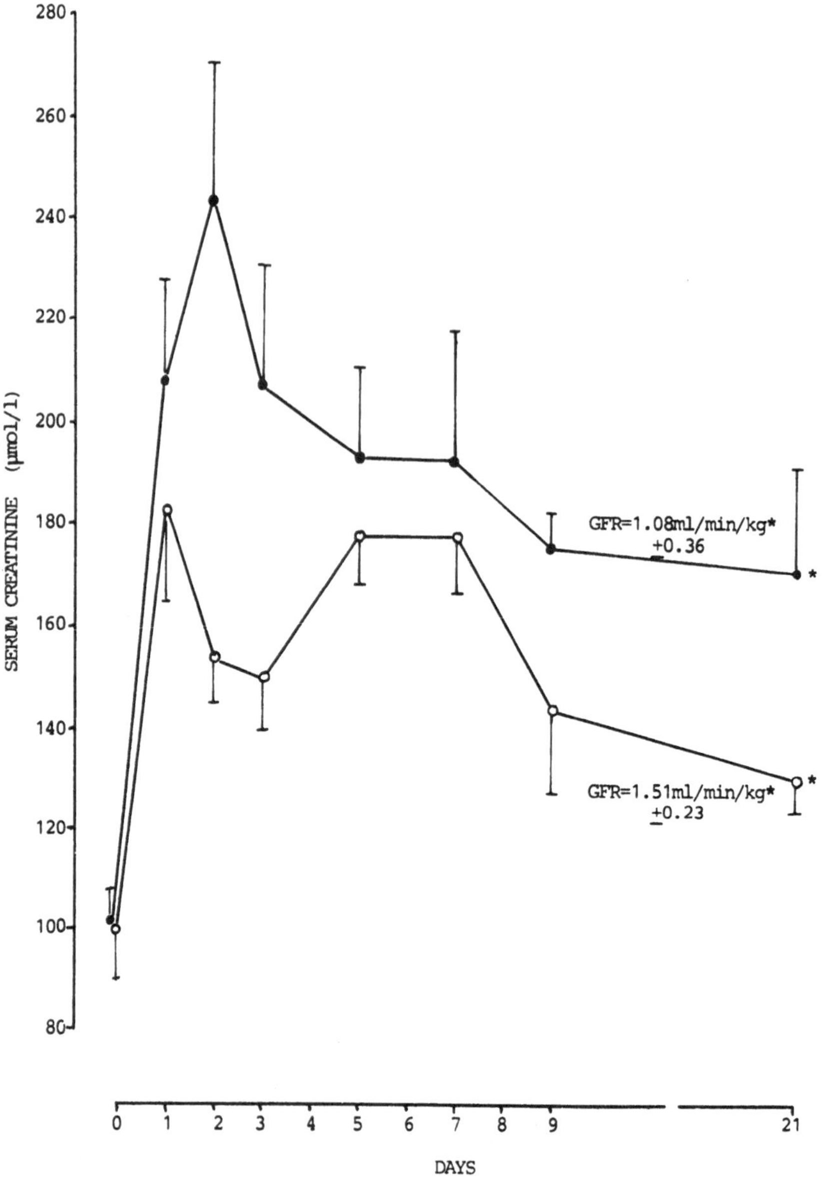

Figure 10.4 Effects of 75 min WI. For key see legend to Figure 10.1.
* Indicates a significant difference between paired results ($p < 0.05$)

DISCUSSION

Prostacyclin pre-treatment appeared to have a beneficial effect on kidneys subjected to 30 or 45 min WI but a deleterious effect on kidneys subjected to 60 or 75 min WI. Thus, it would appear that after a critical period of about 60 min WI, the mechanism by which prostacyclin exerts a beneficial effect becomes deleterious to the structural and functional integrity of the kidney. Another explanation of these findings might be that at this critical period a second factor begins to affect the kidney.

Assuming the first of these two possibilities, there are three potentially related explanations. Firstly, in addition to certain anti-inflammatory properties, prostacyclin has pro-inflammatory effects[2]. Secondly, associated with its vasodilator effect, prostacyclin promotes oedema and thus facilitates extravasation[2]. Thirdly, prostacyclin, by inhibiting platelets, would tend to inhibit their possible role in the repair of damaged endothelium[3].

Thus the beneficial effect of inhibiting microvascular obstruction in a kidney with a good potential for spontaneous recovery might, with increasing ischaemic time, be overshadowed by the adverse effects mentioned above in a kidney with a lesser capacity for spontaneous recovery.

Acknowledgements

We thank B. Eaton and L. Armitage for their excellent technical assistance and J. Collett for typing the manuscript.

References

1. Mundy, A. R., Bewick, M., Moncada, S. and Vane, J. R. (1980). Experimental assessment of prostacyclin in the harvesting of kidneys for transplantation. *Transplantation*, **30**, 251
2. Moncada, S. and Vane, J. R. (1979). Pharmacology and endogenous roles of prostacyclin endoperoxides, thromboxane A_2 and prostacyclin. *Pharmacol. Rev.*, **30**, 293
3. Schwartz, S. M., Stomerman, M. B. and Benditt, E. P. (1975). The aortic intima. II. Repair of the aortic lining after mechanical denudation. *Am. J. Pathol.*, **81**, 15

11
Kidney blood flow and microcirculatory changes after autologous kidney transplantation

H. WILMS and E. SINAGOWITZ

The problem of the non-viable renal transplant has not yet been solved. In the renal transplantation centre in Freiburg we observed 12 kidneys which remained functionless in a series of 300 renal transplants. Shock in the donor prior to removal of the kidney, prolonged warm ischaemia, and perfusion damage (in addition to rejection) are considered to be probable causes. On the other hand, little is known about the deleterious effect of a fall in blood pressure in the recipient during the revascularization phase, yet in our patients the systolic blood pressure during the critical phase of re-vascularization varied between 70 and 100 mmHg over a period of approx-imately 45 min. The cause of this was that our patients had been dialysed immediately prior to transplantation, resulting in a latent hypovolaemia. The hypothesis that hypotension might be the cause of transplant failure was supported by the fact that in 8 of the 12 donors the other kidney functioned well after transplantation.

It was our aim to investigate, by means of autologous kidney trans-plantation in dogs, the effect of hypotension (a systolic pressure of 70 mmHg over a period of 45 min) during implantation.

METHODS

We performed 39 autologous renal transplants in dogs. The left kidney was removed and perfused with the Euro-Collins solution (group I). In group II, this was followed by constant perfusion using the Gambro machine. The kidney was then reimplanted end-to-side just above the aortic bifurcation. The contralateral kidney was left *in situ* and the excretory functions of both kidneys were studied individually through ureterocutaneostomies. In half of the animals revascularization was performed at normal blood pressure; in half the blood pressure was lowered to 70 mmHg over a period of 45 min using aortic banding.

We carried out the following measurements during the investigation: (1) renal blood flow with an electromagnetic flowmeter; (2) tissue-PO_2 on the kidney surface with the multiwire-platinum electrode of Kessler and Lübbers[1]. This instrument has eight platinum electrodes which are embedded in glass and isolated through high resistances. The diameter of each individual electrode is $15\,\mu m$. The hemispheric measurement area for each electrode was $20-25\,\mu m$, so that the PO_2 measured was that of only a few cells. Depending on the localization of the electrode cell, areas with high oxygen partial pressures are interspersed among areas having lower values. The sum of approximately 80–100 PO_2 measurements results in a Gaussian distribution curve.

RESULTS AND DISCUSSION

Even under apparently optimal conditions of perfusion and transplantation, the renal blood flow of the transplanted kidney reached only 70–75% of the original value. As expected we found no significant difference between gravity perfusion (group I) and constant perfusion (group II). When the controlled hypotension of 70 mmHg was produced the blood flow fell on average to 25.6% of the original value, as can be seen in column I*b* of Figure 11.1. A flow reduction of this degree is not observed in a normal, non-transplanted kidney, despite compression of the suprarenal aorta.

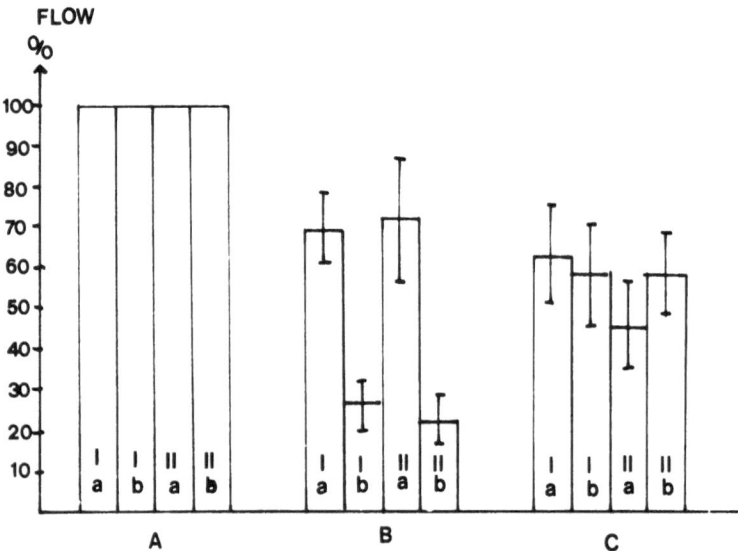

Figure 11.1 Reduction of renal blood flow (RBF) after transplantation: group I: cold preservation; group II: machine preservation – (a) normotension; (b) controlled hypotension after revascularization. (A) before nephrectomy; (B) after revascularization under controlled hypotension; (C) 5 days after transplantation

Before excision for transplantation, the values of renal cortical tissue PO_2 demonstrated a Gaussian distribution curve (lowest portion of Figure 11.2). The mean PO_2 was 50.6 mmHg. Following grafting and re-vascularization with a normal blood pressure, the distribution curve is broadened with some values of PO_2 being zero. However, a Gaussian distribution curve persists, and 4–6 days after transplantation the mean PO_2 fell further to 28.4 mmHg. If the blood pressure was lowered during the revascularization phase, more kidney cortex areas show a PO_2 of zero (Figure 11.2, reading b), and the distribution is no longer Gaussian. This PO_2 histogram must be considered pathological. Similar experimental conditions in non-transplanted kidneys do not change the PO_2 histograms.

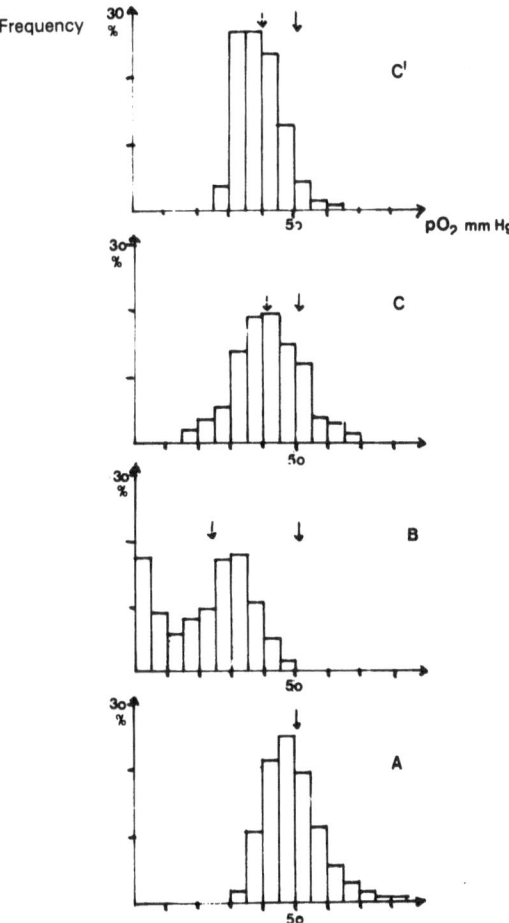

Figure 11.2 PO_2 histograms of the renal cortex: (A) before nephrectomy; (B) after re-vascularization under controlled hypotension; (C) histogram 5 days after transplantation; (C') histogram of the contralateral non-transplanted kidney at the same time as (C)

Our findings indicate that the phase of revascularization must be included, when considering the problem of non-viable kidney transplants. In our opinion, microcirculatory damage is caused by suboptimal perfusion. The measurement of tissue Po_2 using a multiwire surface electrode has been validated in animal experiments, and may serve as a parameter to predict the viability of the transplant.

Reference

1. Kessler, M. and Lübbers, D. W. (1966). Aufbau und Anwendungsmöglichkeiten verschiedener Po_2-Elektroden. *Pflügers Arch.*, **291**, 82

PART III
BIOCHEMICAL AND
PHARMACOLOGICAL
ASPECTS OF
HYPOTHERMIA

12
Future prospects in organ preservation

B. D. ROSS

Organ and tissue preservation is a long-standing dream which has become of practical importance since the advent of immunosuppression allowed transplantation. In addition, preservation of individual cell types, such as the islets of Langerhans, becomes important as various types of 'replacement' surgery are introduced.

The aims of organ preservation have been rather limited; a viable organ maintained for 12–48 h suffices for most practical purposes, and techniques have changed very little in 10 years. The need for improvement is debatable: 'If you could manage a couple of months . . .' was the suggestion of a transplant immunologist, in a recent and casual conversation. But the challenge is real enough; since embryos and whole animals can be preserved under special circumstances, why not whole organs? Much might be learned incidentally about the prevention of ischaemic damage to organs.

This symposium deals with existing methods of organ preservation and is concerned largely with technical detail. To predict new approaches of a theoretical kind is more difficult. However, biochemical studies on whole organs still have something to offer which has not already been used in organ preservation, and this forms the basis of the ideas in this chapter.

Organ preservation demands identification of the effects of anoxia, ischaemia (which differs from anoxia in a number of ways), and possibly also of cooling. The prevention or reversal of, or the avoidance of, any of these noxious stimuli underlie most approaches to organ preservation. Cold storage or homeostatic perfusion are the usual methods employed.

Future prospects depend largely upon the introduction of modifications in these existing methods, but will be much improved by increased understanding of the nature of ischaemic damage. In this chapter I suggest that prevention of, or enhanced recovery from, cell swelling might be achieved by modifications to Na-K-ATPase; that ATP turnover measurements might provide a better indicator of subsequent function than either ATP content or ATP resynthesis. In addition, the possible importance of protecting ischaemic tissues against falling pH is stressed. Finally, non-invasive methods are seen as the best prospect for improving methods of organ preservation since they permit minute-by-minute modification of the environment and monitoring of the outcome of individual transplants.

CELL SWELLING

Cells swell during anoxia and during rewarming, and the 'no-reflow' phenomenon has for long been considered a reasonable explanation for much of the tissue damage which results from ischaemia. Since the sodium pump (Na-K-ATPase) is the regulator of cell volume the properties of the enzyme are of possible importance to organ preservation. The enzyme is membrane-bound, and contains a labile lipid component which can easily be dissociated, with loss of some activity[1]. In addition, the enzyme is inducible, that is to say that its total activity can be increased *in vivo* by new protein synthesis under appropriate conditions. Two approaches to organ preservation suggest themselves on the basis of this information. Prior enzyme induction regimes, applied to the donor organ *in vivo*, are of interest; aldosterone or hyperkalaemia are potent stimuli in experimental animals, effectively increasing ATPase activity in a few hours. The stored organ thus treated may cope more effectively with the problems of restoring cell volume after anoxia. Enzymologists, on the other hand, are familiar with the idea that an enzyme inhibitor, by attaching itself to the active site of the enzyme, may protect the enzyme during isolation procedures. Perhaps a similar approach, using biologically known inhibitors of Na-K-ATPase, such as endigin, toad-skin extract, or human myeloma light-chain[2], may allow a prior treatment of the organ to be preserved, to ensure that Na-K-ATPase is undamaged during the storage period. Even the well-known chemical inhibitors of Na-K-ATPase, ouabain, digitalis and harmaline, may be effective in this respect. A relatively simple experimental system, consisting of isolated membrane vesicles, or artificial liposomes, into which the purified ATPase is incorporated[3], might provide a test system for this idea.

Calcium is closely involved in cell volume control, and leaks out readily from damaged cells. At least one preservation technique, the citrate flushing medium of H. Ross and Marshall, depends upon the inclusion of both a divalent ion, magnesium, and a chelating agent, citrate. The mode of action of this rather effective mixture is still unclear, but could well reside in its capacity to bind intracellular calcium. If so, there are a variety of agents, as yet untried in preservation, including chelating agents, and calcium ionophores, which alter membrane permeability to calcium, and which may therefore exert a preserving effect. Objective tests, in isolated organs, would in this case be of value in determining to what extent calcium efflux was important; ^{45}Ca efflux techniques are readily available, and could be used to follow calcium movements experimentally.

KEY METABOLIC PROCESSES IN PRESERVATION

Most of our existing information comes from studies on kidney preservation, and while it may be unsafe to generalize from this to the preservation of other organs, consideration of what is known will no doubt save some of the years of development which have been invested. What is being preserved? Is it the ATP content of the organ or the ability to re-synthesize ATP from ADP and inorganic phosphorus which determines the outcome of storage? The bulk of literature indicates that if ATP resynthesis can be assured, reasonable preservation follows. Finding a significant amount of ATP after storage may only be a reflection of this fact, since ATP content is a function of both the anoxic ATP hydrolysis and the continuous resynthesis of ATP. A method is required which will permit these synchronous rates to be determined. It can readily be achieved in isolated mitochondria (Chapter 16) and the technique of ^{31}P NMR will probably permit it in whole organs. This is a more sophisticated application of the technique of ^{31}P NMR described in this volume by Sehr et al. (Chapter 13) and Chan et al. (Chapter 14) called 'saturation-transfer' and may permit some advance over the simple enzymatic methods of analysis of adenine nucleotides by being both non-invasive (see below) and dynamic.

ATP synthesis is only one example of a metabolic reaction susceptible to anoxia or rewarming. We really are in the dark as to which of the many reactions affected by anoxia is required for tissue recovery. Glycolysis rate increases in most organs during anoxia; is this a protective reaction, by virtue of the small amount of ATP which is produced in the conversion of glucose to lactate, or is it destructive, on account of the protons (acid!) generated at the same time?

Since the advent of ^{31}P NMR it has been possible to determine tissue pH in whole functioning organs within a matter of minutes. Intrarenal pH falls rapidly during ischaemia (Chapter 13). Preventing the fall in pH by flushing the kidney with a powerful buffer has an important protective effect on renal function, a fact which has been demonstrated both in the isolated perfused kidney[4] and in survival experiments in vivo. Prevention of tissue acidosis, by whatever means, may therefore be of importance in future organ preservation techniques. By extension, preventing or inhibiting glycolysis during the induction of ischaemia may preserve rather than damage tissues. A number of inhibitors of glycolysis are known, which may be of interest in this context. Williams[5] has shown, for example, that inhibiting glycolysis in the isolated heart by means of the non-metabolizable analogue, 2-deoxyglucose, minimizes the fall in pH. This phenomenon has not been studied in organ preservation.

If pH is important in determining the outcome of preservation, then it might be rewarding to consider the pH-sensitive reactions which underlie this fact. Textbooks attest to the fact that many enzymes are inhibited at low pH. It is sufficient here to point out that such information is mis-leading. We may anticipate that only those enzymes which show a change in K_m with acidosis will affect the outcome of anoxia. Such an enzyme is oxo-glutarate dehydrogenase, a key enzyme in the TCA cycle; it is accelerated significantly by acid under conditions obtaining in the cell. It is not, however, sensitive to pH when tested under 'saturating' conditions, such as are reported in tables of pH sensitivity. This therefore is an area for further study which may be of help in predicting successful preservation techniques.

Further, as NMR studies are extended to other organs, the relative pH sensitivity of major metabolic and physiological functions appears to be different. Heart, skeletal muscle, human kidney and rat kidney all appear to achieve different pH minima during anoxia, and individual studies may well be repaid by defining optimum buffers for the preservation of different organs.

AVOIDING THE SCOURGE OF STATISTICS: NON-INVASIVE BIOCHEMICAL TECHNIQUES

The interpretation of experimental and clinical studies on organ preservation has been much hampered by statistics. Is 8/12 better than 5/9 in comparing one preservation method with another? Is $p < 0.05$ relevant to the outcome in an individual patient?

If non-invasive methods of biochemical monitoring were applied to the preserved organ and if predictive tests of function could be devised, the history of the individual preserved organ could be correlated with the outcome in the individual recipient. Better still, the non-invasive monitoring method might be ultimately applied in the recipient to assess the progress of the reimplanted organ. This ambition is still remote, but a number of candidates for non-invasive biochemical monitoring are being studied at present. Surface oxygen electrodes, surface pH measurement, and ^{31}P NMR are all dealt with in this volume. The theoretical basis of NMR is that mobile phosphorus-containing nuclei can be continuously identified and quantified from the radiofrequency signal which is emitted when the biological specimen is held in a powerful and uniform magnetic field. Two features of the technique have led to its application in renal preservation: intracellular pH can be monitored, and ATP can be quantified. These two features are explored in chapters in this volume. More recently, the technique has been extended to permit not only non-invasive monitoring of the whole organ, but focusing of sufficient precision to make it possible that the kidney, for example, can be observed within the body. Application of this method to man awaits the development of magnets large enough to contain the whole patient. It should then be possible to determine ATP content of the kidney reimplanted into the iliac fossa, as an indicator of the effectiveness of renal oxygen delivery.

A further non-invasive technique which promises to be of value in organ preservation is surface or transmission spectroscopy. This method, which has been in the biochemists' armamentarium for many years, allows the state of electron transport and of oxygen delivery to be monitored by recording the relative state of oxidation or reduction of the cytochromes of the electron-transport chain. In the isolated perfused kidney (Balaban, Epstein and Ross, unpublished) some 30% of cytochrome $a–a_3$ is present in the reduced form. We may deduce from this that even the 'normal' kidney is on the brink of anoxia. The ability to follow the degree of cytochrome oxidation during a cycle of preservation and recovery in organ transplantation could provide a very sensitive monitor of pharmacological interventions in clinical practice.

HETEROGENEITY

Perhaps the most remarkable feature of organ preservation is the extreme simplicity of the methods employed and their relative success. No account has been taken, in the preservation of kidney for example, of the many different cell-types represented in the nephron, and glomerulus, not to mention endothelium of blood vessels, interstitial cells and nerves. This may indicate that such variations are unimportant for survival of whole organs, and that the same methods may be expected to apply to other organs as have been worked out for the kidney. For a variety of reasons this is not likely to be true, and progress in organ preservation may depend upon the recognition of the heterogeneity of cell types within the organ to be preserved. In kidney, the poor correlation between enzyme measurements and outcome of preservation can be directly attributed to the heterogeneity of enzyme distribution along the nephron[6]. Thus, N-acetylglucosaminidase (Chapter 34) is representative of a different cell type from lactic dehydrogenase, and may only reflect the state of a small proportion of the nephron (Table 12.1). Function of the kidney, on the other hand, clearly requires the glomerulus, and several different cell types. This is an argument for further studies, first to identify and localize enzymes along the human nephron (information is available to date only for the rat and rabbit!) and then to correlate tests of function with the release of individual enzymes. Such studies are likely to be long-term and extremely tedious, but seem to offer the best hope of a breakthrough from the limited preservation currently available to some more long-term preservation.

Table 12.1 Distribution of enzymes used in diagnosis of renal viability

Enzyme	Location in nephron
Lactic dehydrogenase	distal > proximal
N-acetylglucosaminidase	proximal
Glutamic-oxaloacetate transaminase	distal > proximal
Succinic dehydrogenase	follows mitochondria
5-Nucleotidase	proximal > distal follows luminal membrane

Data from Ref. 6

BIOLOGICAL FACTORS IN PRESERVATION

With the discovery of endorphins, the possibility that there is a 'sleep factor' or even a 'hibernating factor' which permits tissues to survive long periods of ischaemia or reduced temperature without loss of function becomes more hopeful. Only detailed studies in hibernating animals, a topic introduced in Chapter 19, can hope to make this a reality.

CONCLUSIONS

Future prospects in organ preservation lie, as they always have done, in a more complete understanding of the nature of hypoxic damage. Preventing or reversing tissue-acidification may play a crucial role. Recognition of the heterogeneity of preservation and subsequent function will permit more subtle methods of organ preservation and predictive tests to be developed. Finally, in all subjects, new methods provide new subjects for study, and in organ preservation non-invasive methods for continuous biochemical analyses, of tissue oxygenation (surface spectroscopy) and high-energy phosphates (^{31}P NMR) will provide us with new insight. The original articles in this volume indicate to some extent what can be achieved with new techniques. Their application to human organ preservation and transplantation will become urgent only when current preservation times become inadequate by virtue of advances in immunology or long-range transport.

References

1. Jorgensen, P. L. (1980). Energetics of active transtubular transport: Function of the Na-K-ion pump. *Int. J. Biochem.*, **12**, 283
2. Ross, B. D. and Guder, W. G. (eds.) (1980). *Biochemical Aspects of Renal Function*, pp. 291–292. (Oxford: Pergamon Press)
3. Anner, B. M. (1980). Operation of the renal Na-K-ATP'ase pump in artificial membranes. *Int. J. Biochem.*, **12**, 295
4. Bore, P. J., Sehr, P. A., Chan, L., Thulborn, K. R., Ross, B. D. and Radda, G. K. (1981). *Transplant. Proc.*, **13**, 707
5. Williams, S. J. (1980). *D.Phil. thesis,* University of Oxford
6. Ross, B. D. and Guder, W. G. (1982). Heterogeneity and compartmentation in the kidney. In Sies, H. (ed.), *Heterogeneity in Biochemistry*. (New York: Academic Press). (In press)

13
Tissue pH changes in renal preservation

P. SEHR, P. BORE, K. THULBORN, I. PAPATHEOFANIS, L. CHAN
and G. K. RADDA

Ischaemic tissue rapidly becomes acidotic and it has been shown that a fall
in pH has a deleterious effect on a number of tissues, including decreased
oxygen consumption in diaphragm[1] and loss of contractility[2] in association
with the depression of several metabolic processes[3] in myocardium. A
number of studies have sought to correlate tissue pH during ischaemia with
renal viability. Surface pH is easily measured but has not been found to be
consistently helpful[4,5]. The pH on the surface may not be an accurate
reflection of changes within tissue or cells. Other workers have approached
the problem by attempting to modify renal viability by using buffered flush
solutions, but in the absence of measurements of pH a cause-and-effect
relationship cannot be substantiated[6,7]. A major obstacle in this field is the
difficulty in measuring intracellular pH, particularly under conditions of
ischaemia[8,9]. Nuclear magnetic resonance (NMR) spectroscopy using the
^{31}P nucleus has been shown to be a reliable means of measuring pH even
during ischaemia[10-13] since it is able to determine the degree of protonation
of inorganic phosphate[14]. We have measured pH by ^{31}P NMR in three series
of experiments.

Isolated ischaemic rat kidneys were examined at $0\,°C$ after having the
blood flushed out with Perfudex, and at $37\,°C$ with blood *in situ*. Figure
13.1 shows the pH changes in the kidneys at $0\,°C$. The solid line indicates
the exponential decay expected of a first-order reaction. The deviation of
this line from the results suggests that a slower proton-generating process is
present in addition to the one causing the rapid phase of the pH fall. The
curve for kidneys at $37\,°C$ was of similar shape but the rate of pH fall was
an order of magnitude greater. In rats, 60–70 min of warm ischaemia
rendered kidneys non-functional as judged by survival after immediate
contralateral nephrectomy. At $37\,°C$ the pH decreased by 0.45 units in
60–70 min. At $0\,°C$ a decrease in pH of 0.45 units was measured after some
20–24 h. In clinical transplantation, 20–24 h was the maximum acceptable
period of cold ischaemia for Perfudex-flushed kidneys.

In the second series of experiments we used kidneys which had been
removed from rabbits and perfused normothermically with whole blood
derived from a remote animal. In this model the pH changes were similar to

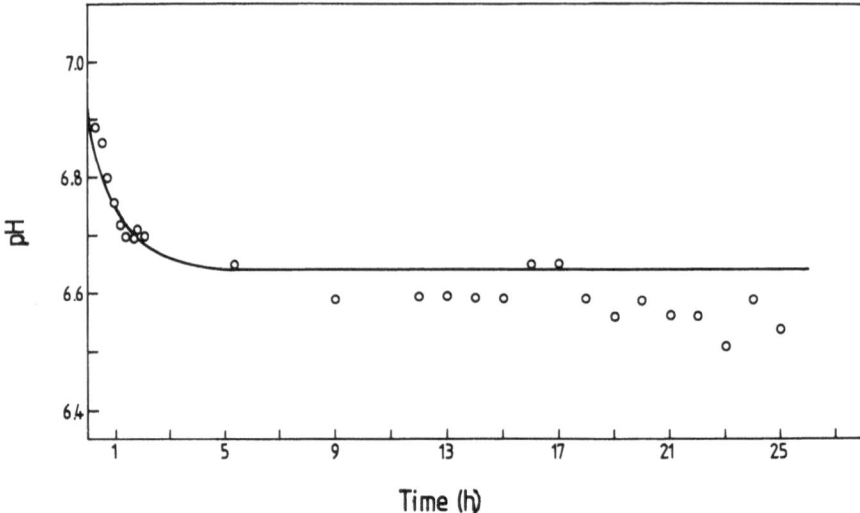

Figure 13.1 Variation of the pH of renal tissue during cold (0°C) ischaemia in a kidney flushed with Perfudex. The solid line represents the exponential change expected of a first-order reaction

those seen in isolated rat kidneys but recovery of pH was observed on restoration of a blood supply even in kidneys which had suffered a period of warm ischaemia that would render them non-functional as judged by parallel survival experiments. These findings suggested that pH recovery was less tightly coupled to viability than was the effect of low pH at the onset of ischaemia and therefore this latter area required further study.

In order to demonstrate a possible harmful effect of acidosis it was first necessary to show that the pH change during ischaemia could be modified. We were able to reduce the pH fall during warm ischaemia by flushing the kidneys with a divalent buffer introduced in high concentration at the onset of ischaemia and at a pH which optimized its buffering capacity (100 mmol/l Bis-Tris-Propane at pH 7.8). The ^{31}P NMR spectra were recorded *in vivo* by placing the NMR coil around the mobilized left kidney. Figure 13.2 shows that the pH fall was reduced from 0.7 units in control animals to 0.4 units in those animals with buffer-flushed kidneys. In a parallel series of survival experiments (rats subjected to 1 h of renal ischaemia at 37 °C and an immediate contralateral nephrectomy) flushing with the above buffer at the onset of ischaemia improved survival from 8% (1/13) in control animals to 50% (7/14) in animals with buffer flushed kidneys.

Similar protective effects of Bis-Tris-Propane have been demonstrated in isolated perfused kidneys at both 37 °C[15] and 0 °C[16]. In concluding that Bis-Tris-Propane protects the ischaemic kidney we recognize the possibility that this action may result from properties other than its buffering capacity.

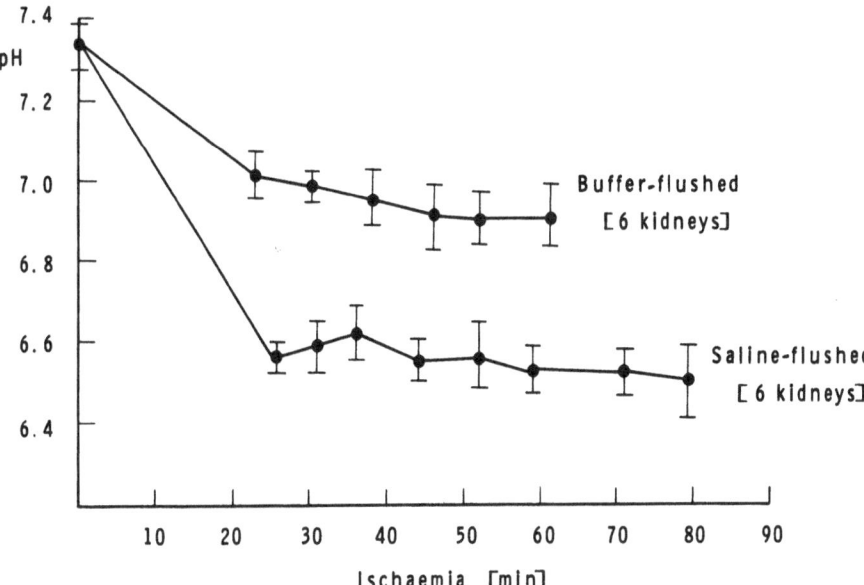

Figure 13.2 Variation of pH in *in vivo* kidneys flushed with either NaCl (150 mmol/l) or Bis-Tris-Propane (100 mmol/l) plus NaCl (100 mmol/l)

References

1. Enerson, D. M. and Berman, H. M. (1966). Effects of hypotonicity, low molecular weight dextran addition and pH changes on oxygen consumption of isolated tissues. *Ann. Surg.*, **163**, 537
2. Poole-Wilson, P. A. and Langer, G. A. (1975). Effect of pH on ionic exchange and function in the rat and rabbit myocardium. *Am. J. Physiol.*, **229**, 570
3. Williamson, J. R., Schaffer, S. W., Ford, C. and Safer, B. (1976). Contribution of tissue acidosis to ischaemic injury in the perfused heart. *Circulation,* **53** (suppl. 1), 1
4. Couch, N. P., Maginn, R. R., Middleton, M. K., Appleton, D. R. and Dmochowski, J. R. (1967). Effects of ischaemic interval and temperature on renal surface hydrogen ion concentration. *Surg. Gynaecol. Obstet.*, **125**, 521
5. Hardie, I. R., Clunie, G. J. A. and Collins, G. M. (1973). Evaluation of a simple means of assessing renal ischaemic injury. *Surg. Gynaecol. Obstet.*, **136**, 43
6. Collins, G. M., Hartley, L. C. J. and Clunie, G. J. A. (1971). Kidney preservation for transportation. 5. Comparison of perfusates for hypothermic storage. *Med. J. Aust.*, **1**, 1171
7. Lannon, S. G., Bickis, I. and Dossetor, J. B. (1971). Viability testing of kidneys for transplantation. *Invest. Urol.*, **9**, 180
8. Cohen, R. D. and Iles, R. A. (1975). Intracellular pH: measurement, control and metabolic interrelationships. *Crit. Rev. Clin. Lab. Sci.*, **6**, 101
9. Poole-Wilson, P. A. (1978). Measurement of myocardial intracellular pH in pathological states. *J. Molec. Cell. Cardiol.*, **10**, 511
10. Radda, G. K. and Seeley, P. J. (1979). Recent studies on cellular metabolism by nuclear magnetic resonance. *Ann. Rev. Physiol.*, **41**, 749
11. Gadian, G. D., Radda, G. K., Richards, R. E. and Seeley, P. J. (1979). ^{31}P NMR in living tissue. In Shulman, R. G. (ed.), *Biological Applications of Magnetic Resonance*, pp. 463–535. (New York: Academic Press)

12. Garlick, P. B., Radda, G. K. and Seeley, P. J. (1979). Studies of acidosis in the ischaemic heart by phosphorus nuclear magnetic resonance. *Biochem. J.*, **184,** 547
13. Bailey, I. A., Williams, S. R., Radda, G. K. and Gadian, D. G. (1981). The activity of phosphorylase in total global ischaemia in the rat heart; a ^{31}P NMR study. *Biochem. J.*, **196,** 171
14. Garlick, P. B., Radda, G. K. and Seeley, P. J. (1979). Studies of acidosis in the ischaemic heart by phosphorus nuclear magnetic resonance. *Biochem. J.*, **184,** 547
15. Bore, P. J., Sehr, P. A., Chan, L., Thulborn, K. R. and Radda, G. K. (1981). The importance of pH in renal preservation. *Transplant. Proc.*, **13,** 707
16. Thulborn, K. R., Chan, L., Radda, G. K., Bore, P. J. and Ross, B. D. (1982). Maintenance of physiological pH during hypothermic storage of ischaemic rat kidney. (In preparation)

14
Study of human kidneys prior to transplantation by phosphorus nuclear magnetic resonance

L. CHAN, M. E. FRENCH, D. G. GADIAN, P. J. MORRIS,
G. K. RADDA, P. J. BORE, B. D. ROSS and P. STYLES

The possible applications of phosphorus nuclear magnetic resonance (NMR) to medicine are only just beginning to be explored[1]. It is a non-invasive method of analysing many aspects of energy metabolism of living intact cells because it can be used to detect adenosine triphosphate and diphosphate (ATP and ADP), phosphorylated sugar (sugar P) including adenosine monophosphate (AMP) and inorganic phosphate (P_i)[2,3]. Furthermore, the intracellular pH can also be determined simultaneously by measuring the frequency of the P_i peak. This technique has been used to determine adenine nucleotide content and intrarenal pH in kidneys from experimental animals, and has contributed to an understanding of the effects of ischaemia and preservation for transplantation[4,5]. With the development of a new wide-bore (20 cm) magnet (Oxford Research System, TMR-32), it is now possible to examine whole human kidneys *in vitro* and human limbs *in vivo*.

We report the results of a pilot NMR study of human kidneys which had been cooled after nephrectomy and then stored in ice. We asked the following questions:

(1) Is ATP detectable in human kidneys by NMR during cold ischaemia?
(2) Do NMR spectra alter predictably with the cold ischaemic time?
(3) Does the type of flushing solution alter the NMR spectra?
(4) Are changes in the normal tissue in tumour-bearing kidneys similar to those which occur in cadaver donor kidneys?
(5) Does the level of ATP (and P_i) *in vitro* correlate with early graft function?

METHODS

Seven kidneys removed because they contained tumours, and two cadaver kidneys which were not transplanted were first examined. Four of the tumour-bearing kidneys were cooled by flushing with normal saline solution at 4 °C. The remainder were cooled with hypertonic citrate solution (26.5 mmol/l potassium citrate, 26.5 mmol/l sodium citrate, 35 mmol/l magnesium sulphate and 130 mmol/l mannitol) at 4 °C. The kidneys were then prepared as though they were to be transplanted by removing excess fat, and enclosing them in three sterile polythene bags which were then stored in ice. The core temperatures of the normal and neoplastic parts of the first two kidneys were measured with a thermometer and were found to decrease to 10 °C or less at the end of flushing with 250 ml perfusate (< 5 min). Seven cadaver kidneys, after flushing with cold hypertonic citrate solution, have also been examined on at least one occasion before transplantation. Initial function of these kidneys was assessed in order to place them in ranking order.

Kidneys were kept at 0 °C by placing them in a transparent plastic box in which they were surrounded by ice. The box was then positioned in the centre of the bore of a TMR-32 magnet with the kidney positioned on top of a 2 cm radius, two-turn radiofrequency coil. ^{31}P NMR spectra were obtained at 32.5 MHz by the Fourier transform method using 60–960 radio-frequency pulses at either 2 or 8 s intervals. For accurate pH determination, field drift was corrected by obtaining proton NMR spectra immediately before and after accumulation of each ^{31}P NMR spectrum. In the intervals between analysis, kidneys were stored in ice in a large Thermos flask. Spectra were analysed by measuring the area or the height of each peak. Both gave the same relative concentrations. In the final results, spectra were analysed by measuring the peak heights (of the γ, α and β phosphates of ATP, sugar P and P$_i$) and expressing the height of each peak as a percentage of the sum of the peak heights. By measuring the position of the P$_i$ peak on the X axis (i.e. its frequency), the pH was determined using a standard calibration curve at 0 °C. The proton NMR signal from tissue water was used as the reference.

RESULTS

Is ATP detectable in human kidneys during cold ischaemia?

In as short a time as 4 min, peaks corresponding to the β, α and γ phosphate of ATP, sugar P and P$_i$ were visible (Figure 14.1). Better results were obtained using longer accumulation times. Hitherto only rat kidneys have been examined during ice storage by NMR spectroscopy[4,5]. In these, the ATP peaks were not observed after the first hour of cold ischaemia.

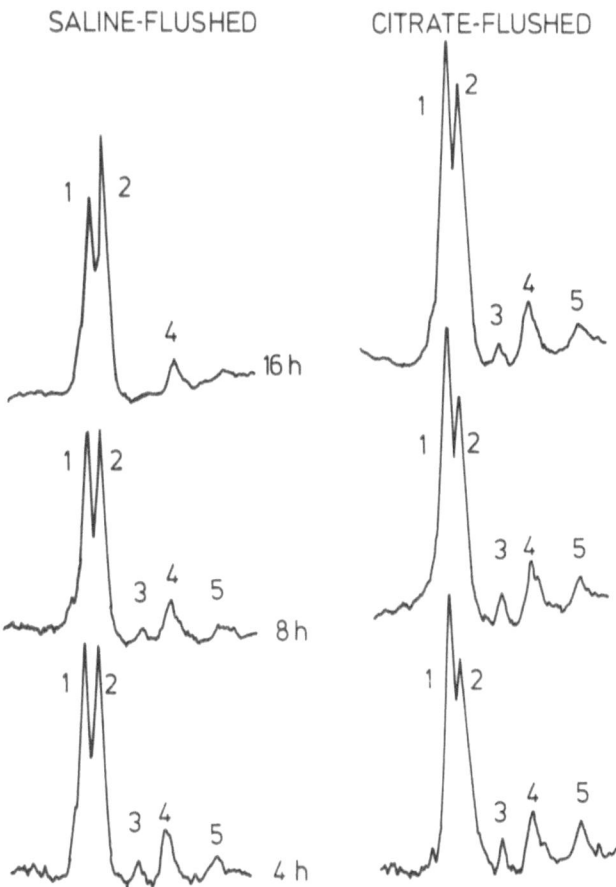

Figure 14.1 ^{31}P NMR spectra of single human kidneys flushed with saline or hypertonic citrate solutions after 4, 8 and 16h of cold ischaemia. 1: sugar phosphate, 2: inorganic phosphate, 3: γ phosphate of ATP + ADP, 4: α phosphate of ATP + ADP and NAD, 5: β phosphate of ATP

Do NMR spectra alter predictably with the period of cold ischaemia?

The time courses of changes were followed by studying the normal tissue of kidneys that contained tumours, and two cadaver kidneys from a donor who was subsequently found to have had malignant hypertension. The changes in ATP, P_i and sugar P levels with time after citrate flushing for five such kidneys are shown in Figure 14.2. Because the P_i level rises with time $(100 - P_i)\%$ was plotted to simplify presentation.

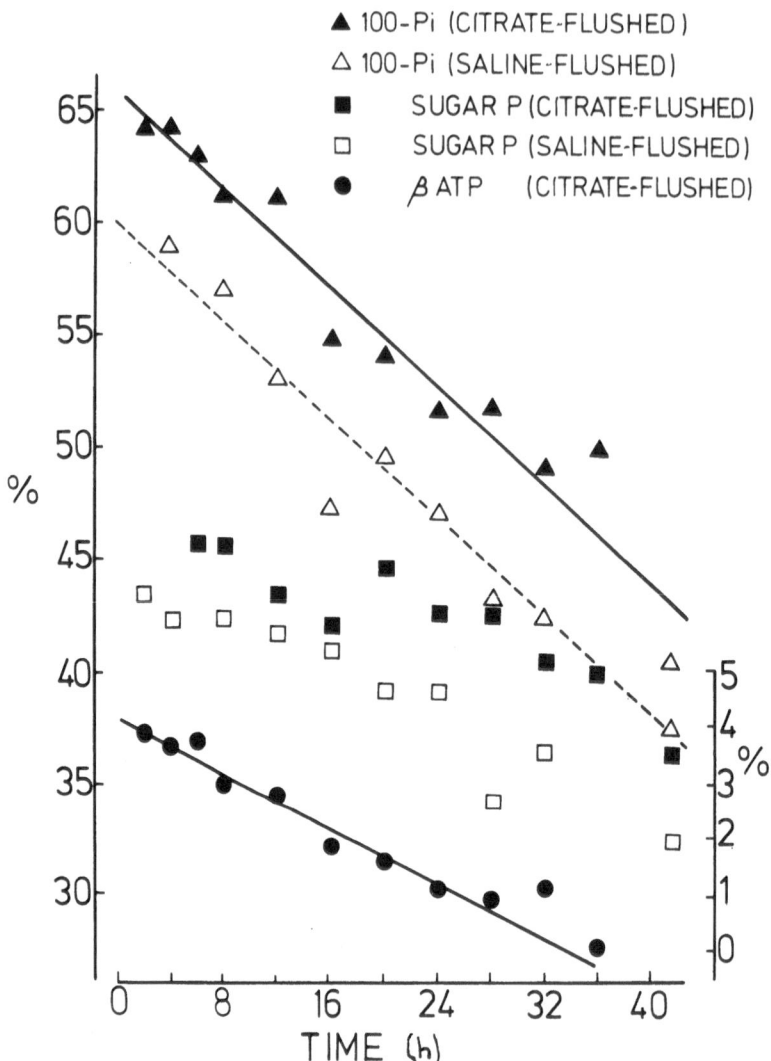

Figure 14.2 NMR spectroscopic analysis of the effect of time on the relative proportions (%) of phosphate metabolites of saline or citrate flushed kidneys during cold ischaemia. Right hand scale: β-ATP %, left hand scale: sugar P % and $(100 - P_i)$

Does the type of flushing solution used to cool kidneys alter the NMR spectra?

The results from the saline flushed kidneys are shown by the open symbols and the dotted line in Figure 14.2. $(100 - P_i)$ and sugar P levels were consistently lower in such kidneys than those flushed with hypertonic citrate. ATP levels were also lower but are not shown as the results were very scattered.

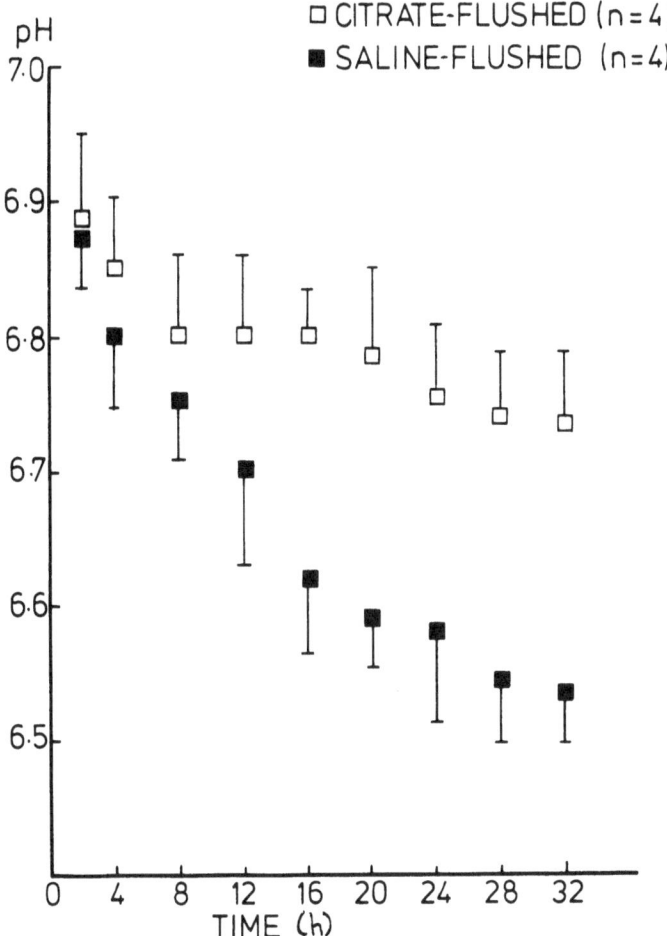

Figure 14.3 The change of pH with time of saline or citrate flushed human kidneys during cold ischaemia. pH values are expressed as mean and one standard deviation (vertical bar). From 12 h onward the differences were statistically significant ($p < 0.05$)

The spectra from representative kidneys are shown in Figure 14.1. At 16 h, peak 5 (β phosphate of ATP) is absent in the saline-flushed kidney, but is present in the citrate-flushed kidney. It should also be noted that peak 2 (P_i) gradually increases in height relative to peak 1 (sugar P). The two peaks are of equal height by 4 h in the saline-flushed kidney, but even after 16 h in the corresponding citrate-flushed kidney peak 2 has not reached the height of peak 1.

The detectable difference between citrate and saline flushing was shown even more convincingly by measuring the pH (Figure 14.3). Within 12 h the pH in saline-flushed kidneys was lower than that in citrate-flushed kidneys at 32 h.

Are changes in the normal tissue in tumour-bearing kidneys similar to those which occur during cold storage of cadaver donor kidneys?

Because the spectra from renal tumours differ significantly from those of normal kidneys[6], care was taken to place the coil under the normal portion of the kidney tissue. These spectra were then compared with those obtained from the seven transplant kidneys. The results were essentially the same.

Does the level of ATP (and P_i) in vitro correlate with early graft function?

ATP is detectable in human kidneys, and its signal decreases gradually with time whilst the P_i signal rises progressively. It seems highly probable that either ATP content (and hence P_i) or pH determined by NMR spectroscopy might be used to predict kidney viability. If this were true, one would expect high ATP and low P_i levels to predict good early graft function. In this preliminary report therefore the seven transplants for which data are available were placed in two ranking orders. Kidneys were examined 4 h after donor nephrectomy and shortly before transplantation. Kidneys were ranked according to their initial ATP concentration and also according to their final P_i concentration. After transplantation their initial function was assessed by initial urine output, sodium reabsorption, creatinine clearance and requirements for dialysis. The results (Table 14.1) suggest that high ATP levels and low P_i during cold ischaemia predict good early graft function.

Table 14.1 Ranking orders of initial function and NMR spectra during cold ischaemia of seven transplanted kidneys.

	Best ⟶ Worst function
Initial function	2 3 9 6 10 5 1
NMR data	2 3 & 6 5 & 9 10 1

Initial function based on tubular reabsorption of Na$^+$, urine output and creatine clearance. NMR data based on ATP and inorganic phosphate levels in kidneys during the cold ischaemic period. The numbers refer to the code number of the kidney (1 = the first kidney to be examined by NMR spectroscopy prior to transplantation).

DISCUSSION

Phosphorus nuclear magnetic resonance examination of the human kidney is feasible without prejudice to its survival. The major advantage of this non-invasive technique is in following the dynamic changes of the important phosphorus metabolites in the organ during the period of cold ischaemia.

It is important to note that narrow NMR signals are obtained only from mobile compounds, and therefore signals may not be obtained from metabolites that are strongly immobilized by binding to macromolecules or membranes. The levels that we quote here therefore represent the concentrations of mobile metabolites, and could in principle differ from values obtained by freeze-extraction procedures, which measure the total cellular amounts of the metabolites. In fact, we have found that the general pattern of changes in adenine nucleotide levels during hypothermic storage is comparable to that obtained by other workers using the conventional quick-frozen sample in experimental animals[7,8]. However, higher ATP levels were obtained with the human kidneys than those observed in the previous NMR study of rat kidneys during the period of cold ischaemia[4]. In view of the possible species difference in biochemical behaviour, results from experimental animals may not apply to human kidneys.

Despite the small number of kidneys examined, the five questions asked in the introduction can be answered 'yes' with varying degrees of certainty. The confirmation that ^{31}P NMR spectroscopy can predict how cadaver donor kidneys function immediately after transplantation is now an urgent task. If such confirmation is obtained it will give a new impetus to the study of organ preservation. It will also make it possible and worthwhile to re-examine which factors in the donor and recipient can improve or impair early graft function.

Acknowledgements

We are grateful to Mr J. C. Smith and Mr G. J. Fellows for permission to examine kidneys removed from their patients. This work was supported by the Medical Research Council and Science Research Council.

References

1. Gadian, D. G. (1982). *NMR and its Applications to Living Systems.* (Oxford: Oxford University Press)
2. Gadian, D. G., Radda, G. K., Richards, R. E. and Seeley, P. J. (1979). ^{31}P NMR in living tissue: the road from a promising to an important tool in biology. In Shulman, R. G. (ed.), *Biological Applications of Nuclear Magnetic Resonance,* pp. 463–535. (New York: Academic Press)
3. Gadian, D. G. and Radda, G. K. (1981). NMR studies of tissue metabolism. *Ann. Rev. Biochem.,* **50,** 69
4. Sehr, P. A., Bore, P. J., Papatheofanis, J. and Radda, G. K. (1979). *Br. J. Exp. Pathol.,* **60,** 632
5. Bore, P. J., Sehr, P. A., Chan, L., Thulborn, K. R., Ross, B. D. and Radda, G. K. (1981). *Transplant. Proc.,* **13,** 707
6. Chan, L., French, M. E., Gadian, D. G. and Radda, G. K. (1982). Phosphorus magnetic resonance study of renal cell carcinoma. (In preparation)
7. Collins, G. M., Taft, P., Green, R. D., Rurprecht, R. and Halasz, N. A. (1977). *World J. Surg.,* **1,** 237
8. Southard, J. H., Benzig, K. A., Hoffman, R. M. and Belzer, F. O. (1977). *Transplant. Proc.,* **9,** 1535

15
Effects of hypothermia on anabolic and catabolic processes and on oxygen consumption in perfused rat livers

F. A. ZIMMERMANN, H. G. DIETZ, Ch. O. KÖHLER, N. KILIAN,
J. KOSTERHON and R. SCHOLZ

Hypothermia prolongs the viability of isolated organs by reducing metabolic activity. On the other hand hypothermia also creates risks. The swelling of cells under hypothermic conditions is a well-recognized problem[1,2]. Little is known as to what extent metabolic processes are influenced by low temperatures and whether these changes are identical in the different processes or not. The intermediary metabolism of homeo-thermic animals is based on a constant body temperature. Transferring an organ to hypothermia interferes profoundly with the biochemical reactions and their equilibria, yet these reactions are responsible for the viability of an organ and its various functions. It is impossible to predetermine when the products of such harmful events have accumulated to the point of 'no return'. Since the limits of empirical animal experience for organ preservation may have been reached, it became necessary to return to basic principles of physiology and biochemistry during low-temperature conditions. The aim of our studies was to investigate the influence of hypothermia on the velocity of the basic pathways of intermediary metabolism.

METHODS

Isolated liver perfusion

The perfusion apparatus is shown in Figure 15.1. The operative technique has been reported elsewhere[3]. Isolated livers from male Wistar rats were perfused with a non-recirculating normo-osmolalic Krebs-bicarbonate buffer through the portal vein. The buffer was oxygenated and its temperature regulated in a silastic tube oxygenator and heat exchanger[4]. The liver was kept in an isolated chamber. Its temperature and the temperature of the perfusate were identical. The livers were cooled in

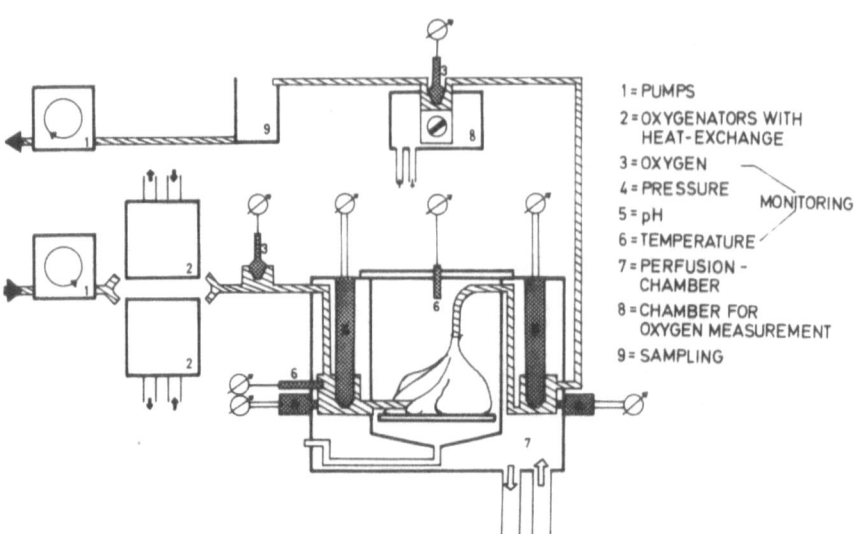

Figure 15.1 Perfusion apparatus. The perfusate is oxygenated with O_2:CO_2 (95:5). The effluent is cooled to a constant temperature (1 °C) in a special box (8). The Clark electrode is calibrated at this temperature

70 min from 37 °C to 1 °C and rewarmed at the same velocity. The effluent was collected in single fractions. The metabolites in the samples were measured using standard enzymatic-photometry tests. For measuring CO_2 production the fractions were acidified, and the CO_2 was trapped in phenylethylamine and measured by liquid scintillation spectrometry. The rates of the processes were calculated from the porta-caval differences of the concentrations of metabolites, the perfusion flow and the wet liver weight. For calculating the CO_2 production the specific activity of [1-^{14}C]octanoate was employed.

Measurement of oxygen consumption

The Clark platinum electrode for oxygen measurement is extremely sensitive to temperature changes, but in our system the effluent in which the electrode was placed was cooled immediately beyond the liver to a constant low temperature, and the standardizing and measuring temperatures were identical. Figure 15.2 shows the theoretical solubility of oxygen in saline expressed by the Bunsen coefficient under constant pressure and temperature (□ — □). The curve (○—○) shows the oxygen solubility measured in the effluent without employing our system to stabilize temperatures. The third curve (△ — △) shows the solubility of oxygen measured in saline using our device at a constant low temperature and is similar to the theoretical coefficient.

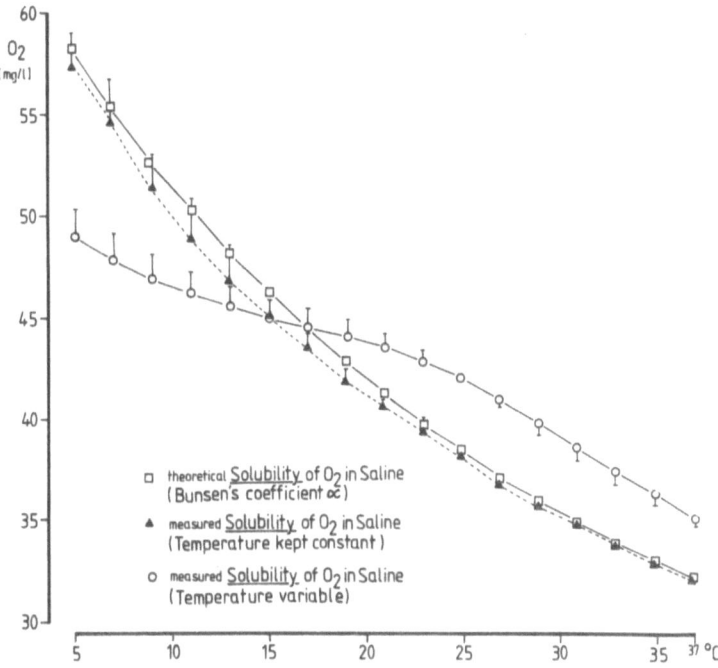

Figure 15.2 Solubility of oxygen in saline. Pressure constant at 760 Torr

Theoretical considerations

The Arrhenius equation[5] describes the relation between reaction velocity and temperature. Metabolic rates were plotted as the logarithm versus the reciprocal of the absolute temperature: The graphical plot has a slope of $E_a/2.3R$. It is assumed that the velocity constant corresponds to the maximal velocity of a process, and this requirement is fulfilled in our experiments. The expected relationship for biological systems is linear from the freezing point to the temperature of protein denaturation. From the slopes we calculated the Q_{10} for each process.

Results

Various catabolic and anabolic processes have been investigated so far[4], located in different subcellular compartments of the cells. Glycolysis, whose enzymes are located in the cytosol, exhibits a linear Arrhenius plot. The activation energy is 59 kJ/mol and is constant between 37 °C and 1 °C. The situation in mitochondrial processes is different. The plot of keto-genesis and $^{14}CO_2$ production from [1-^{14}C]octanoate shows a 'break' at 22 °C. The activation energies increase below this temperature to 105 kJ/mol (Figure 15.3). Urea production seems to be temperature-independent between 37 °C and 30 °C. It shows a 'break' in its plot at 18 °C, unlike other mitochondrial processes. Even more complicated is the situation in processes, whose sequential reactions take place in different cell compartments, and which therefore require transport for the exchange of metabolites. Figure 15.4 shows glucose synthesis from lactate and pyruvate. The Arrhenius plot exhibits two 'breaks', the first at 22 °C, the second at 11 °C. The activation energies increase from 50 kJ/mol to 150 kJ/mol in two steps. Oxygen consumption of a perfused rat liver is expressed in μgram atom/g/h. At 37 °C the liver utilizes some 280 μgram atom/g in 1 h. The oxygen consumption drops to a fifth at 20 °C and to 5% at 10 °C, and does not decrease linearly. There is a 'break' in its plot at 22 °C. The activation energy increases to 125 kJ/mol below this temperature (Figure 15.5). Finally, it has to be stressed that the same plot is obtained in all experiments whether the liver is being cooled or rewarmed.

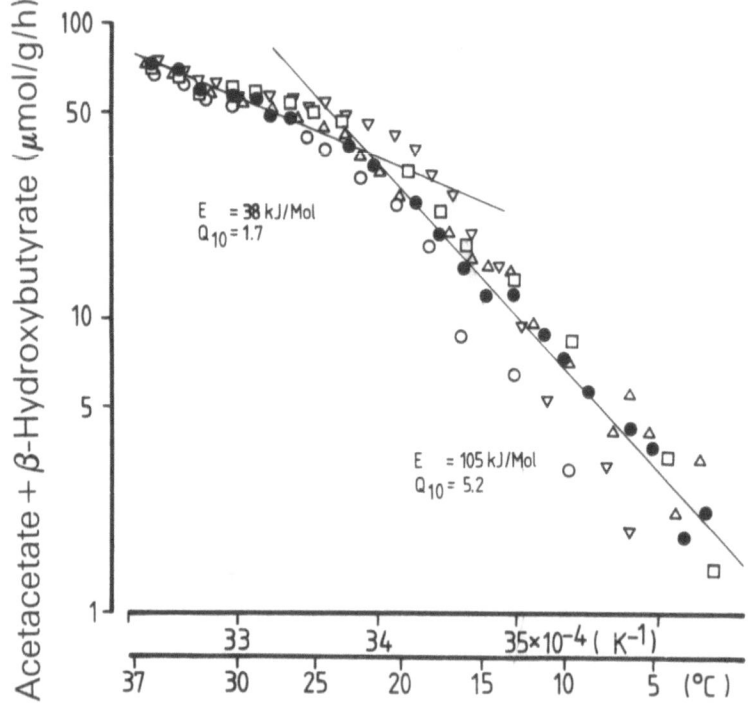

Figure 15.3   Ketogenesis from [1-14C]octanoate (0.5 mmol/l). The rate of ketogenesis is calculated from the β-hydroxybutyrate and acetoacetate production. The symbols show five different experiments. Ordinate: logarithm of reaction velocity; abscissa: reciprocal of absolute temperature. The regression slope is calculated. The $^{14}CO_2$ production is identical

DISCUSSION

The integrity and the co-ordination of metabolism is a prerequisite for the

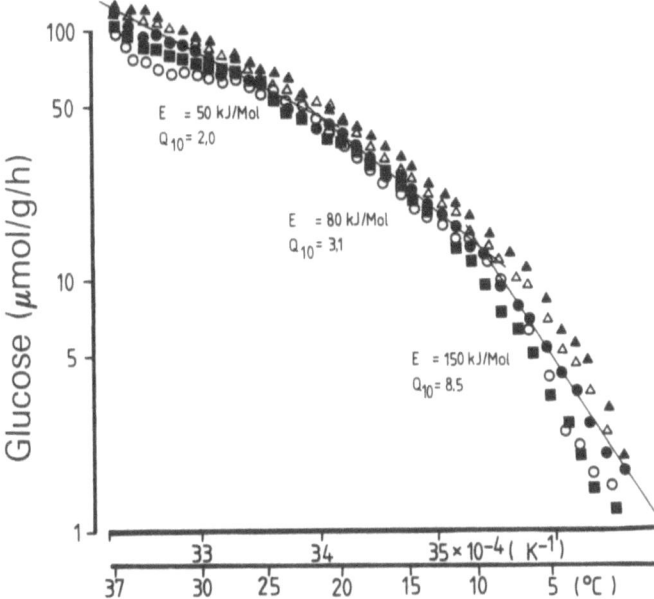

Figure 15.4 Glucose production in perfused livers from fasted rats. Glucose synthesis from lactate (4 mmol/l) and pyruvate (0.5 mmol/l). The symbols show five different experiments. The regression slope is calculated

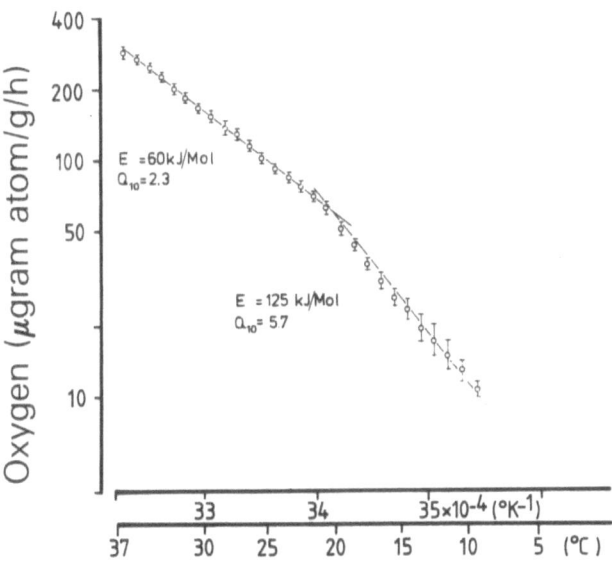

Figure 15.5 Oxygen consumption of perfused livers from fed rats. The mean ± SD of seven experiments is given. Ordinate: logarithm of oxygen consumption (μgram atom/g/h). Abscissa: reciprocal of absolute temperature

viability of an organ. As we have shown, metabolic processes are influenced by hypothermia in different ways. Furthermore, within a single process temperature-dependence can change in processes where enzymes are associated with mitochondrial membranes.

The interpretation of discontinuities in some plots is difficult and different explanations can be given:

(1) In some processes a single step may limit the overall velocity. This rate-limiting step may change and another one become limiting at a different temperature.

(2) The process, or part of it, may not function maximally in a certain temperature range, but that is the prerequisite condition for the Arrhenius equation.

(3) Because 'breaks' are observed only in processes in which regulating enzymes are bound to mitochondrial membranes, these breaks may be due to changes in the membranes themselves.

At a certain temperature a transition from a liquid-crystalline state to a solid gel state occurs in the lipid portion of the subcellular membranes. This change is probably responsible for the different behaviour of soluble enzyme systems and membrane-associated enzyme systems. Thus, the result would be the accumulation or depletion of metabolites at the point of entry into mitochondria. Accordingly, the phase transitions or shape changes in the subcellular membranes could cause metabolic imbalance and provide one component of the hypothermic injury suffered by homeothermic cells and organs stored for transplantation purposes.

References

1. Belzer, F. O., Hoffman, R., Huang, J. and Downes, G. (1973). Endothelial damage in perfused dog kidney and cold sensitivity of vascular Na-K-ATPase. *Cryobiology,* **9,** 457
2. Martin, D. R., Scott, D. F., Downes, G. D. and Belzer, F. O. (1972). Primary cause of unsuccessful liver and heart preservation: cold sensitivity of the ATPase system. *Ann. Surg.,* **175,** 111
3. Scholz, R., Hansen, W. and Thurman, R. G. (1973). Interaction of mixed function oxidation with biosynthetic processes. I. Inhibition of gluconeogenesis by aminopyrine in perfused rat liver. *Eur. J. Biochem.,* **38,** 64
4. Zimmermann, F. A., Dietz, H. G., Sippell, W. G., Hollmann, G. and Scholz, R. (1976). Temperaturabhängigkeiten von Stoffwechselgrößen in der perfundierten Rattenleber. *Res. Exp. Med.,* **168,** 57
5. Arrhenius, S. (1915). *Quantitative Laws in Biological Chemistry.* (London: G. Bell & Sons)

16
Mechanism of loss of mitochondrial functions during hypothermic storage of kidneys

J. H. SOUTHARD, R. M. HOFFMANN and F. O. BELZER

The limitations of obtaining good-quality, long-term (> 5 days) kidney preservation are not known. We have shown that hypothermic preservation of kidneys results in a loss of mitochondrial energy-linked functions[1,2]. The exact mechanism for the loss of mitochondrial function during preservation is not known.

In this study we compare the effects of ageing kidney cortex homogenates and mitochondria at 0–4 °C to the effects of 3 days of hypothermic perfusion and cold storage on respiratory activity. Ageing the freshly prepared subcellular fractions produces changes in mitochondrial activity that are remarkably similar to the changes induced by preservation and suggest the existence of similar mechanisms for the loss of mitochondrial energy-linked processes.

METHODS

Adult mongrel dog kidneys were used in all studies. Perfusion preservation was done as described previously[3]. The perfusate was a human serum albumin-based perfusate containing sodium gluconate (90 mmol/l) in place of chloride (see Chapter 35). Cold storage (3 days) was done at 6–8 °C using Collins' C3 solution[4].

A homogenate of kidney cortex tissue (20% w/v) was prepared in ice-cold sucrose 0.25 mol/l; *tris*-Cl 20 mmol/l; pH 7.4 or in the same medium containing 1 g/dl defatted bovine serum albumin (BSA) and filtered through four layers of gauze. Mitochondria were isolated from the homogenate by the procedure of Johnson and Lardy[5]. Respiratory activity was determined on homogenates and mitochondria at 30 °C as described previously[1]. The respiratory control ratio (RCR) is calculated from the ratio of the rate of respiration with substrate + ADP to the rate of respiration in the presence of substrate alone (mitochondria) or substrate + oligomycin (homogenates). Mitochondrial (0.8–1.6 mg protein/ml) free fatty acids were determined by the colourimetric procedure of Novak[6] using palmitic acid as a standard.

Experimental values reported were obtained from at least three separate experiments (three different kidneys) for controls, perfused and cold stored kidneys.

RESULTS

Our previous results on the effects of preservation on respiratory activity and energy metabolism were obtained using, primarily, homogenates of dog kidney cortex tissue[1]. We have used homogenates because mitochondrial functional integrity (i.e. RCR) can easily be determined without isolating the mitochondria by differential centrifugation, if selective mitochondrial inhibitors are used. Furthermore, we felt that the isolation procedure for mitochondria may result in the isolation of only one type of mitochondria (i.e. intact) and not structurally damaged (i.e. swollen) organelles. The experimental data reported in Table 16.1 compare the effects of perfusion preservation and cold storage on the respiratory activity obtained in homogenates to that obtained in isolated mitochondria. In general, perfusion preservation and cold storage result in a loss of respiratory activity and decrease in the RCR. The degree of respiratory activity loss, as determined in homogenates, is very similar to the degree of loss as determined in isolated mitochondria. Thus, either system can be used to accurately reflect the effects of preservation on certain mitochondrial-linked functions.

Mitochondria isolated from perfused kidneys contain 56% more (114.0 ± 10 nmol/mg protein) free fatty acids than controls (72.8 ± 7.0 nmol/mg protein); those from cold-stored kidneys contain 121% more (161.2 ± 30.0 nmol/mg protein). This increase in the levels of free

Table 16.1 Comparison of the effects of preservation of dog kidneys on respiratory activity in homogenates and isolated mitochondria

| Substrate | Respiration rates (percentage of control) | | | |
| | Perfused | | Cold stored | |
	Homogenate	Mitochondria	Homogenate	Mitochondria
P+M	100 ± 38	62 ± 21	113 ± 31	171 ± 31
P+M−ADP	46 ± 17	50 ± 21	56 ± 15	52 ± 13
P+M−DNP	49 ± 19	50 ± 18	44 ± 18	55 ± 14
P+M−RCR	3.4	3.9	3.6	1.7
Suc	80 ± 5.0	76 ± 18	42 ± 17	32 ± 18
Suc−ADP	49 ± 7.0	61 ± 21	51 ± 5.0	53 ± 26
Suc−DNP	49 ± 6.0	51 ± 14	76 ± 6.0	69 ± 12
Suc−RCR	3.3	4.0	1.7	1.5

Experimental methods are described in the text. P + M = pyruvate + malate; Suc = succinate, DNP = dinitrophenol, RCR = respiratory control ratio. Results are means with standard error of the mean

fatty acid is greater than required to bring about uncoupling[7], an observation that we have also made using fresh dog kidney mitochondria titrated with oleic acid (unpublished observation).

Ageing homogenates or mitochondria at 0–4 °C for 24 h induces changes in respiration that are related to the formation of free fatty acids[8–10]. The changes in respiratory activity induced by ageing are very similar to the effects of preservation on respiratory activity in homogenates (Table 16.2) and mitochondria (results not shown). Ageing, perfusion and cold storage all induce a similar degree of loss in the capability of ADP to maximally stimulate respiration. A similar loss in the rate of DNP-stimulated respiration is also observed. The only major difference in the effects of these storage conditions is on the resting rate of respiration. Both ageing and cold storage result in a stimulation of the resting rate of respiration (oligomycin-sensitive), whereas perfusion results in no change or a decrease. The results suggest that a similar, although not exactly the same, mechanism may be involved in the effects of ageing and preservation on mitochondria.

Table 16.2 The effects of ageing and preservation on respiratory activity in homogenates (percentage of control)

Respiration	Aged	Perfused	Cold store
Pyruvate + malate respiration			
Resting rate	200 ± 14	100 ± 15	13 ± 31
ADP-stimulated	43 ± 23	46 ± 17	56 ± 15
DNP-stimulated	40 ± 19	49 ± 19	44 ± 8
Succinate respiration			
Resting rate	27 ± 9	20 ± 17	58 ± 17
ADP-stimulated	55 ± 3	57 ± 7	51 ± 10
DNP-stimulated	52 ± 6	59 ± 3	80 ± 4

Experimental methods are described in Methods section of text

The effects of BSA on the RCR of mitochondria and homogenates prepared from preserved kidneys were compared to the effects in aged homogenates and mitochondria. The effects of ageing on mitochondria are reversed or prevented by chelation of free fatty acids by BSA. In our studies, BSA prevented the loss of respiratory control in aged mitochondria and homogenates by 80–90%. BSA also reverses the loss of RCR in mitochondria from cold-stored kidneys (RCR = 1.7 in controls to 4.4 with BSA). This is indirect evidence that free fatty acids are involved in the uncoupling of mitochondria in preserved kidneys. The restoration of coupling by BSA is due to a decrease in the resting rate of respiration. BSA had no effect on restoring maximal rates of respiration (ADP- or DNP-stimulated) after cold storage or perfusion, indicating that both cause irreversible changes in mitochondria.

DISCUSSION

Perfusion and cold storage of kidneys for 3 days leads to irreversible changes in mitochondrial-catalysed reactions, including a loss of maximal ADP- and DNP-stimulated respiration. The data presented suggest that these irreversible changes are due to elevated levels of free fatty acids in the mitochondria of preserved kidneys. This conclusion is also supported by the observation that BSA reversed the effects of cold storage on the resting rate of respiration and the RCR. In addition, the effects of cold storage and perfusion on mitochondrial activity are similar to the effects induced by ageing which are due to free fatty acids. These changes are also similar to those obtained by adding free fatty acids directly to mitochondria.

A mechanism responsible for the loss of mitochondrial activity during preservation can be postulated from these results. Preservation results in a loss of ATP which initiates a chain of events that is catastrophic to the kidney. The loss of ATP causes membrane instability[11] and activation of membrane-bound phospholipases. This results in the production of large quantities of free fatty acids and degradation of the structural components of membranes. The free fatty acids become distributed in membrane systems including the mitochondria, suppressing adenine nucleotide translocase activity[12] and inducing uncoupling of mitochondria. Cold storage and perfusion cause additional changes in mitochondria including structural changes and changes in the permeability of the mitochondrial membrane due to the presence of free fatty acids and active phospholipases. A consequence of increased membrane permeability is the loss of cofactors involved in electron transport which leak out of the mitochondria, reducing the capacity for maximal electron transport. Similar changes may also occur in other membrane systems. These changes are irreversible and reperfusion of the organ does not regenerate viability. The suppression of loss of mitochondrial activity during preservation may be a critical factor in increasing preservation quality and/or duration.

Acknowledgement

This work was supported by NIH Grant AM18624.

References

1. Southard, J.H., Senzig, K.A., Hoffmann, R.M. and Belzer, F.O. (1980). Toxicity of oxygen to mitochondrial respiratory activity in hypothermically perfused canine kidneys. *Transplantation*, **29**, 459
2. Southard, J.H., Senzig, K.A., Hoffmann, R.M. and Belzer, F.O. (1977). Energy metabolism in kidneys stored by simple hypothermia. *Transplant. Proc.*, **9**, 1535
3. Huang, J.S., Downes, G.L. and Belzer, F.O. (1971). Utilization of fatty acids in perfused dog kidneys. *J. Lipid Res.*, **12**, 622
4. Collins, G.M., Hartley, L.C.J. and Clunie, G.J.A. (1972). Kidney preservation for transportation. Experimental analysis of optimal perfusate composition. *Br. J. Surg.*, **59**, 187

5. Johnson, D. and Lardy, H. (1967). Isolation of liver and kidney mitochondria. *Methods Enzymol.,* **10,** 94
6. Novak, M. (1965). Colorimetric ultramicro method for the determination of free fatty acids. *J. Lipid Res.,* **6,** 431
7. Boime, I., Smith, E.E. and Hunter, F.E. Jr. (1968). Stability of oxidative phosphorylation and structural changes of mitochondria in ischemic rat liver. *Arch. Biochem. Biophys.,* **128,** 704
8. Chan, S.H.P. and Higgins, E. Jr. (1978). Uncoupling activity of endogenous free fatty acids in rat liver mitochondria. *Can. J. Biochem.,* **56,** 111
9. Scarpa, A. and Lindsay, J.G. (1972). Maintenance of energy-linked functions in rat liver mitochondria aged in the presence of nupercaine. *Eur. J. Biochem.,* **27,** 401
10. Carafoli, E. and Gazzotti, P. (1970). Loss and maintenance of energy-linked functions in aged mitochondria. *Biochem. Biophys. Res. Commun.,* **39,** 842
11. Wilkinson, J.H. and Robinson, J.M. (1974). Effect of ATP on release of cellular enzymes from damaged cells. *Nature (Lond.),* **249,** 662
12. Shug, A.L., Sharago, E., Bittar, N., Folts, J.D. and Koke, J.R. (1975). Acyl-CoA inhibition of adenine nucleotide translocation in ischemic myocardium. *Am. J. Physiol.,* **228,** 689

17
Depletion of CoA in dog kidneys during hypothermic perfusion

S. SKREDE, G. LANDE, O. SLAATTELID and A. FLATMARK

A major problem in kidney preservation is the maintenance of adequate adenine nucleotide pools[1-3]. Loss of adenine nucleotides can be counteracted by the addition of proper precursors, e.g. adenosine[1]. Kidneys perfused hypothermically are able to oxidize short-chain fatty acids[4-6], and are better preserved when such substrates are present in the perfusate[5]. Fatty acids and acetoacetate are in fact the main exogenous fuels of respiration in kidney cortex[7]. Since the metabolism of fatty acids and ketone bodies is critically dependent on the reserves of CoA in the tissue, we performed studies on the content of CoA in the renal cortex during hypothermic perfusion.

METHODS

The study comprised two series (A and B) of mongrel dogs weighing 15–20 kg each, 12 in A, and 10 in B. Anaesthesia and surgical procedures were as described previously[6]. One kidney was removed first and served as control. In study A, biopsies from cortex of the perfused kidney (see below) were taken after 24 h, and in a few cases also at other intervals. The kidney was reimplanted[5] after 72 h. Perfusion[5,6] was performed in a Gambro machine (Gambro, Lund, Sweden), using 600 ml of perfusate that was continuously equilibrated with O_2 (97%) and CO_2 (3%).

Table 17.1 shows the composition of five different solutions used in study B. In study A, solution E 1 was the basis for the perfusate in each of three subgroups. Wedge-shaped biopsies (3–4 mm deep, wet weight after removal of capsule about 50 mg) were removed with a scalpel. CoA is rapidly degraded in homogenized tissues[8,9], hence special precautions were taken[10]. Homogenates were prepared rapidly in chilled NaCl solution (150 mmol/l) with added L-tartrate (25 mmol/l) and EDTA (5 mmol/l) and were frozen rapidly.

On removal the control kidneys were immediately flushed free of blood with ice cold NaCl (150 mmol/l) and weighed. Cortical tissue was gently

Table 17.1 Composition of solutions for kidney perfusion

		Solutions				
	Unit	E 1	E 2	I 1	I 3	K 2
Albumin*	g/l	47	47	47	47	47
Na$^+$	mmol/l	146	146	30	30	10
K$^+$	"	6.7	6.7	124	124	188
Mg^{2+}	"	8.3	8.3	10	10	10
Cl$^-$	"	125	125	15	15	50
HCO$_3^-$	"	21	21	20	20	20
Phosphate	"	—	—	2	2	2
SO$_4^{2-}$	"	8.3	8.3	30	30	10
Citrate^{3-}	"	—	—	30	30	50
Glucose	"	—	10	10	10	10
Adenosine	"	—	1.0	—	1.0	1.0
Pantethine (SS)	"	—	0.5	—	0.5	0.5
l-methionine	"	—	1.0	—	1.0	1.0
Caprylic acid	"	—	5.0	—	5.0	5.0
l-carnitine	"	—	0.08	—	0.08	0.08

Perfusates resembling extracellular fluid are indicated by the abbreviation E, those more comparable to intracellular fluid by I, and that with a very high potassium concentration by K
* Bovine, 'fatty acid free' (Sigma)

homogenized in sucrose (70 mmol/l), mannitol (220 mmol/l), HEPES (2 mmol/l), L-tartrate (25 mmol/l) and EDTA (5 mmol/l) at pH 7.4. The 'nuclear' (N-) fraction was obtained at 6600 g min, the mitochondrial fraction at 100 000 g min, the 'lysosomal' (L-) fraction at 250 000 g min and the 'microsomal' (P-) fraction at 6×10^6 g min. After deproteinization and hydrolysis of CoA esters[9,11], the total CoA was estimated by the CoA-dependent incorporation of radioactive carnitine into palmitoyl carnitine[11]. Protein was estimated by a Lowry method.

RESULTS

Gain of kidney weight during perfusion

Avoidance of tissue swelling is an important goal in kidney preservation[2,3]. Table 17.2 shows that perfusion fluids with an 'intracellular' electrolyte composition (I 1 and I 3) did not induce swelling. Solutions of an 'extra-

Table 17.2 Gain of weight during 48 h perfusion of dog kidneys

	Solutions				
	E 1	E 2	I 1	I 3	K 2
Weight before perfusion (g)	51.3	69.6	63.5	62.7	60.9
Weight after perfusion (g)	58.1	78.8	63.2	63.0	69.9
Weight change (%)	+13.2	+10.4	−0.5	+0.4	+14.9

The solutions are described in Table 17.1; the results are means of experiments with two dogs

cellular' type (E1 and E2) or with high potassium content (K2) caused 10–15% gain of weight.

Depletion of CoA during perfusion

Table 17.3 shows total CoA in kidney cortex during perfusion with the 'extracellular' solution E1 (cf. Table 17.1). E1 was tested without additions, with substrate (DL-β-hydroxybutyrate) or with chlorpromazine – the latter agent added to counteract phospholipid degradation previously observed[6]. In all three subgroups, CoA decreased to about two-thirds of the initial amounts. This observation led us to investigate if this decrease affected more than one cellular pool of CoA.

Table 17.3 Content of CoA (nmol/mg protein) in biopsies from the renal cortex during hypothermic perfusion

Additions to the perfusate	No. of dogs	Time (h)	
		0	24
None	5	2.4 (0.5)	1.7 (0.2)
DL-β-hydroxybutyrate (10 mmol/l)	4	2.4 (0.6)	1.6 (0.3)
Chlorpromazine (6.7 mg/l)	3	2.1 (0.4)	1.7 (0.7)

Solution E1 (cf. Table 17.1) was used for perfusion; the values are arithmetical means (and SD)

A rather large fraction of CoA was recovered from the N ('nuclear') fraction (Table 17.4), which may be explained by the presence of unbroken cells in this fraction. It was essential, however, that the homogenization was gentle enough to maintain the integrity of mitochondria and lysosomes – (CoA is more easily lost from kidney mitochondria than from liver mitochondria[8]). During perfusion for 48 h with the 'basic' solutions E1 and I1 the CoA in the mitochondria and in the particle-free supernatant – roughly corresponding to cytosol – both decreased significantly.

With the 'enriched' solutions E2 and I3, the decrease of the cytosolic CoA pool was reversed, but not the decrease of the mitochondrial or the N-fraction CoA pool.

Preliminary observations (Halvorsen, O., personal communication) indicate that high potassium concentrations stimulate the activity of pantothenate kinase – the first, rate-limiting step[12] in the biosynthesis of CoA. The perfusion solution K2 (Table 17.1) with 'artificially high' potassium concentration was therefore designed. Table 17.4 shows that with this solution, no decrease of the total content of CoA occurred. The increase of cytosolic CoA with K2 was more pronounced than with E2 or I3, and also the mitochondrial CoA pool was maintained. K2 is the only solution tested so far that has preserved mitochondrial CoA.

Table 17.4   Content of CoA (nmol/g wet weight)* in subcellular fractions from the cortex of kidneys perfused for 48 hours (P) and control kidneys (C)

	Solutions				
	E 1	E 2	I 1	I 3	K 2
Total homogenate					
C	258	214	200	216	198
P	133	131	153	121	184
'Nuclear' fraction					
C	58	63	42	61	53
P	40	41	43	28	34
Mitochondrial fraction					
C	46	50	40	50	45
P	32	32	30	30	46
Lysosomal fraction					
C	0.7	1.2	0.6	1.0	0.7
P	0.6	1.0	0.7	0.7	0.7
Microsomal fraction					
C	0.3	0.2	0.5	0.1	0.3
P	0.3	0.2	0.2	0.3	0.4
Supernatant ('particle-free')					
C	37	30	33	28	37
P	25	37	29	43	55

The solutions are shown in Table 17.1; the values are means of results from two dogs
* The wet weight is not corrected for weight gain (cf. Table 17.2)

DISCUSSION

Maintenance of the renal adenine nucleotide levels appears related to the efficiency of different methods of preservation[1,2]. To our knowledge the present report is the first one to demonstrate that CoA may be depleted during hypothermic perfusion. This loss probably discloses a new, important problem in renal preservation. If the levels of CoA are critically lowered, the metabolism of the most important substrates for the renal cortex (fatty acids and ketone bodies[7]) will suffer. This may affect the viability of the kidney.

CoA may also be regarded as a marker of nucleotide metabolism in general, since adequate reserves of ATP are required for its synthesis[12]. It has recently been shown that mitochondria synthesize CoA with 4-phosphopantetheine as the first precursor[13]. The present study shows that it is more difficult to maintain the mitochondrial than the cytosolic pool of CoA, and it is known that the loss of mitochondrial function can be limiting in preservation[14]. Among the solutions tested by us, only that with very high potassium concentration (K 2) preserves the mitochondrial pool of CoA. High potassium concentrations may stimulate CoA biosynthesis at the pantothenate kinase level (Halvorsen, O., personal communication), but it is not at all clear if this explains their apparently beneficial effect. Prevention of kidney swelling was obtained by solutions with impermeant anions and an 'intracellular' electrolyte composition (I 1 and I 3) – not

136

unlike those recommended by Collins *et al.*[15]. Reimplantation experiments will be performed, where such solutions and media with high potassium concentration are compared with solutions with an 'extracellular'[5,6] electrolyte composition.

References

1. Buhl, M. R., Kemp, E. and Kemp, G. (1979). Purine nucleotide and nucleoside administration to kidneys: the effect on tolerance to ischaemia. In Pegg, D. E. and Jacobsen, I. A. (eds.) *Organ Preservation II*, pp. 247–252. (Edinburgh: Churchill Livingstone)
2. Pegg, D. E. (1978). An approach to hypothermic renal preservation. *Cryobiology*, **15**, 1
3. Belzer, F. O. and Southard, J. H. (1980). The future of kidney preservation. *Transplantation*, **30**, 161
4. Pettersson, S., Claes, G. and Scherstén, T. (1974). Fatty acid and glucose utilization during continuous hypothermic perfusion of dog kidney. *Eur. Surg. Res.*, **6**, 79
5. Slaattelid, O., Flatmark, A. and Skrede, S. (1976). The importance of perfusate content of free fatty acids for kidney preservation. *Scand. J. Clin. Lab. Invest.*, **36**, 239
6. Skrede, S. and Slaattelid, O. (1979). Fatty acid metabolism during hypothermic perfusion of the isolated dog kidney. *Scand. J. Clin. Lab. Invest.*, **39**, 765
7. Weidemann, M. J. and Krebs, H. A. (1969). The fuel of respiration of rat kidney cortex. *Biochem. J.*, **112**, 149
8. Bremer, J., Wojtczak, A. and Skrede, S. (1972). The leakage and destruction of CoA in isolated mitochondria. *Eur. J. Biochem.*, **25**, 190
9. Skrede, S. (1973). The degradation of CoA. Subcellular localization and kinetic properties of CoA- and dephospho-CoA pyrophosphatase. *Eur. J. Biochem.*, **38**, 401
10. Skrede, S. and Halvorsen, O. (1979). Increased biosynthesis of CoA in the liver of rats treated with clofibrate. *Eur. J. Biochem.*, **98**, 223
11. Skrede, S. and Bremer, J. (1970). The compartmentation of CoA and fatty acid activating enzymes in rat liver mitochondria. *Eur. J. Biochem.*, **14**, 465
12. Abiko, Y. (1975). Metabolism of coenzyme A. In Greenberg, D. M. (ed.), *Metabolic Pathways*. Vol. 7, pp. 1–25, (New York: Academic Press)
13. Skrede, S. and Halvorsen, O. (1979). Mitochondrial biosynthesis of CoA. *Biochem. Biophys. Res. Commun.*, **91**, 1536
14. Southard, J. H., Senzig, K. A., Hoffmann, R. M. and Belzer, F. O. (1980). Toxicity of oxygen to mitochondrial respiratory activity in hypothermically perfused canine kidneys. *Transplantation*, **29**, 459
15. Collins, G. M., Bravo-Shugarman, M. and Terasaki, P. J. (1969). Kidney preservation for transportation. *Lancet*, **2**, 1219

18
Renal viability testing during preservation by metabolic parameters

J. H. FISCHER, I. HANSEN-SCHMIDT, D. KULUS and W. ISSELHARD

Many attempts have been made to find a method for renal viability testing during the preservation period. Most of the techniques have turned out to be of rather limited value. Because of the central importance of the energy metabolism for the survival of cells in unphysiological situations, the substances of the energy-distributing system (in the kidney, mainly the adenine nucleotides) as well as the metabolites of the glycolytic pathway (the only way for energy production in anaerobiosis) should be excellent parameters for viability[1-4]. Our experience includes experiments on several species (dogs, rats and guinea pigs) as well as different preservation techniques (normothermic ischaemia, hypothermic ischaemia, continuous hypothermic perfusion or retrograde oxygen persufflation (ROP)[5-8]).

METHODS

Dog experiments

Canine kidneys were flushed with Collins' solution C2 for 5 min and from a height of 100 cm after 2 min ischaemia or after 30 min of 'normothermic' ischaemia (NI) at 31–32 °C. The organs were then preserved by hypothermic ischaemic storage (HIS) or retrograde oxygen persufflation (ROP). For ROP, gaseous oxygen was administered via the renal vein at a pressure of 50–60 mmHg, leaving the organ through opened capsular veins[5,6]. A third group of organs was continuously perfused with an oxygenated albumin perfusate after a flush with Ringer's solution to which mannitol had been added[7].

After various preservation periods the kidneys were transplanted to the neck of the donor animal and the immediate function determined up to 3 h post-transplant by measurements of inulin and PAH clearances. (For technical details see refs. 5 and 6.) Tissue samples from the renal cortex were taken by a wedge incision and immediately frozen in liquid oxygen using the freeze–stop method[9]. The time between the beginning of the incision and freezing was about 5 sec. The samples were freed from adhering perfusate and capsular tissue in liquid oxygen and after weighing they were freeze-dried at $-30\,°C$ for at least 72 h. The samples were then homogenized and deproteinized in at least 10 ml of $\frac{1}{2}$ molar perchloric acid per g wet tissue at 0–4 °C. Following centrifugation and neutralization of the supernatant with 2 molar KOH the concentrations of adenine nucleotides and lactate in the tissue extracts were determined enzymatically.

Rat and guinea pig experiments

The kidneys were flushed with Collins' solution at the same pressure as the canine kidneys, and stored in this solution for 4 and 24 h. The organs were then frozen[9], freed of capsular and medullary tissue and then treated further like the samples of canine kidneys.

RESULTS AND DISCUSSION

The immediate function of the preserved canine kidneys after autotransplantation is shown in Figure 18.1. Figure 18.2 shows the initial changes of adenine nucleotide content of canine renal cortex together with energy charge potentials (ECP) after 2 min of NI and 5 min of reperfusion with Ringer's solution equilibrated with room air. The graph shows a rapid change during ischaemia and reoxygenation of all components except the total nucleotide content. Figures 18.3–18.6 show the changes of SAN, ATP, ECP and lactate content of canine kidney cortex during preservation,

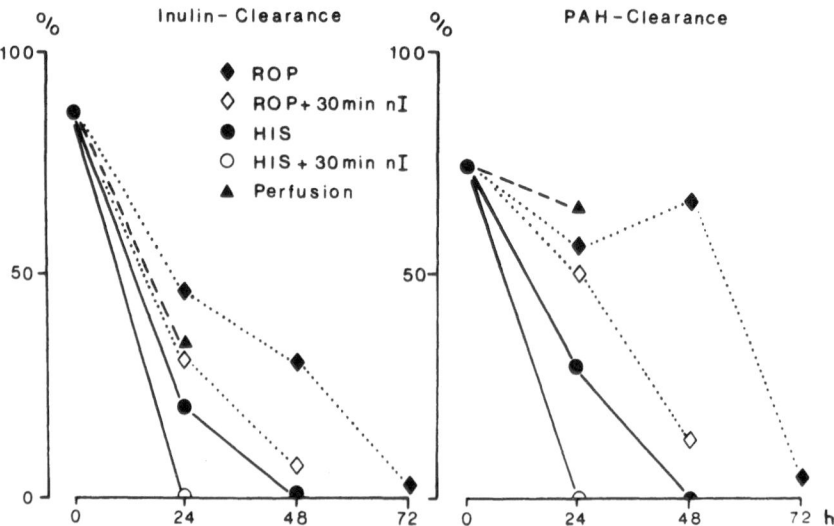

Figure 18.1 Immediate function of canine kidneys after preservation at 6 °C. Inulin and PAH clearances are in percentages of the function of the normal contralateral kidney (mean values, $n = 4$–6 per group)

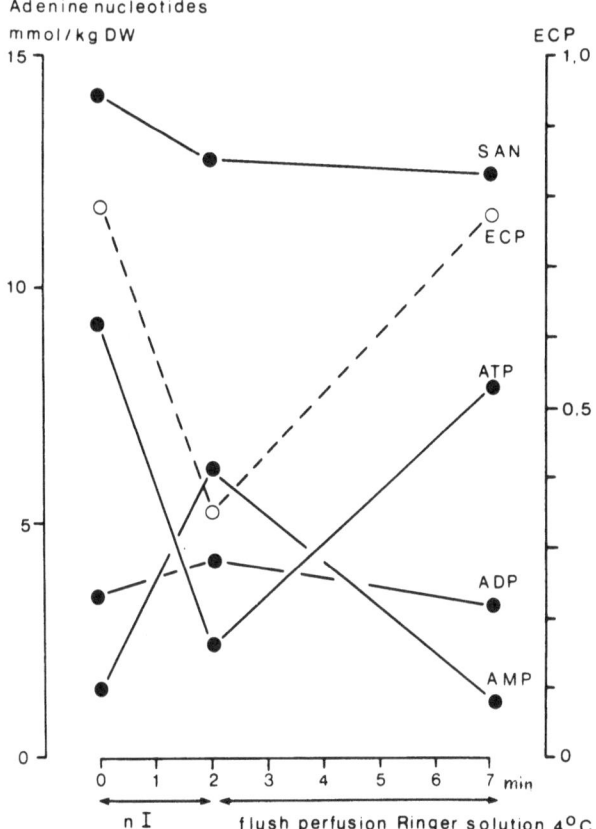

Figure 18.2 Adenine nucleotide content of canine kidney cortex, after 2 min of normo-thermic ischaemia (NI) and after a subsequent 5 min of hypothermic perfusion (mean values, $n = 4-8$ per group)

and Figure 18.7 shows the adenine nucleotide values following preservation of dog, rat and guinea pig kidneys for up to 24 h.

The results can be summarized as follows: the ATP content gives some information only when combined with the total nucleotide content (SAN) or the energy charge potential (ECP). The energy charge potential reflects the instantaneous effectiveness of the aerobic metabolic pathways[10] and thus the quality of preservation in fully oxygenated conditions (continuous perfusion or retrograde oxygen persufflation). It varies within a few minutes of change of oxygen administration or can be influenced by lack of adequate substrates. In hypothermic ischaemic storage it gives no information during preservation but during the period of post-transplant recovery it might reflect the quality of reperfusion.

The total adenine nucleotide content of the kidney changes in good correlation with viability in normo- and hypothermic ischaemia, during perfusion and ROP, but the absolute values indicating loss of viability are

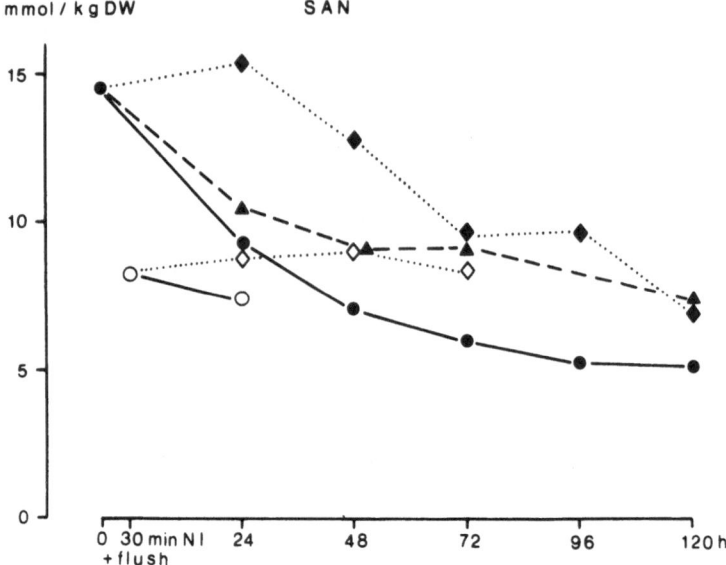

Figure 18.3 Total adenine nucleotide content (SAN) of canine kidneys during HIS or ROP with or without initial normothermic ischaemia and continuous perfusion (symbols identical to Figure 18.1) (mean values, $n = 5–11$ per group)

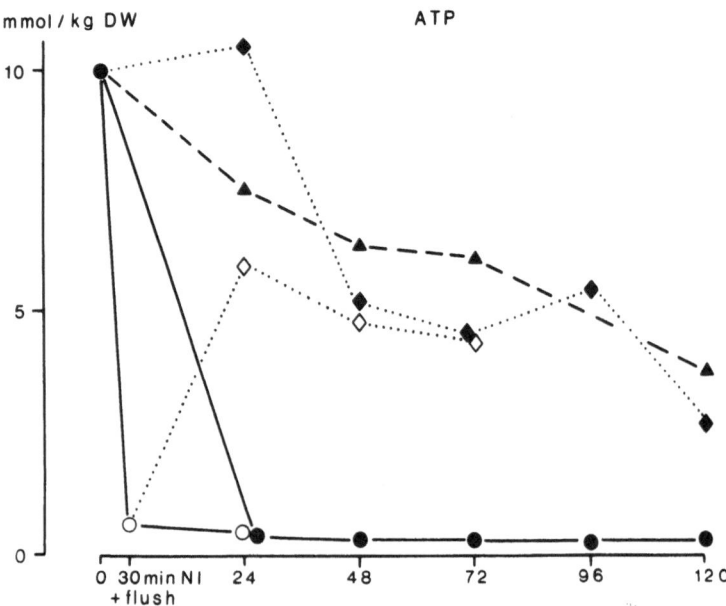

Figure 18.4 ATP content of the same kidneys as in Figure 18.3

VIABILITY TESTING BY METABOLIC PARAMETERS

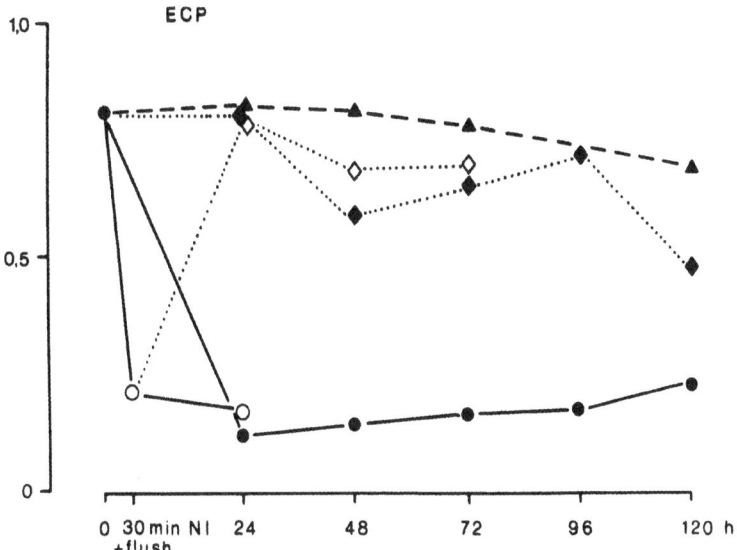

Figure 18.5 Energy charge potential (ECP = (ATP + ½ADP)/SAN) of the same kidneys as in Figure 18.3

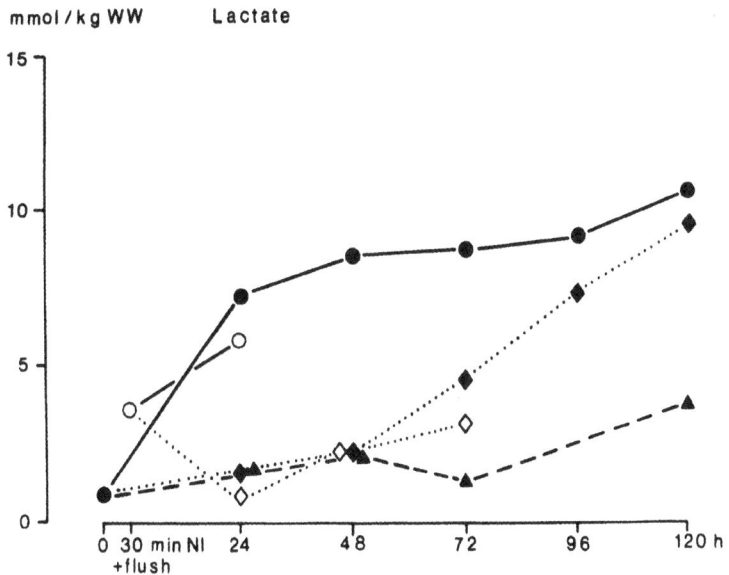

Figure 18.6 Lactate content of the same kidneys as in Figure 18.3

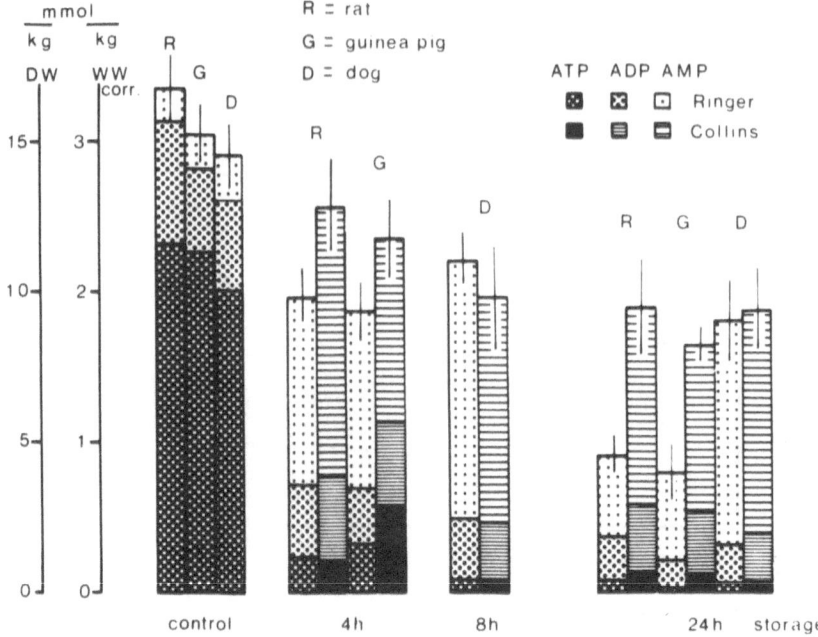

Figure 18.7 ATP, ADP, AMP and mean value ± SD of SAN of the cortex of rat ($n = 35$), guinea pig ($n = 54$) and dog ($n = 28$) kidneys after flush and hypothermic ischaemic storage. (Adenine nucleotide content in mmol/kg dry weight and mmol/kg corrected wet weight (WW corr.) i.e. the wet weight with 20% dry matter)

different in the different forms of preservation. Any change of the preservation conditions, including pre-damage by normothermic ischaemia, results in an impairment of the correlation, and in HIS substantial species differences exist.

The lactate level reflects defects in aerobic metabolism during preservation by ROP or continuous perfusion, but the rate of lactate accumulation is low and non-predictive if the preservation period is preceded by normothermic ischaemia. Thus SAN, ECP or lactate are reliable parameters of renal viability if there is no damage to the organ before preservation and if the preservation conditions do not change.

References

1. Calman, K. C. (1974). The prediction of organ viability. I. An hypothesis. *Cryobiology*, **11**, 6
2. Collins, G. M., Taft, P., Green, R. D., Ruprecht, R. and Halasz, N.A. (1977). Adenine nucleotide levels in preserved and ischemically injured canine kidneys. *World J. Surg.*, **1**, 237
3. Plachta, N., Rowinski, W., Ryffa, T., Ruka, M. and Stepkowski, S. (1978). Correlation of *in vitro* viability assays with the life supporting function of the ischemically damaged kidney. *Acta Med. Pol. Vars.*, **19**, 35

4. Southard, J. H., Senzig, K. A., Hoffmann, R. M. and Belzer, F. O. (1977). Energy metabolism in kidneys stored by simple hypothermia. *Transplant. Proc.,* **9**, 1535

5. Fischer, J. H., Czerniak, A., Hauer, U. and Isselhard, W. (1978). A new simple method for optimal storage of ischemically damaged kidneys. *Transplantation,* **25**, 43

6. Fischer, J. H., Czerniak, A., Kulus, D., Hansen-Schmidt, I. and Isselhard, W. (1979). Persufflations-Konservierung von Nieren in intrazellulären Lösungen über 48 und 72 Stunden. In Schellerer, W. and Schildberg, F. W. (eds.) *Chirurgie aktuell. Vol. 5. Aktuelles aus der Abdominal und Unfallchirurgie,* p. 257

7. Fischer, J. H., Armbruster, D., Grebe, W., Czerniak, A. and Isselhard, W. (1980). Effects of differences in substrate supply on the energy metabolism of hypothermically perfused canine kidneys. *Cryobiology,* **17**, 135

8. Fischer, J. H., Kulus, D., Hansen-Schmidt, I. and Isselhard, W. (1981). Adenine nucleotide levels of canine kidneys during hypothermic aerobic or anaerobic storage in Collins' solution. *Eur. Surg. Res.,* **13**, 181

9. Wollenberger, A., Ristau, O. and Schoffa, G. (1960). Eine einfache Technik der extrem schnellen Abkühlung grösserer Gewebsstücke. *Pflügers Arch Ges. Physiol.,* **270**, 399

10. Atkinson, D. E. (1968). The energy charge of the adenylate pool as a regulatory parameter. Interaction with feedback modifiers. *Biochemistry N. Y.,* **7**, 4030

11. Fischer, J. H., Marsen, S., Fabri, P. and Isselhard, W. (1979). Renal energy metabolism during hypothermic storage - comparative experiments on dogs, rats and guinea pigs. *Eur. Surg. Res.,* **11** (suppl. 2), 85

19
Hibernatory animals as a model for hypothermic organ preservation

C. J. GREEN, B. D. ROSS, B. J. FULLER, J. T. BROSNAN, M. LOWRY, M. STUBBS and E. SHOEBRIDGE

The ability of true hibernators to 'store' their organs for long periods at temperatures of about 4 °C may be one avenue worth exploring in an attempt to improve organ storage techniques.

As far as we know, hibernatory animals have not previously been used as a model for *in vitro* storage during hypothermia. We are setting up a range of experiments to compare tissue function during summer with that in the winter months when the animals may be either in deep hibernation at 4 °C, maintained in an ambient temperature of 4 °C but active and awake, or active at an ambient temperature of 22 °C. These are being compared with similar studies in non-adapted rats, with the aim of finding a dialysable factor which will produce hibernatory behaviour and cold tolerance when injected into normal rats. Very preliminary results of some pilot studies are reported here.

In December 1980, fourteen 13-lined ground squirrels were placed in a cabinet at 4 °C; ten went into hibernation, some within 48 h and the remainder by the end of 2 weeks. The other four did not hibernate, but tolerated the cold temperature with no apparent alteration to their body temperature or behavioural activity. In April they were returned to the normothermic colony. The ten hibernators remained torpid for 7–12 days, then became hyperactive for 2–7 days before another bout of torpor set in. Arousal and return to torpor occurred in 3–4 h and 12–24 h respectively. One animal even returned to torpor at the end of April after a long period (14 days) of activity.

The action of anaesthetic agents was assessed both during normal activity and hibernation. Fentanyl-fluanisone-diazepam proved more effective than pentobarbitone sodium or ketamine-xylazine just as we have found in other rodent species[1]. Even when the body temperature of the hibernators was as low as 4 °C they still required about 70% of the normothermic pentobarbitone dosage before reflex response to pain was eliminated. Renal autografting was performed by standard end-to-end microsurgical techniques on the renal artery and vein, but the ureteral lumen proved too small even for these techniques, so ureteric drainage was constructed directly into the bladder by ureterocystotomy.

Whole kidney and liver segments were freeze-clamped *in situ* in anaesthetized animals. These tissues were then assayed for ATP, ADP, AMP and the K : Na ratio. Isolated renal cortical tubules were prepared after the techniques of Tange *et al.*[2]. Isolated hepatocytes were prepared by the technique of Berry and Friend[3]. For enzyme distribution studies, mitochondria were separated from the supernatant by sucrose centrifugation. The ^{31}P NMR technique was used to measure adenine nucleotides and pH, the anaesthetized squirrels being placed intact into the core of the magnet. Renal function was assessed on an *in vitro* system, previously described for use with rats[4]. Function was then measured whilst varying the perfusion temperature between 4 °C and 37 °C.

Nucleotide analysis (Table 19.1)

Although the numbers are too small for statistical analysis, we found in both liver and kidney tissues that the hibernator had higher total adenine nucleotides and energy charge than its non-hibernating fellows, but perhaps most interesting, the levels of ATP in both the liver and the kidney of the hibernator were double those in the others. The $K^+ : Na^+$ ratio in the hibernator livers was about double that in the non-hibernators but was similar in the kidneys.

Table 19.1 Adenine nucleotide levels in liver (L) and kidney (K) from torpid and non-torpid ground-squirrels (μmol/g dry weight tissue)

Animal status	ATP		ADP		AMP		Total		Energy charge*		$K^+ : Na^+$	
	L	K	L	K	L	K	L	K	L	K	L	K
Summer non-torpid	–	4.20	–	2.11	–	0.83	–	7.14	–	0.74	–	1.1
Winter non-torpid	2.39	2.38	2.57	1.88	0.11	0.46	5.07	4.72	0.73	0.70	1.1	1.0
Winter non-torpid	2.55	2.61	1.95	1.93	0.04	0.35	4.54	4.89	0.73	0.73	1.8	1.0
Winter torpid	6.88	5.10	1.33	0.99	0.59	0.38	9.47	6.47	0.80	0.87	3.1	1.0

$$* \text{ Energy charge} = \frac{ATP + \frac{1}{2}ADP}{\text{Total AN}}$$

Gluconeogenesis

In the liver, rapid rates of gluconeogenesis were demonstrated and hibernation did not modify these. Lactate yielded similar rates as pyruvate, and high rates could also be obtained with propionate and glycerol. In the kidney, very high rates of glucose synthesis were measured, the rate from glycerol being remarkable.

Urea synthesis and ammonia genesis

In the liver, alanine and glutamine both caused urea synthesis but no change in either the endogenous or the maximum rates were associated with hibernation. Ammonia was produced from alanine and glutamine in the kidney and here there was a possible increase in the rate observed in hibernators.

Ketogenesis

A high endogenous rate of ketogenesis was stimulated 2.5 times with butyrate, but oleate had no effect. Hibernators were no different from non-hibernators. Blood glucose levels fell during hibernation whilst ketone levels were elevated.

Enzyme markers

Concentrations of lactic dehydrogenase (LDH), glutamate dehydrogenase (GLDH) and phosphoenolpyruvate carboxykinase (PEPCK) were used as enzyme markers of the sites and distribution of gluconeogenesis. In the liver very high total PEPCK levels were detected and, although these were increased by fasting, they were not altered by hibernation. However, interesting changes in the distribution between mitochondria and cytosol were observed: for example in the liver from hibernators, the concentrations of PEPCK in the cytosol increased 10-fold relative to mitochondria (an increase similarly observed during fasting). In normothermic liver the enzyme was primarily mitochondrial. This suggests that during hibernation, gluconeogenesis will proceed most efficiently with pyruvate and analine as substrates. Again very high PEPCK activity, equally distributed between mitochondria and cytosol, was measured in the kidneys of normothermic animals. As in the liver, this distribution changed during hibernation until the enzyme was found predominantly in cytosol.

Adenine nucleotides

Incubated liver cells exhibited a 4–7-fold increase in ATP concentration during hibernation, just as had been seen in freeze-clamped tissues. Incubated kidney cells from hibernating squirrels exhibited a rise in ATP relative to other nucleotides, but this was less marked than in the liver cells. Using non-invasive ^{31}P NMR, high ATP levels were measured in hibernator brain and the pH remained within normothermic physiological limits.

CONCLUSIONS

From our initial studies, we can state that it is technically feasible to isolate, cannulate and perfuse ground-squirrel kidneys for *ex vivo* functional assessment. It is also possible to store and autograft their kidneys by micro-surgical techniques.

Very high metabolic rates can readily be measured in isolated cells from liver and kidney but there are interesting adaptations during hibernation, for example in the redistribution of the enzymes of gluconeogenesis, which may indicate a switch of preferred substrates. Similarly, high oxidative metabolism was demonstrated in the brain of hibernators. Perhaps most intriguing, ATP levels were significantly increased in hibernator tissues.

The natural history of these animals also suggests manoeuvres which might help us to store organs for longer periods. Perhaps perfusion at low pressure pulsed at one or two per minute to dilate the capillary bed, the use of buffers efficient at low temperatures, and above all brief rewarming periods interspersed with the cold, might prove effective.

However most of the evidence suggests that true hibernators are highly adapted at a cellular level, particularly in terms of membrane fluidity and maintenance of pH, and it would be difficult to translate this to organ storage without a period of prior donor adaptation. Nevertheless, we feel encouraged to do further studies in case cold tolerance should be latent in all mammals.

Acknowledgement

Part of this work was funded by a grant from the National Kidney Research Fund.

References

1. Green, C. J. (1979). *Animal Anaesthesia*. (London: Laboratory Animals Ltd.)
2. Tange, J. D., Ross, B. D. and Ledingham, J. G. (1978). Effects of analgesics and related compounds on renal metabolism in rats. *Clin. Sci. Mol. Med.,* **53,** 485
3. Berry, M. N. and Friend, D. S. (1976). High yield preparation of isolation rat liver cells: a biochemical and fine structural study. *J. Cell. Biol.,* **43,** 506
4. Ross, B. D., Epstein, A. and Leaf, E. P. (1973). Sodium resorption in the perfused rat kidney. *Am. J. Physiol.,* **225,** 1165

20
Pharmacological factors in organ preservation

N. A. HALASZ

This chapter will deal with pharmacological considerations involved in organ preservation, mainly with material published within the last 10 years.

The models in which the effectiveness of pharmacological agents is studied are of great importance. Species-related differences in response are legion, the effects of shock in the donor far exceed the effects of an equivalent period of warm ischaemia, and manipulations affecting warm ischaemic injury will not necessarily have a comparable effect on preservation injury; qualitative as well as quantitative differences exist between the two.

VASOSPASM AND ITS CONTROL

The importance of this topic is mainly a geographical one. Many centres around the world today use heart-beating cadavers which have been maintained in the best possible physiological state. In other areas the organ recovery operation is not initiated until 'clinical death' has occurred, some 15–30 min after discontinuing ventilatory support. In view of this difference in approach, the incidence and severity of vasospasm varies greatly. After long perfusions, with plasma as a perfusate, the elaboration of angiotensin has been demonstrated[1], but for most intents and purposes the heart-beating donor avoids problems due to vasospasm.

When circumstances likely to cause vasospasm exist, it can be prevented by pharmacological pretreatment. Chlorpromazine was the first agent used for this purpose. Løkkegaard showed good protection of pig kidneys from the effects of 60 min of warm ischaemia by pretreating with this agent[2]. Turner et al. confirmed these findings, showing that chlorpromazine allowed cold storage of dog kidneys with consistent success for 24 h (when added to the serum used for flushing), while six out of ten kidneys failed without this agent[3]. The thesis that the effects of chlorpromazine are primarily vascular is supported by a later report of Løkkegaard et al.[4]. They could show no effect of the drug on the [^{125}I]hippuran uptake of kidney slices studied with or without prior warm ischaemia.

Pryor *et al.*[5] induced death by hypoxia in pigs, comparable to the conservative donor approach. Survival was clearly better in recipients of kidney homografts taken from animals pretreated with phenoxybenzamine intravenously.

Dhabuwala *et al.* compared the effects of warm ischaemia with those of shock and hypercarbia on rat kidneys[6]. They found that warm ischaemia was a weak inducer of vasospasm compared to the other two. Dopamine produced far better protection than did phenoxybenzamine, but the former drug was used with volume replacement and the latter without. Therefore, no definitive conclusion can be reached. Eliahou *et al.* studied the role of β_1 receptors in the rat kidney after 70 min of warm ischaemia and found that practolol did provide some protection of kidneys when used as pre- and post-treatment[7]. In a similar model, Solez made the interesting observation that kidneys exposed to a warm ischaemic insult *in situ* were significantly protected by propranolol, but that transplanted ones were not so protected[8]. Denervation of the transplant was thought to eliminate the neurogenic renin secretion which occurred in the innervated kidney. Stowe *et al.* also showed some protective effects of propranolol after short storage at 25 °C[9].

Papaverine was studied by Valido in rats[10], with kidneys exposed to 60 min of warm ischaemia *in situ*. Survival was not significantly affected, but there was significant delay in the onset and severity of the uraemia.

In our studies of rabbit kidneys after a 1 h warm ischaemic insult (without subsequent preservation), chlorpromazine, phenoxybenzamine and dopamine pretreatment did not protect renal function, short or long term[11]. Propranolol did allow a more speedy recovery of renal function. These studies must be evaluated in terms of the sluggish vasomotion of rabbit kidneys. The pig probably is a better predictor of the behaviour of human kidneys.

In summary, both β- and α-active agents can prevent or reverse the vasospasm produced by agonal processes and thereby permit better perfusion dynamics and early function. However, as Miller *et al.* pointed out[12], the most significant determinant of ultimate function is the length of warm ischaemia. This produces effects over and above those of vasospasm, which vasoactive drugs therefore cannot forestall or reverse.

STEROIDS

A broad spectrum of theoretical reasons exist for employing steroids in organ preservation. Several studies sought to evaluate the effects of adding steroids to flush or perfusion solutions. Starling *et al.*[13] added methylprednisolone (MP), 350 mg/l, to a Krebs/dextran perfusate, used for 24 h preservation of dog kidneys at 10 °C. The release of the lysosomal enzymes cathepsin D and β-glucuronidase was diminished, but the increase in vascular resistance observed in the control kidneys was not prevented. Tremann *et al.* added various amounts of MP to cryoprecipitated plasma used for preserving canine kidneys for 5 h[14]. 2.66 g/l halved the survival and caused significant vascular injury, especially in the glomerular and post-glomerular capillaries. Borderline injury was produced with 1.33 g/l. Rashid *et al.,* using Ursol as a flushing solution, preserved canine kidneys for 20 h with or without the addition of 1.0 g/l of MP to the flush[15]. Significant diminution in glomerular filtration rate, effective renal plasma flow and urine production occurred in the MP-flushed group, in these acute short-term studies. Dvorak *et al.*[16] studied the haemodynamic and histological effects of steroids on 20 h perfusions of dog kidneys. 0.192 g/l of MP was well tolerated, but 3.27 g/l or 6.35 g/l induced vascular changes in the glomeruli and the periglomerular capillaries, tubular occlusion and epithelial cell damage. At the higher range of MP, damage became irreversible after 4 h. Toledo-Pereyra reported the effects of adding MP to a plasma protein fraction used for perfusion preservation of dog kidneys[17]. Vascular resistance increased and subsequent survival diminished when the MP concentration was higher than 1.0 g/l.

As pretreatment, Miller and Alexander[18] administered MP to dogs prior to a 2 h warm ischaemic injury. The drug had to be given 2 h prior to the induction of ischaemia in order to be effective. It then lowered mortality from 80% to 20%. Chatterjee and Berne studied a similar model[19]. The kidneys were left *in situ* with immediate contralateral nephrectomy. Five of seven control animals died of uraemia, whereas those pretreated with 60 mg/kg of MP 90 min prior to clamping the vessels all survived (7/7).

Corticosteroids can be given to the donor along with cytotoxic drugs to diminish the load of passenger lymphocytes, or can be given in order to protect the kidney from a subsequent warm ischaemic insult. Two of the studies quoted show that the latter indeed can be accomplished, using doses which correspond to about 4.0 g in the average adult human, and provided that the steroid is administered 90–120 min prior to the onset of ischaemia. When steroids are added to the perfusate (usually to 'protect' the kidney but occasionally for immunological benefit), it would appear that even 1.0 g/l is damaging, and that the concentration best be kept below 300 or 350 mg/l. Whether even this concentration is indicated is unclear.

PROSTAGLANDINS

Two recent reports are of interest here, one dealing with pretreatment of donor animals and one with post-treatment. Mundy *et al.*[20] pretreated dogs with PGI_2 (prostacyclin) prior to 45 min of warm ischaemia. This prostaglandin lowered blood pressure by 25% yet increased renal blood flow by 50% prior to clamping. All the experimental and control dogs survived, but in the group treated with PGI_2 the creatinine had returned to normal by day 2, whereas it was still elevated on day 21 in the control animals. Casey *et al.*[21] gave PGE_1 or PGI_2 to dogs after 1 h of renal warm ischaemia. Histologically both of these agents protected the kidney almost completely against the damaging effects of warm ischaemia. On the other hand, no protective effect whatsoever could be demonstrated in terms of renal function, renal blood flow or the distribution of injected microspheres. This may be a reflection of late administration of the agents. If indeed vascular protection was expected, it might have been better to prime the animals with the drug(s) prior to reperfusing the ischaemic kidneys.

ALLOPURINOL

This xanthine oxidase inhibitor prevents the irreversible degradation of purine nucleotides. Vasko et al.[22] reported that when dogs were treated with it 2 days prior to, on the day of, and then daily after a 2 h warm ischaemic injury to the kidney, four out of four dogs survived, whereas five out of five not receiving allopurinol died (immediate contralateral nephrectomy).

Toledo-Pereyra et al.[23,24] studied dog kidneys exposed to 1 h of 25 °C 'warm ischaemia', then preserved for 24 h by perfusion and finally re-implanted with immediate contralateral nephrectomy. Treatment with oral allopurinol did not significantly alter the 25% control survival rate. With allopurinol added to the perfusate, 80% of the dogs survived. When the oral treatment was combined with adding allopurinol to the perfusate, survival was 100%. All of these perfusates contained 500 mg/l of methyl-prednisolone.

Owens et al. evaluated the effects of allopurinol on canine kidneys exposed to 2 h of haemorrhagic hypotension[25]. The kidneys were re-implanted as allografts. In the control group of 11, none survived 5 days. When the donors were treated with allopurinol, 10 out of 18 lived 5 days and had a significantly lower creatinine on day 1 than the control group (3.5 vs 6.0 mg/dl).

Murdock and Cho studied the effect of allopurinol on dog kidneys exposed to 60 min of warm ischaemia[26]. They added allopurinol to the perfusate and administered it postoperatively for 10 days. No kidneys exposed to 1 h of warm ischaemia supported life, whether treated with allo-purinol or not.

Fernando et al. could demonstrate no protective effect pretreating rat kidneys exposed to 60 min of warm ischaemia in situ[27].

Chatterjee and Berne[28,29] studied the effect of allopurinol on dog kidneys exposed to 1.5–2.0 h of warm ischaemia in situ. Six of eight control animals died of uraemia; in the treated group, only three of eight died.

In a randomized double-blind study by Toledo-Pereyra et al., 34 cadaver kidneys were perfused, one-half with and one-half without allopurinol added to the perfusate[30]. Perfusion characteristics, enzyme release, the need for post-transplantation dialysis and long-term function of the kidneys were entirely comparable. None of these donors was in shock prior to or during donation, and warm ischaemia was less than 5 min in all cases.

In summary, allopurinol may have a protective effect on ischaemically injured kidneys. The more important question, namely whether it can also protect kidneys during long periods of preservation (> 72 h), has not been studied, and needs an answer.

FUROSEMIDE

Panijayanond *et al.* preserved kidneys from hydrated dogs, with no mannitol pretreatment or warm ischaemia using C4 flush for 48 h[31]. There was a significant mortality after reimplantation and immediate contralateral nephrectomy, and a maximum creatinine in the survivors of 11.2 ± 1.7 mg/dl. 40 mg/l of furosemide added to the flush made no difference. When 1.0 mg/kg furosemide was given to the dogs 10 min prior to nephrectomy as well as added to the flush solution, there was no mortality in 12 animals, and the maximum creatinine was significantly lower, i.e., 4.0 ± 1.1 mg/dl. This last result must be compared with a report of no deaths and a maximum creatinine of 2.5 ± 0.5 mg/dl after 48 h storage using C2 solution (differing only in the absence of phenoxybenzamine and low-dose procaine from C4)[32]. These latter dogs had been pretreated with mannitol and hydrated, but received no furosemide. Therefore, it is entirely possible, indeed likely, that Panijayanond's results were dependent on ideal donor preparation and the harvesting of an actively diuresing kidney, rather than on a specific pharmacological protective effect of furosemide.

Fernando *et al.* evaluated the effects of adding 1.0 g/l of furosemide to a Brunius–Gelin flush solution in dog kidneys which were either immediately reimplanted or preserved for 5 h in the cold[33]. No comment is made as to the state of hydration of the animals, and mannitol was not given prior to nephrectomy. It was found that the renal blood flow and cortical flow (by ^{133}Xe) was maintained at about normal levels when furosemide was added to the flush, but diminished by one-third to one-half in its absence. Once again, one has to wonder about the effect of the quality of donor preparation in these animals.

Vanherweghem *et al.* studied the effects of furosemide on the function of kidneys after a 20–26 h period of cold preservation after flushing with C2[34]. Hydration was not specified and mannitol was not given. Furosemide was administered after preservation into the Nizet (warm) perfusion system, which was used to evaluate renal function. No improvement in RBF, GFR or in PAH transport could be shown by adding furosemide.

In some recent studies, using an *ex vivo* rabbit kidney model, Green *et al.* evaluated the effects of various pharmacological agents on renal function subsequent to 1 h of warm ischaemia (without subsequent preservation)[11]. In this system furosemide did have a modest protective effect when given prior to ischaemia; none when given after it. This protection was significantly inferior to that provided by mannitol.

MAGNESIUM

The vasomotor effects of this agent were analysed by Levowitz *et al.* in intact dog kidneys[35]. 0.4 mmol/min of Mg infused into the renal artery was able to block the vasoconstrictive effects of norepinephrin, angiotensin and pitressin. Unfortunately, it is not known whether this effect is modified by hypothermia. Osias et al.[36] studied the effects of $MgCl_2$ administered intravenously to rats after 30 min of warm renal ischaemia. No beneficial effects could be demonstrated, whereas $MgCl_2$ with ATP improved GFR significantly and maintained a normal BUN. The vascular component of the action of Mg was eliminated by Downes et al.[37], who studied its effects in flush solutions on the function of kidney slices. These studies, carried out in dog kidneys, showed that Mg did not prevent potassium loss when added to C3 flush solution. However, it did markedly diminish or inhibit cellular swelling.

Watkins et al. evaluated the role of Mg in well-hydrated and mannitolized dog kidneys[38]. The organs were removed, flushed and re-implanted after 24 h. The removal of Mg from C5 flush solution had no harmful effects. Jensen and Kemp compared the effectiveness of Collins' solution with and without $MgSO_4$ in rabbit kidneys undergoing 24 h preservation[39]. Mg made no difference in these studies. Green and Pegg[40], also working in rabbits, compared various 'intracellular' renal preservation solutions containing between 1.0 and 36.0 mmol/l of magnesium ion. No specific effects could be attributed to Mg, but anions in their flush solutions differed at the various Mg concentrations, therefore the latter was not the sole variable. Similarly, Mg could not be shown to have a consistent effect in our studies either, even using a constant anion composition in ex vivo, plug-in rabbit kidneys after 24 h of preservation[32]. In contrast, Jablonski et al., using the rat kidney and a 24 h storage period, found that 20.0 mmol/l of Mg in the flush solution was far superior to 1.0 mmol/l[41]. It is important to emphasize, however, that their solution was based on citrate, and in this setting Mg may have a very different role to play than in other solutions.

In summary, there is no clear evidence of a beneficial effect of magnesium in organ preservation.

SPECIFIC TOXICITIES

Procaine has been added to the perfusate of flush solutions for many years for the potential spasmolytic effect it might exert on the renal vasculature. This is a largely empirical move, and the minimum effective dose (if there is indeed one) has not been defined. At the other extreme, it has been shown by Collins et al. that when added to the C2 flush solution in amounts over 0.5 g/l and then used for preserving dog kidneys for 48 h, this amount is clearly associated with inferior function[42].

Problems which may arise from the use of various plastics for tubing, containers, etc. have been studied by Pegg et al.[43]. Polyvinylchloride (PVC) was found to be the source of two rather specific problems: firstly, toxic plasticizers were found to be released by a variety of different brands and batches of PVC; secondly, this plastic has a high affinity for free fatty acids and tends to adsorb them out of the perfusate. In addition, PVC shares a deleterious characteristic with silicone rubber and with polyethylene, namely a high permeability to gases. They all interfere with control of the partial pressures within a recirculating perfusate. None of these three problems was observed to occur with polyamide (nylon).

DISCUSSION AND SUMMARY

It is regrettable that a large proportion of the experimental work dealing with organ preservation is unstandardized, and often incompletely documented. Therefore, results are not comparable, and conclusions often cannot be transferred from one set of experiments to another, even within the same species. One aspect to which this observation applies particularly is the casual preparation of animals prior to the harvesting of organs. A plea is therefore made here:

(1) to assure ample hydration and optimal renal function in donors (preparation to include the administration of mannitol 15 min prior to cross-clamping[11]);
(2) to clearly include the specific details of donor preparation in reports and publications.

In more general terms, it seems to this reviewer that it is erroneous to view organ preservation as an isolated episode. Instead, one should look at the continuum of risks to which a transplanted organ is exposed:

(1) in-host injury (shock, acidosis, nephrotoxic drugs, etc.);
(2) harvesting injury (warm ischaemia);
(3) injury produced by imperfect (inadequate or incomplete) preservation;
(4) specific injury produced by preservation (dys-preservation: mechanical or perfusion endothelial damage, immunological injury by perfusate, etc.);
(5) in-recipient injury (triggered by any of the above factors via continued vasospasm, platelet aggregation on damaged intima, etc.).

It is often difficult to isolate and specify the type of injury involved. However, it is critical to at least attempt to undertake this dissection in order to be able to deal with the causes of failed preservation. Pharmacological intervention can then be rational and specific rather than of the shotgun or polypharmacy type, which so often characterized early attempts in this field.

In regard to category 5 above, it is entirely possible that pharmacological manipulation of the recipient will have a role to play in the future. Since vascular injury is one of the two major components of damage observed in preserved organs, it is reasonable to expect that manipulations of platelet function, endothelial integrity, vascular smooth muscle, etc. may come to be important in allowing a graft to reconstitute itself under the protective umbrella of such short-term pharmacological intervention.

Looking then at the continuum of the care of preserved organs, pharmacological intervention may be indicated at a variety of stages: as pre-treatment of the donor prior to harvesting, as the addition of drugs to perfusates and flushing solutions, and as the treatment of recipients of preserved organs. This chapter has attempted to define our understanding of the indications for and limitations of these interventions.

References

1. Belzer, F.O. and Southard, J.H. (1980). The future of kidney preservation. *Transplantation,* **30,** 161
2. Løkkegaard, H., Bilde, T., Gyrd-Hansen, N., Jaglicic, D., Jensen, E., Nerstrøm, B. and Rasmussen, F. (1973). The effect of chlorpromazine on preservation of kidneys with one hour of warm ischaemia. *Acta. Med. Scand.,* **193,** 65
3. Turner, M.D., Hicks, F.F., Hicks, J.S. and Warren, R.B. (1969). The use of metabolic inhibitors in hypothermic kidney storage. *J. Surg., Res.,* **9,** 665
4. Løkkegaard, H., Bilde, T. and Dahlager, J.I. (1979). Experimental and clinical studies of extended renal preservation by simple hypothermia. In Pegg, D.E. and Jacobsen, I.A. (eds.) *Organ Preservation II,* p. 102. (London: Churchill Livingstone)
5. Pryor, J.P., Keaveny, T.V., Reed, T.W. and Belzer, F.O. (1971). Improved immediate function of experimental cadaver renal allografts by elimination of agonal vasospasm. *Br. J. Surg.,* **58,** 184
6. Dhabuwala, C.B., Bird, M. and Salaman, J.R. (1979). Relative importance of warm ischaemia, hypotension, and hypercarbia in producing renal vasospasm. *Transplantation,* **27,** 238
7. Eliahou, H.E., Solomon, S., Iaina, A., Oshman, R. and Serban, I. (1978). Alleviation of acute anoxic renal failure in rats by β_1-adrenergic blockade with practolol. *Israel J. Med. Sci.,* **14,** 274
8. Solez, K., Freshwater, M.F. and Chi-Tsung, S. (1977). The effect of propranolol on post-ischemic acute renal failure in the rat. *Transplantation,* **24,** 148
9. Stowe, N., Emma, J., Magnusson, M., Loening, S., Yarimizu, S., Ocon, J., Khairallah, P. and Straffon, R. (1978). Protective effect of propranolol in the treatment of ischemically damaged canine kidneys prior to transplantation. *Surgery,* **84,** 265
10. Valido, A., Lopez-Novoa, J.M. and Hernando, L. (1977). Papaverine effect on post-ischemic acute renal failure in rats. *Biomedicine,* **27,** 278
11. Green, R.D., Boyer, D., Halasz, N.A. and Collins, G.M. (1979). Pharmacological protection of rabbit kidneys from normothermic ischemia. *Transplantation,* **28,** 131
12. Miller, H.C., Alexander, J.W., Smith, E.J. and Fidler, J.P. (1974). Salutary effect of phentolamine (Regitine) on renal vasoconstriction in donor kidneys. *Transplantation,* **17,** 201
13. Starling, J.R., Rudolf, L.E., Ferguson, W. and Wangensteen, S.L. (1973). Benefits of methylprednisolone in the isolated perfused organ. *Ann. Surg.,* **177,** 566
14. Tremann, J.A., Haines, J.G., Bleifuss, J.H., Agodoa, L.C.Y. and Marchioro, T.L. (1975). The effect of high dose steroid and cyclophosphamide on perfused canine renal homografts. *Transplantation,* **19,** 520
15. Rashid, H.A., Panner, B.J. and Linke, C.A. (1975). Effect of pharmacological doses of methylprednisolone on preservation of renal function. *J. Surg. Res.,* **18,** 21
16. Dvorak, K.J., Braun, W.E., Magnusson, M.O., Stowe, N.T. and Banowsky, L.H.W. (1976). Effect of high doses of methylprednisolone on the isolated, perfused canine kidney. *Transplantation,* **21,** 149
17. Toledo-Pereyra, L.H., Oh, H.K. and Dienst, S.G. (1978). Optimal dose of methyl-prednisolone during renal hypothermic pulsatile perfusion. *Transplantation,* **25,** 342
18. Miller, H.C. and Alexander, J.W. (1973). Protective effect of methylprednisolone against ischemic injury to the kidney. *Transplantation,* **16,** 57
19. Chatterjee, S.N. and Berne, T.V. (1975). Use of cellular membrane stabilizers to prevent ischemic damage to the kidneys. *Surg. Forum,* **26,** 335

20. Mundy, A. R., Bewick, M., Moncada, S. and Vane, J. R. (1980). Experimental assessment of prostacyclin in the harvesting of kidneys for transplantation. *Transplantation*, **30**, 251
21. Casey, K. F., Machiedo, G. W., Lyons, M. J., Slotman, G. J. and Novak, R. T. (1980). Alteration of postischemic renal pathology by prostaglandin infusion. *J. Surg. Res.*, **29**, 1
22. Vasko, K. A., DeWall, R. A. and Riley, A. M. (1972). Effect of allopurinol in renal ischemia. *Surgery*, **71**, 787
23. Toledo-Pereyra, L. H. and Najarian, J. S. (1973). Total recovery of ischemic kidneys treated with allopurinol before transplantation. *Surg. Forum*, **24**, 302
24. Toledo-Pereyra, L. H., Simmons, R. L. and Najarian, J. S. (1974). Effect of allopurinol on the preservation of ischemic kidneys perfused with plasma or plasma substitutes. *Ann. Surg.*, **180**, 780
25. Owens, M. L., Lazarus, H. M., Wolcott, M. W., Maxwell, J. G. and Taylor, J. B. (1974). Allopurinol and hypoxanthine pretreatment of canine kidney donors. *Transplantation*, **17**, 424
26. Murdock, M. I. and Cho, S. I. (1975). The lack of beneficial effect of allopurinol on renal preservation. *Transplantation*, **19**, 353
27. Fernando, A. R., Griffiths, J. R., O'Donoghue, E. P. N., Ward, J. P., Armstrong, D. M. G., Hendry, W. F., Perrett, D. and Wickham, J. E. A. (1976). Enhanced preservation of the ischemic kidney with inosine. *Lancet*, **1**, 555
28. Chatterjee, S. N. and Berne, T. V. (1975). Use of cellular membrane stabilizers to prevent ischemic damage to the kidneys. *Surg. Forum*, **26**, 335
29. Chatterjee, S. N. and Berne, T. V. (1976). Protective effect of allopurinol in renal ischemia. *Am. J. Surg.*, **131**, 658
30. Toledo-Pereyra, L. H., Simmons, R. L., Olson, L. C. and Najarian, J. S. (1977). Clinical effect of allopurinol on preserved kidneys. *Ann. Surg.*, **185**, 128
31. Panijayanond, P., Cho, S. I., Ulrich, F. and Nabseth, D. C. (1973). Enhancement of renal preservation by furosemide. *Surgery*, **73**, 368
32. Collins, G. M., Green, R. C. and Halasz, N. A. (1979). Importance of anion content and osmolarity in flush solutions for 48 and 72 hr hypothermic kidney storage. *Cryobiology*, **16**, 217
33. Fernando, O. N., Newman, S. P., Hird, V. M., Sampson, D. G., Read, P. R., Moorhead, J. F., Williams, H. S. and Hopewell, J. P. (1974). Enhancement of renal blood flow in transplanted dog kidneys following perfusion with frusemide. *Scot. Med. J.*, **19**, 50
34. Vanherweghem, J. L., Vereerstraeten, P. and Toussaint, C. (1974). In vitro performances of stored canine kidneys: effects of furosemide. *Nephron*, **12**, 140
35. Levowitz, B. S., Goldson, H., Rashkin, A., Kay, H., Valcin, A., Mathur, A. and LaGuerre, J. N. (1970). Magnesium ion blockade of regional vasoconstriction. *Ann. Surg.*, **172**, 33
36. Osias, M. B., Siegel, N. J., Chaudry, I. H., Lytton, B. and Baue, A. E. (1977). Post-ischemic renal failure. *Arch. Surg.*, **112**, 729
37. Downes, G., Hoffman, R., Huang, J. and Belzer, F. O. (1973). Mechanism of action of washout solutions for kidney preservation. *Transplantation*, **16**, 46
38. Watkins, G. M., Prentiss, N. A. and Couch, N. P. (1971). Successful 24-hour kidney preservation with simplified hyperosmolar hyperkalemic perfusate. *Transplant. Proc.*, **3**, 612
39. Jensen, E. H. and Kemp, E. (1972). Kidney preservation. III. The importance of the composition of perfusion fluids in the transplantation of rabbit kidneys. *Scand. J. Urol. Nephrol.*, **6**, 284
40. Green, C. J. and Pegg, D. E. (1979). Mechanism of action of 'intracellular' renal preservation solutions. *World J. Surg.*, **3**, 115
41. Jablonski, P., Howden, B., Marshall, V. and Scott, D. (1980). Evaluation of citrate flushing solution using the isolated perfused rat kidney. *Transplantation*, **30**, 239
42. Collins, G. M. and Halasz, N. A. (1975). Composition of intracellular flush solutions for hypothermic kidney storage. *Lancet*, **1**, 220
43. Pegg, D. E., Fuller, B. J., Foreman, J. and Green, C. J. (1972). The choice of plastic tubing for organ perfusion experiments. *Cryobiology*, **9**, 569

21
Effect of chlorpromazine on the contractile function and metabolic status of continuously perfused and ischaemic hearts

G. E. THOMAS, S. LEVITSKY and H. FEINBERG

Cardiac surgical procedures that require a period of ischaemia, e.g. coronary bypass, entail a significant risk of myocardial damage. Reperfusion of ischaemic myocardium may aggravate ischaemic damage by inducing a further drop in ATP, a rise in diastolic pressure and a loss of compliance. In part, the compliance loss has been attributed to Ca^{2+} accumulation during reperfusion, particularly into mitochondria[1]. Recently pretreatment (30 min before sacrifice) of rats with chlorpromazine (CPZ) (30 mg/kg, i.p.) was shown to reverse the loss of liver mitochondrial function seen after 3 h of ischaemia[2]. In particular the 4-fold increase in mitochondrial Ca^{2+}, seen after reperfusion in the untreated animals, did not occur in the CPZ-treated rats.

We treated rabbits with CPZ in the same manner as Mittnacht *et al.*, 1979[2] treated rats (30 mg/kg i.p., 30 min before sacrifice) and studied its effect on ameliorating ischaemia-induced changes in contractility of perfused hearts. A fluid-filled balloon was placed in the left ventricle and the hearts were perfused via a cannula placed in the aorta with Krebs–Ringers (Ca^{2+}, 1.25 mmol/l; glucose, 11 mmol/l) at 37 °C, at constant perfusion pressure (80 mmHg) and heart rate (95 beats/min). Ventricular isovolumic pressure, dP/dt and coronary flow were measured. Untreated (UT) and CPZ-treated hearts were perfused for 30 and 150 min and were then frozen in liquid N_2 (using a Wollenberger clamp) for later ATP and CP analysis[3]. Another group of UT and CPZ-treated animals were perfused for 30 min, made totally ischaemic (at 27 °C) for 90 min, and then reperfused for 30 min.

CPZ treatment had little effect on contractile parameters (peak isovolumic pressure, diastolic pressure at constant volume, dP/dt) during 30–150 min of continuous perfusion. ATP and CP levels were decreased during continuous perfusion but were not significantly different as between

161

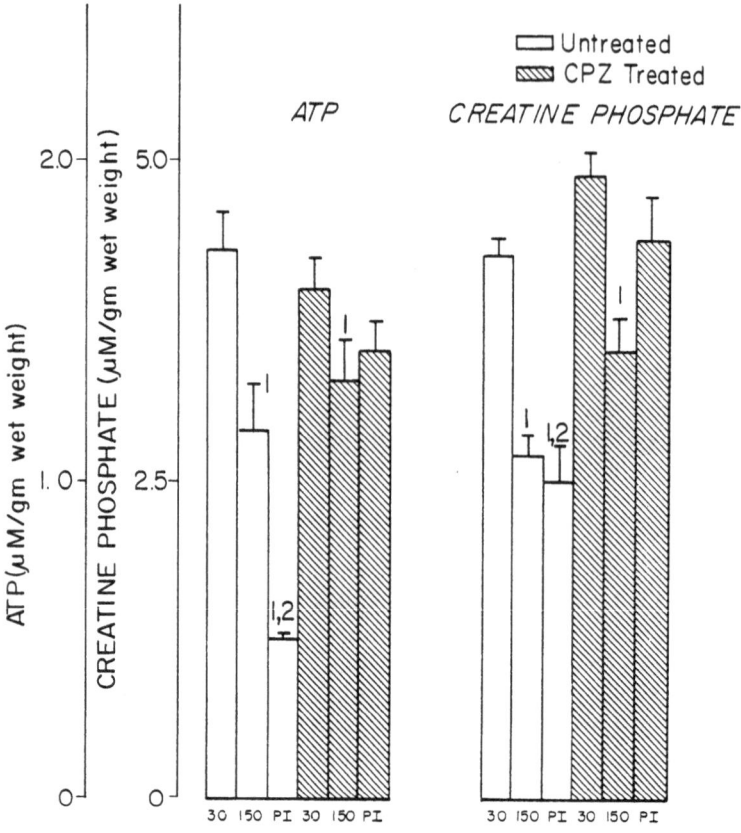

Figure 21.1 ATP and creatine phosphate concentrations of untreated and chlorpromazine-treated hearts at 30 and 150 min of continuous perfusion and at post-ischaemia (PI)

the UT and CPZ-treated hearts (Figure 21.1). Ischaemia for 90 min followed by reperfusion resulted in a significant loss of dP/dt, developed pressure (peak isovolumic minus diastolic pressure) and coronary flow in the untreated group (Figure 21.2). On the other hand the CPZ-treated group exhibited pre-ischaemic levels of dP/dt and developed pressure. Compliance was measured (end-diastolic pressure (EDP) at three different balloon volumes) and it was found that EDP was greater at all balloon volumes in the UT group while the CPZ-treated hearts exhibited an increase in compliance (Figure 21.3). ATP and CP did not decrease in the post-ischaemic period in the CPZ-treated group while a profound fall was seen in the UT group (Figure 21.1). At present we have no explanation for the compliance increase in the CPZ-treatment group.

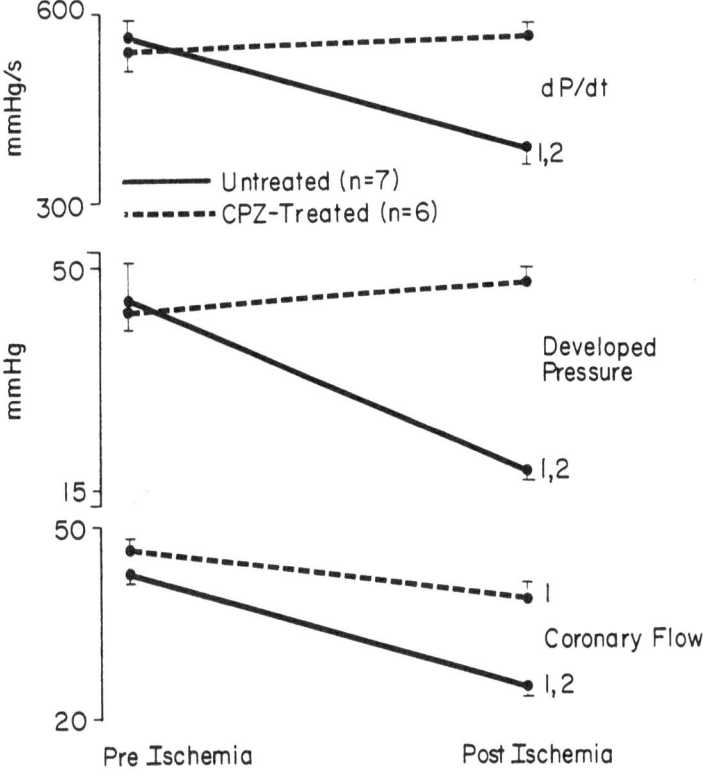

PRETREATMENT WITH CHLORPROMAZINE

———— Untreated (n=7)
·------- CPZ-Treated (n=6)

dP/dt

Developed
Pressure

Coronary Flow

Pre Ischemia   Post Ischemia

*MEAN ± STANDARD ERROR OF MEAN
1-SIGNIFICANT DIFFERENCE WITHIN GROUP (p<0.05)
2-SIGNIFICANT DIFFERENCE BETWEEN UNTREATED AND
   CPZ-TREATED HEARTS (p<0.05)

Figure 21.2 Contractile function and coronary flow of untreated and CPZ-treated hearts during pre- and post-ischaemia

We conclude that CPZ treatment confers significant protection against ischaemia-induced loss of cardiac contractility, compliance and high-energy phosphates.

References

1. Shen, A.C. and Jennings, R.B. (1972). Kinetics of calcium accumulation in acute myocardial ischemic injury. *Am. J. Pathol.,* **67,** 441
2. Mittnacht, S. Jr, Sherman, S.C. and Farber, J.C. (1979). Reversal of ischemic mitochondrial dysfunction. *J. Biol. Chem.,* **254,** 9871
3. Holland, C.E., Feinberg, H., Levitsky, S., Buinevicius, Z. and Wright, R.N. (1978). Serial myocardial biopsies using an improved microfluorometric assay. *J. Surg. Res.,* **25,** 342

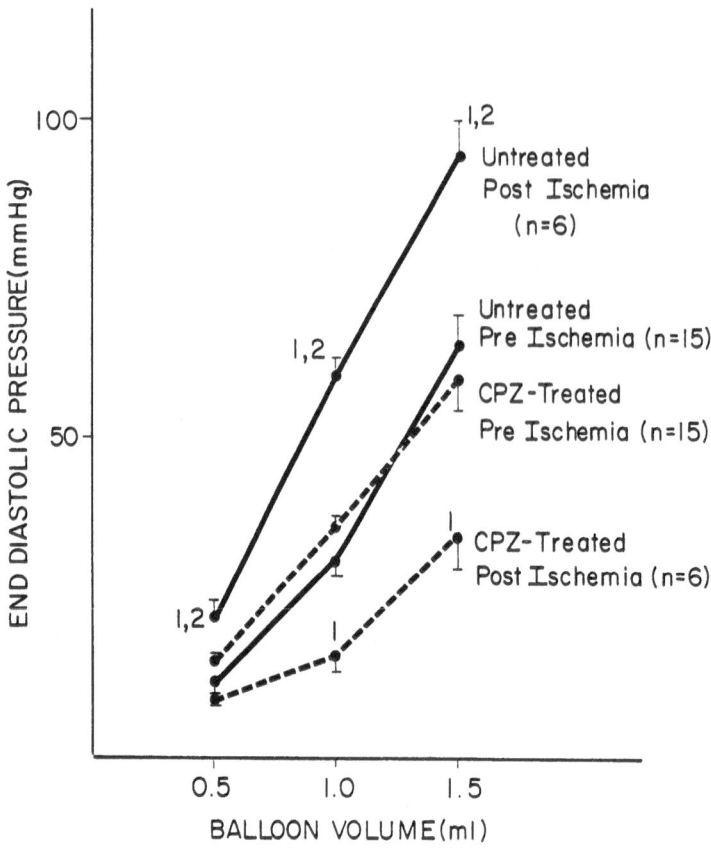

Figure 21.3 The effect of ischaemia and chlorpromazine treatment on ventricular compliance

PART IV
PRESERVATION BY INITIAL PERFUSION AND HYPOTHERMIA

22
Flush preservation

G. M. COLLINS

Tolerance of the kidney to normothermic ischaemia would appear to be in the range of 1–2 h[1,2]. In general, it has been found that the protection afforded by simple cooling is related to the reduction in temperature[3], the maximum preservation time by ice immersion being in the range of 12–24 h[4,5]. This period, however, falls short of that theoretically attainable considering the degree of metabolic suppression produced by cooling to 0 °C[6,7]. This relative failure of ice immersion to reach its full theoretical potential may be explained by two considerations. First, surface cooling is an inefficient method for reducing the core temperature of a large organ[8]. The detrimental effects of even a short period of normothermic ischaemia on kidneys subsequently preserved by simple hypothermia is well recognized[9,10]. Secondly, cooling itself has an adverse effect on cell physiology which can be minimized by the use of appropriate flush solutions.

Historically, the development of modern flush solutions began with the observation reported by Keeler and his colleagues in 1966[11]. They perfused rat kidneys with 0.9% sodium chloride at 0 °C and found a 50% loss of tissue potassium within 30 min and a 16% loss of magnesium over 3 h. There was a concurrent 73% gain in water and 172% gain in sodium. Postulating that kidney damage might result from these ionic exchanges, they perfused dog kidneys with solutions containing elevated concentrations of potassium and magnesium. Subsequently Martin and colleagues confirmed Keeler's findings[12] while investigating continuous low-flow perfusion as a method for kidney preservation[13]. Eight hours of perfusion with an extracellular solution led uniformly to non-viable kidneys whereas similar perfusion with a simulated intracellular solution was highly successful.

Prompted by these reports, we undertook experiments which showed that an intracellular type solution (solution C4) was capable of preserving canine kidneys for up to 30 h[5]. Numerous studies subsequently confirmed the value of hyperosmolar, hyperkalaemic, hypermagnesaemic flush solutions for the storage of rabbit, pig, dog, and human kidneys for periods of up to 72 h[14-24]. Many cadaveric kidneys have been successfully re-implanted after storage times in the range of 1–2 days[14,25-27], and in one case after 61 h (Barry, J., personal communication).

Although the efficacy of this method is well established, the optimal composition and precise mode of action of flush solutions remain controversial. In the first place, the value of the pharmacological additives in C4, namely heparin, procaine and phenoxybenzamine, is now rather questionable[19]. Heparin is presumably unnecessary in the presence of high concentrations of phosphate which chelates calcium ions, and phenoxy-benzamine tends to form a precipitate in the solutions and thus lose activity. The procaine content of C3-4, originally 0.1 g/100 ml, was later empirically increased 10-fold[28] with the intention of counteracting the potential effects of agonal vasospasm[29] in cadaver donors. However, we subsequently demonstrated in an experimental study that procaine in that concentration was detrimental[30], perhaps because of conversion to para-aminobenzoic acid[19].

The major hypotheses under consideration to explain the mode of action of intracellular flush solutions include: (1) conservation of cell energy substrates, (2) control of cell swelling as a result of the content of poorly permeant anions and non-electrolytes, and (3) avoidance of any adverse effects produced by changes in intracellular ion content.

CONSERVATION OF CELL ENERGY

It has long been recognized that the maintenance of normal cell volume is an energy-requiring process dependent on cellular respiration[31,32] to support active membrane transport mechanisms, principally extrusion of sodium ions[33,34]. Thus lowering the extracellular sodium content to 10 mmol/l (the concentration present in the C2 solution) can be expected to reduce the level of kidney cortical slice respiration by one-third[35]. Certainly cooling alone markedly reduces energy requirements[36] but significant levels of active transport persist even at 0 °C[37,38]. Thus the prospect of additional energy conservation by manipulation of perfusate composition is theoretically tenable. In this connection Shumakow et al.[24] reported that the amount of lactic acid in the washout solution after 24 h kidney storage was three times as high for a kidney preserved in saline as for one preserved with an intracellular type solution.

Because of its key role in cellular energy exchange, derangement of adenine nucleotide (AN) metabolism might be expected to have an important bearing on the outcome of organ ischaemia and preservation. Indeed, there would appear to be a reasonably good correlation between viability and breakdown of adenine nucleotide[1,7,39,40]. Furthermore, there have been a number of reports describing enhanced viability as a result of the administration of agents designed to improve AN regeneration[41-47]. Following flush cooling and cold storage, it has been reported that higher AN levels reflect a better quality of preservation using an intracellular solution than with Ringer's lactate or saline[1,40,48]. The inference is that intracellular solutions do indeed conserve intracellular energy substrates.

Despite these promising experimental data, the significance of the correlation between AN levels and organ viability has been seriously questioned. Farber reported that cellular ATP levels could be selectively reduced to one-quarter or one-third of normal by the administration of ethionine or fructose without producing irreversible changes[49] and we have demonstrated that ischaemically injured kidneys perfused *in vitro* with 5 mmol/l adenosine could regenerate AN as well as fresh ones[50]. In other studies we have found no correlation between the protection from ischaemia afforded by mannitol administration and AN levels[51]. Prior administration of inosine and allopurinol did not improve function. Even when inosine administration has been found to provide some protection from ischaemia, this effect appeared not to depend on enhanced AN levels[52]. In the setting of hypothermic organ storage the correlation between function and conservation of AN is likewise imperfect. Although AN levels are generally higher during continuous perfusion preservation than with flush cooling, they tend to remain stable over a period of days whereas organ function after reimplantation falls progressively with time[1]. With flush cooling the energy-conserving effect cannot be ascribed solely to hyperkalaemic depression of transmembrane ion transport since hyperosmolar sodium-based solutions seem to be capable of conserving tissue AN levels to a similar extent[1]. Others have also reported poor correlation between quality of preservation with flush solutions and AN conservation[53].

It appears reasonable to conclude that conservation of cellular energy substrate and preservation of AN metabolism are not major factors in the protection from organ ischaemia afforded by pharmacological agents, continuous perfusion or flush solutions.

PREVENTION OF CELL SWELLING

Under normal conditions the stability of cell volume is maintained by the active extrusion of sodium ions which establishes a Donnan equilibrium balancing that of the intracellular protein anions[54]. When the sodium pump is inhibited by hypoxia, cold, or metabolic inhibitors, sodium ions enter the cell and other ions diffuse down their electrochemical gradients so that the protein Donnan effect becomes dominant, resulting in swelling of the cell and intracellular organelles[31,32,54,55]. The extent of these effects in response to cold stress depends on the sensitivity of the sodium pump to hypothermic depression. This varies both with the particular organ studied, the kidney appearing to be more resistant than either the liver or the heart[36], and within animal species. Among the latter, the sodium pump of hibernating animals tends to be especially cold-resistant[56]. The marked temperature sensitivity of the membrane adenosine triphosphatase of vascular endothelium[57] is of particular significance for whole organ preservation since swelling of these cells would tend to amplify and prolong the parenchymal cell ischaemia into the recovery phase by interfering with the restoration of blood flow to the organ. Much importance has been attached to this possibility and it has been called the 'no-reflow' phenomenon[55,58]. The well-recognized increase in renal vascular resistance following ischaemia is an example of this effect[50,59].

The importance of these concepts for organ preservation with flush solutions has been emphasized by several workers[50,60-63]. Acquatella *et al.*[61] conducted canine kidney preservation experiments in order to determine what flush solution composition would best maintain the normal tissue electrolyte content and cell morphology during storage at 4 °C for up to 48 h. With Ringer's lactate there was an immediate 50% increase in cell water reaching 100% by 48 h. Histological examination revealed a corresponding increase in cell size, with evidence of ruptured cells. Sodium and chloride content increased three-fold and potassium level decreased to a similar extent during 48 h storage. The addition of 200 millimolar glucose to the Ringer's lactate, rendering it hypertonic, almost completely prevented the gain in tissue water, somewhat reduced that of sodium and chloride but had no effect on the loss of potassium ions from the cells. With a hyperosmolar glucose–potassium chloride solution, intracellular sodium and potassium levels remained close to normal but cell swelling still occurred due to an influx of freely diffusible chloride ions. This could be prevented by substituting the poorly permeant sulphate for chloride ions in the hyperkalaemic solution. The preservation of cell morphology and electrolyte content with this last flush solution provides a direct demonstration of the beneficial effects on cell physiology of the major components of an intracellular type flush solution, namely, preservation of cell volume, morphology and electrolyte content within normal limits during hypothermic storage.

The influence of flush solution osmolarity on organ function was studied by Downes[62] and Pegg[63]. Both groups of workers showed that an extracellular type of flush solution could be used for organ storage provided that it contained a poorly permeant non-electrolyte for the prevention of cell swelling. Sucrose appeared to be superior to glucose for this purpose. Southard and Belzer have argued against the use of hyperosmolar solutions on the grounds that the initial shrinkage produced may disrupt renal architecture and the non-electrolytes may slowly enter the cells during the storage period[64,65]. Instead, they recommend reliance on impermeant anions to prevent cell swelling in an isosmotic solution. These data are basically in agreement with our own findings of satisfactory 48 h renal preservation using a solution containing sodium as the principal cation together with a poorly permeant anion and non-electrolyte[28,30]. Clearly control of cell swelling is a major factor in the action of flush solutions for hypothermic kidney storage. Whether the important focus for this action is the vascular endothelium, the parenchymal cells or both cannot yet be determined.

MAINTENANCE OF INTRACELLULAR IONIC COMPOSITION

The importance of attempting to maintain intracellular ionic composition during hypothermic storage is not universally accepted[62,63]. It has been argued that ionic exchange in the cold ought to be readily reversed when normothermic conditions are restored[66] and that the benefit of flush solution results entirely from the presence of impermeant solutes[67]. Specifically, the question raised is whether there is any advantage to utilizing increased concentrations of intracellular cations in these solutions.

Flushing with hyperkalaemic solutions lacking impermeant solutes has been shown to cause cell swelling and to be harmful[68,69]. Although this effect may be readily understood in terms of unrestricted entry of potassium chloride into the cell, it is more difficult to explain the findings of Pegg and Gallant[70] and Green and Pegg[67]. These workers compared two hyperosmolar solutions, WF2 and WF4, and found that although cell swelling was controlled better by the latter solution, which contained approximately 70 mmol/l each of potassium and sodium chloride, renal function was better with the former which contained only 4 mmol potassium and 140 mmol of sodium chloride per litre. It should be noted, however, that the lowest serum creatinine levels after 24 and 48 h preservation were reported for the group flushed with the C4 solution. Furthermore, the majority of flush solutions which have been found to work well experimentally and clinically have been characterized by elevated concentrations of intracellular cations. It is presumed that there may be some biochemical advantage to the prevention of exchange of extracellular sodium for intracellular potassium[71].

We have reported experiments designed to analyse the specific effects of individual cations and anions by formulating a series of flush solutions in which the electrolyte content was systematically varied but the osmolarity was kept constant at 320 mosmol/l by the addition of mannitol and glucose[2,30]. In these studies, elevated concentrations of both potassium and magnesium conferred a significant advantage whereas the species of impermeant anion – whether phosphate, citrate, or sulphate – did not seem to matter.

Two components of flush solutions which are most controversial at the present time are magnesium and citrate. Some have reported the inclusion of magnesium in flush solutions to be of benefit[53,72] whereas others have found it to be of no value[19,21,67,73,74] apart from an osmotic effect[62]. The theoretical advantages of inclusion of magnesium include its actions as a metabolic inhibitor[74], vasodilator[75], preserver of intracellular potassium[67] and its ability to inhibit the rigidizing effect of calcium binding to the membrane of ATP-depleted red cells[63]. On the other hand it has the potential disadvantages of forming insoluble precipitates within the kidney[15,76,77]. The use of citrate as a major anion in a flush solution was first proposed by Ross and others[22] as a result of an experiment in which the citrate solution was found to yield better 72 h kidney preservation than either C2 or Sacks' solutions. In our study, however, the results were essentially similar whether sulphate, phosphate, or citrate served as the principal anion. It was originally claimed that the citrate anion had some special metabolic properties to account for the efficacy of the Ross solution[78]. However, substitution of a non-metabolizable analogue, tricarballylate, gave equal results provided that the reduced buffering power of this agent was compensated by the addition of 10 millimolar HEPES to the solution[53]. This finding indirectly supports a preference which we have had for the use of phosphate, since within the physiological pH range the citrate anion is inferior in its buffering capacity.

EMPIRICAL FINDINGS

Several new formulations of intracellular-type flush solutions have been described which differ from C2 principally in having a higher osmolarity and in the type of impermeant anion or non-electrolyte used. The hyperosmolar solution described by Acquatella et al.[61] was later tested by Schloerb et al.[79] for 48 h canine kidney preservation with indifferent results, only 25% of kidneys providing life-sustaining function. Sacks et al.[18] substantially increased the osmolarity of the C2 solution to 432 mosmol/l using mannitol and reported successful 72 h canine preservation for the first time with this method. However, both we and others have subsequently been able to achieve this period of preservation with the C2 solution which has an osmolarity of only 320 mosmol/l. It is possible that a very high osmolarity is beneficial only for kidneys subjected to a period of warm ischaemia prior to preservation[10,80]. On the other hand, it appears that markedly hypertonic solutions may be detrimental in fresh kidney storage[53,72]. In fact, when compared directly with C2, Sacks' solution proved to be inferior as judged by whole organ function[30,81]. The hypertonic citrate solution has been mentioned above. Although Ross[22] found this solution to be superior to both C2 and Sacks' solutions, others have disagreed with these findings[30,82].

Another hypertonic, hyperkalaemic solution has been described by Vij et al.[82] which appeared to be about equal to Collins' and Sacks' solutions for storage of fresh and ischaemically injured kidneys. This solution is unique in containing 7% albumin and in having a very high osmolarity (465 mosmol/l). No doubt the latter is required to compensate for the use of highly permeant chloride as the principal anion.

The latest addition to this list of intracellular flush solutions is one described by Fahy et al.[83] called RPS-2. This differs from the other solutions in being isotonic (290 mosmol/kg) and in containing only a moderately elevated potassium concentration (42 mmol/l). This solution was reported to be superior to C2 for maintaining rabbit tissue slice Na/K ratios during hypothermic storage. Recent work in our laboratory has confirmed Fahy's observations when comparing the efficacy of RPS-2 and C2 solution for 24 h rabbit kidney preservation.

CLINICAL APPLICATION OF FLUSH SOLUTIONS

There is still some controversy concerning the relative merits of flush cooling and hypothermic perfusion for clinical use. Logistic considerations clearly favour ice storage. Nevertheless, there remains a degree of scepticism, particularly in the USA, regarding the efficacy of this method and many transplant centres are reluctant to accept kidneys stored by the cold flush technique for more than a few hours[84]. Experience with human kidney preservation indicates that when kidneys have been removed without warm ischaemia ice storage can be used successfully for periods of up to 30h or even more[24-26,85]. In fact Barry et al.[14] in the USA using C2 with magnesium, and Squifflet et al.[27] in Europe using Euro-Collins' (no magnesium) have both reported a substantial number of kidneys preserved for 40-50h with excellent initial and long-term function. Clinical comparisons between perfused and flush-cooled kidneys have usually failed to demonstrate any advantage for the former[26,86-90].

Sensitivity of flush-preserved kidneys to preceding warm ischaemia is an issue frequently raised when comparing ice storage and perfusion preservation[9,10,91,92], although not all experimental data support this concept[93,94]. Clinical experience indicates that a period of warm ischaemia has an adverse effect on early renal function by either method[26] and that long-term function does not appear to suffer when flush-cooled kidneys are compared with those preserved by perfusion[26,95].

Acknowledgement

This work was supported by the Veterans Administration Medical Research Service and the PHSAM 20193 and 26324.

References

1. Collins, G. M., Taft, P. M., Green, R. D. et al. (1977). Adenine nucleotide levels in preserved and ischemically injured canine kidneys. World J. Surg., 1, 237
2. Madden, J. L. (1968). Renal artery and supra renal aortic occlusion. An experimental study. Arch. Surg., 97, 853
3. Stueber, P. J., Kovacs, S., Koletsky, S. et al. (1958). Regional renal hypothermia. Surgery, 44, 77
4. Fisher, E. R., Copeland, C. and Fisher, B. (1967). Correlation of ultrastructure and function following hypothermic preservation of canine kidneys. Lab. Invest., 17, 99
5. Collins, G. M., Bravo-Shugarman, M. B. and Terasaki, P. I. (1969). Kidney preservation for transportation. 3. Initial perfusion and 30-hour ice storage. Lancet, 2, 1219
6. Schirmer, H. K. A. and Walton, K. N. (1964). The effect of hypothermia upon respiration and anaerobic glycolysis of dog kidneys. Invest. Urol., 1, 604
7. Buhl, M. R. and Jørgensen, S. (1975). Breakdown of 5' adenine nucleotides in ischemic renal cortex estimated by oxypurine excretion during perfusion. Scand. J. Clin. Lab. Invest., 35, 211
8. Kerr, W. K., Kyle, V. N., Keresteci, A. G. et al. (1960). Renal hypothermia. J. Urol., 81, 236
9. Hartley, L. C., Collins, G. M. and Clunie, G. J. (1971). Kidney preservation for transportation. 7. Function of 29 human cadaver kidneys preserved with an intracellular perfusate. N. Engl. J. Med., 285, 1049
10. Halasz, N. A. and Collins, G. M. (1976). Forty-eight hour kidney preservation. A comparison of flushing and ice storage with perfusion. Arch. Surg., 111, 175
11. Keeler, R., Swinney, J., Taylor, R. M. R. et al. (1966). The problem of renal preservation. Br. J. Urol., 38, 653

12. Martin, D. C., Smith, G. and Fareed, D. O. (1970). Experimental renal preservation. *J. Urol.*, **103**, 681

13. Hermann, T. J. and Turcotte, J. G. (1969). Preservation of canine kidneys by hypothermia and low flow perfusion with a bloodless perfusate. *Arch. Surg.*, **98**, 121

14. Barry, J. M., Farnsworth, M. A. and Bennett, W. M. (1978). Human kidney preservation by flushing with intracellular solution and cold storage. *Arch. Surg.*, **113**, 830

15. Liu, W. P., Humphreys, A. L., Russell, R. *et al.* (1971). 48-hour storage of canine kidneys after brief perfusion with Collins' solution. *Ann. Surg.*, **173**, 748

16. Løkkegaard, H. and Nerstrøm, B. (1973). Clinical experiences with preservation of necrokidneys. The effect of pretreatment with chlorpromazine and the use of a perfusate which mimics the intracellular ion composition. *Acta Med. Scand.*, **194**, 5

17. Diethelm, A. G., Sterling, W. A., Balch, C. M. *et al.* (1976). Preservation of cadaver kidneys using hypothermic/hyperosomolar/intracellular washout solution. *Transplantation*, **21**, 417

18. Sacks, S. A., Petritsch, P. H. and Kaufman, J. J. (1973). Canine kidney preservation using a new perfusate. *Lancet*, **1**, 1024

19. Watkins, G. M., Prentiss, N. A. and Couch, N. P. (1971). Successful 24-hour kidney preservation with simplified hyperosmolar hyperkalemic perfusate. *Transplant. Proc.*, **3**, 612

20. Kreis, H., Lacombe, M., Ciancioni, C. *et al.* (1972). 48-hour kidney preservation (initial perfusion with potassium and magnesium-rich solution). *Rev. Eur. Etudes Clin. Biol.*, **17**, 192

21. Jensen, E. H. and Kemp, E. (1972). Kidney preservation. 3. The importance of the composition of perfusion fluids in the transplantation of rabbit kidneys. *Scand. J. Urol. Nephrol.*, **6**, 284

22. Ross, H., Marshall, V. C. and Escott, M. L. (1976). 72-hour canine kidney preservation without continuous perfusion. *Transplantation*, **21**, 498

23. Dahlager, J. I. and Bilde, T. (1976). The integrity of tubular cell function after preservation in Collins' or Sacks' solution. *Transplantation*, **21**, 365

24. Shumakov, V. I., Onishchenko, N. A. and Stengold, E. S. (1974). Clinical experience of kidney storage by a non-perfusion technique for periods up to 59 hours. *Trans. Am. Soc. Artif. Int. Organs*, **20**, 545

25. Kreis, H., Noel, L. H., Moreau, J. F. *et al.* (1977). Biologic, pathologic, and radiologic studies of cadaver kidneys preserved in Collins' solution. *Transplant. Proc.*, **9**, 1611

26. Opelz, G. and Terasaki, P. I. (1976). Kidney preservation: perfusion versus cold storage – 1975. *Transplant. Proc.*, **8**, 121

27. Squifflet, J. P., Pirson, Y., Gianello, P. *et al.* (1982). Safe preservation of human renal cadaver transplants by Euro-Collins' solution up to 50 hours. *Transplant. Proc.* (In press)

28. Collins, G. M., Hartley, L. C. and Clunie, G. J. (1972). Kidney preservation for transportation. 8. Experimental analysis of optimal perfusate composition. *Br. J. Surg.*, **59**, 187

29. Pryor, J. P., Keaveny, V., Reed, T. *et al.* (1971). Improved immediate function of experimental cadaver renal allografts by elimination of agonal vasospasm. *Br. J. Surg.*, **58**, 184

30. Collins, G. M. and Halasz, N. A. (1976). Forty-eight hour ice storage of kidneys: importance of cation content. *Surgery*, **79**, 432

31. Leaf, A. (1959). Maintenance of concentration gradients and regulation of cell volume. *Ann. NY Acad. Sci.*, **72**, 396

32. Mudge, G. H. (1951). Electrolyte and water metabolism of rabbit kidney slices: effect of metabolic inhibitors. *Am. J. Physiol.*, **167**, 206

33. Whittam, R. and Willis, J. S. (1963). Ion movements and oxygen consumption in kidney cortex slices. *J. Physiol.*, **168**, 158

34. Blond, D. M. and Whittam, R. (1964). The regulation of kidney respiration by sodium and potassium ions. *Biochem. J.*, **92**, 158

35. Reichmann, K., Hardie, I. R., Clunie, G. J. *et al.* (1972). In vitro analysis of the cation content of solutions for kidney storage. *Cryobiology*, **9**, 296

36. Martin, D. R., Scott, D. F., Downes, G. L. *et al.* (1972). Primary cause of unsuccessful liver and heart preservation. Cold sensitivity of the ATPase system. *Ann. Surg.*, **175**, 111

37. Lambotte, L. (1973). Persistence of active and passive ionic transport during low temperature liver preservation. *Surgery*, **73**, 8
38. Burg, M. B. and Orloff, J. (1964). Active cation transport by kidney tubules at 0 °C. *Am. J. Physiol.*, **207**, 983
39. Gerlach, E., Deuticke, B., Dreisback, R. H. *et al.* (1963). Zum verhalten von nucleotiden und ihren dephosporylierten abbauprodukten in der niere bei ischamie und kurzzeitiger post-ischamisher wiederdurchbluntung. *Pflugers Arch.*, **278**, 296
40. Collste, H. (1972). Preservation of kidneys for transplantation. *Acta. Chir. Scand.*, **425**, (suppl.), 31
41. Calman, K. C. (1974). The prediction of organ viability. 2. Testing an hypothesis. *Cryobiology*, **11**, 7
42. Cunningham, S. K., Keaveny, T. V. and Fitzgerald, P. (1974). Effect of allopurinol on tissue ATP, ADP, and AMP concentrations in renal ischemia. *Br. J. Surg.*, **61**, 562
43. Valeri, C. R. and Zaroulis, C. G. (1972). Rejuvenation and freezing of outdated stored human red cells. *N. Engl. J. Med.*, **287**, 1307
44. Crowell, J. W., Jones, C. E. and Smith, E. E. (1969). Effect of allopurinol on hemorrhagic shock. *Am. J. Physiol.*, **216**, 744
45. Fernando, A. R., Griffiths, J. R., O'Donoghue, E. P. N. *et al.* (1976). Enhanced preservation of the ischemic kidney with inosine. *Lancet*, **1**, 555
46. Buhl, M. R., Kemp, E. and Kemp, G. (1977). Inosine in preservation of rabbit kidneys for transplantation. *Transplant. Proc.*, **9**, 1603
47. Osias, M. B., Siegel, N. J., Chaudry, I. H. *et al.* (1977). Postischemic renal failure. Accelerated recovery with adenosine triphosphate–magnesium chloride infusion. *Arch. Surg.*, **112**, 729
48. Warnick, C. T. and Lazarus, H. M. (1979). The maintenance of adenine nucleotide levels during kidney storage in intracellular solutions. *Proc. Soc. Exp. Biol. Med.*, **160**, 453
49. Farber, E. (1973). ATP and cell integrity. *Fed. Proc.*, **32**, 1534
50. Collins, G. M., Green, R. D. and Halasz, N. A. (1979). In vitro regeneration of adenine nucelotide by ischemically injured kidney. *World J. Surg.*, **3**, 367
51. Collins, G. M., Green, R. D., Carter, J. N. and Halasz, N. A. (1981). Adenine nucleotide levels and recovery of function after renal ischemic injury. *Transplantation*, **31**, 295
52. Buhl, M. R., Kemp, E. and Kemp, G. (1977). Inosine in preservation of rabbit kidneys for transplantation. *Transplant. Proc.*, **9**, 1603
53. Jablonski, P., Howden, B., Marshall, V. and Scott, D. (1980). Evaluation of citrate flushing solution using the isolated perfused rat kidney. *Transplantation*, **30**, 239
54. Jamison, R. L. (1974). The role of cellular swelling in the pathogenesis of organ ischemia. *West J. Med.*, **120**, 205
55. Flores, J., Dibona, D. R., Beck, C. H. *et al.* (1972). The role of cell swelling in ischemic renal damage and the protective effect of hypertonic solute. *J. Clin. Invest.*, **51**, 118
56. Willis, J. S. (1966). Characteristics of ion transport in kidney cortex of mammalian hibernators. *J. Gen. Physiol.*, **49**, 1221
57. Belzer, F. O., Hoffman, R., Huang, J. *et al.* (1972). Endothelial damage in perfused dog kidney and cold sensitivity of vascular Na-K-ATPase. *Cryobiology*, **9**, 457
58. Glauman, B. and Trump, B. F. (1975). Studies on the pathogenesis of ischemic cell injury. 3. Morphological changes of the proximal pars recta tubules of the rat kidney made ischemic in vivo. *Virchow's Arch. Pathol.*, **19**, 303
59. Bilde, T. (1976). Vascular resistance in hypothermically perfused kidneys damaged by warm ischemia. *Scand. J. Urol. Nephrol.*, **10**, 43
60. Southard, J. H. and Belzer, F. O. (1980). Control of canine kidney cortex slice volume and ion distribution at hypothermia by impermeable anions. *Cryobiology*, **17**, 540
61. Acquatella, H., Gonzalez, M. P., Morales, J. M. *et al.* (1972). Ionic and histologic changes in the kidney after perfusion and storage for transplantation. *Transplantation*, **14**, 480
62. Downes, G., Hoffman, R., Huang, J. *et al.* (1973). Mechanism of action of washout solutions for kidney preservation. *Transplantation*, **16**, 46
63. Pegg, D. E. (1978). An approach to hypothermic renal preservation. *Cryobiology*, **15**, 1
64. Belzer, F. O., Hoffmann, R. M. and Southard, J. H. (1978). Kidney preservation. *Surg. Clin. N. Am.*, **58**, 261

65. Belzer, F.O., Hoffmann, R.M., Senzig, K.A. *et al.* (1979). Perfusion preservation of canine kidneys. In Pegg, D.E. and Jacobsen, I.A. (eds.) *Organ Preservation II*, p. 207. (Edinburgh: Churchill-Livingstone)

66. Whittembury, G. (1965). Sodium extrusion and potassium uptake in guinea pig kidney cortex slices. *J. Gen. Physiol.*, **48**, 699

67. Green, C.J. and Pegg, D.E. (1979). Mechanism of action of 'intracellular' renal preservation solutions. *World J. Surg.*, **3**, 115

68. Trump, B.F. and Ginn, F.L. (1968). Studies of cellular injury in isolated flounder tubules. 2. Cellular swelling in high potassium media. *Lab. Invest.*, **18**, 341

69. Gordon, E.E. and Maier, D.M. (1964). Effect of ionic environment on metabolism and structure of rat kidney slices. *Am. J. Physiol.*, **207**, 71

70. Pegg, D.E. and Gallant, M. (1977). Water and electrolyte contents and extracellular space of rabbit kidneys after perfusion and storage for 24 hours at 4°C. *Cryobiology*, **14**, 568

71. Blond, D.M. and Whittam, R. (1965). Effects of sodium and potassium ions on oxidative phosphorylation in relation to respiratory control by a cell-membrane adenosine triphosphatase. *Biochem. J.*, **97**, 523

72. Collins, G.M., Green, R.D. and Halasz, N.A. (1979). Importance of anion content and osmolarity in flush solutions for 48 to 72 hour hypothermic kidney storage. *Cryobiology*, **16**, 217

73. Dreikorn, K., Horsch, R. and Röhl, L. (1980). 48 to 96-hour preservation of canine kidneys by initial perfusion and hypothermic storage using the Euro-Collins solution. *Eur. Urol.*, **6**, 221

74. Sacks, S.A., Woo, Y.C., Smith, R.B. *et al.* (1978). Magnesium: not essential for renal preservation by initial perfusion and hypothermic storage. *Transplant. Proc.*, **10**, 287

75. Levowitz, B.S., Goldson, H., Rashkin, A. *et al.* (1970). Magnesium ion blockade of regional vasoconstriction. *Ann. Surg.*, **172**, 33

76. Netto, I.C.V., Basso, A.G. and Cockett, A.T.K. (1973). Renal preservation. A modified solution for 18 hours of protection. *Urology*, **2**, 389

77. Welch, L.T. and Flanigan, W.J. (1973). Kidney preservation. *Lancet*, **2**, 1444

78. Ross, B., Bishop, M. and Marshall, V. (1979). Metabolic aspects of renal preservation using the isolated perfused rat kidney. In Pegg, D.E. and Jacobsen, I.A. (eds.) *Organ Preservation II*, p. 220. (Edinburgh: Churchill-Livingstone)

79. Schloerb, P.R., Postel, J., Moritz, E.D. *et al.* (1975). Hypothermic storage of the canine kidney for 48 hours in a low chloride solution. *Surg. Gynecol. Obstet.*, **141**, 545

80. Grundmann, R., Strumper, R., Kurten, K. *et al.* (1978). Nierenkonservierung durch hypotherme lagerung nach Collins und Sacks: der einffuss von 0–30 min warmer ischamie auf die erreichbare konservierungszeit. *Langenbecks Arch. Chir.*, **346**, 11

81. Chatterjee, S.N. and Berne, T.V. (1975). Failure of 48 hours of cold storage of canine kidneys using Sacks' solution. *Transplantation*, **19**, 441

82. Vij, D., Chee, M. and Toledo-Pereyra, L.G. (1980). Failure of hypertonic citrate solution to preserve canine renal transplants after 24 hours of hypothermic storage. *Transplantation*, **29**, 90

83. Fahy, G.M., Hornblower, M. and Williams, H. (1979). An improved perfusate for hypothermic renal preservation. I. Initial in vitro optimization based on tissue electrolyte transport. *Cryobiology*, **16**, 618

84. Magnusson, M.O. and Stowe, N.T. (1976). Controversy in organ preservation. *Urol. Clin. N. Am.*, **3**, 491

85. Løkkegaard, H., Bilde, T. and Dahlager, J.I. (1979). Experimental and clinical studies of extended renal preservation by simple hypothermia. In Pegg, D.E. and Jacobsen, I.A. (eds.) *Organ Preservation II*, p. 102. (Edinburgh: Churchill Livingstone)

86. Clark, E.A., Terasaki, P.I., Opelz, G. *et al.* (1974). Cadaver kidney failures at one month. *N. Engl. J. Med.*, **291**, 1099

87. Collins, G.M. and Halasz, N.A. (1979). Experimental and clinical results with intracellular washout solutions. In Pegg, D.E. and Jacobsen, I.A. (eds.) *Organ Preservation II*, p. 68. (Edinburgh: Churchill-Livingstone)

88. Scott, D.V., Whiteside, D., Redhead, J. *et al.* (1974). Ice storage versus perfusion for preservation of kidneys before transplantation. *Br. Med. J.*, **4**, 76

89. Cho, S. I., Bradley, J. W. and Nabseth, D. C. (1975). Graft survival of perfused *vs* non-perfused cadaver kidneys. *Surg. Forum,* **26,** 351

90. Barry, J. M., Metcalfe, J. B., Farnsworth, M. A. *et al.* (1980). Comparison of intracellular flushing and cold storage to machine perfusion for human kidney preservation. *J. Urol.,* **123,** 14

91. Johnson, R. W. G., Anderson, M., Morley, A. R. *et al.* (1972). Twenty-four hour preservation of kidneys injured by prolonged warm ischemia. *Transplantation,* **13,** 174

92. Belzer, F. O. and Kountz, S. L. (1970). Preservation and transplantation of human cadaver kidneys: a two year experience. *Ann. Surg.,* **172,** 394

93. Løkkegaard, H., Bilde, T., Gyrd-Hansen, N. *et al.* (1971). Kidney preservation for 24 hours after one hour of warm ischemia. *Acta Med. Scand.,* **190,** 451

94. Noble, M. J., Magnusson, M. O., Stowe, N. T. *et al.* (1980). Preservation of ischemically damaged canine kidneys: cold storage versus perfusion. *Invest. Urol.,* **17,** 503

95. Slooff, J. J. H., VanDerWijk, J., Rijkmans, B. G. and Kootstra, G. (1978). Machine perfusion versus cold storage for preservation of kidneys before transplantation. *Arch. Chir. Neerl.,* **30,** 83

23
The effect of cooling rate in flush preservation of rabbit kidneys

I. A. JACOBSEN, J. CHEMNITZ and E. KEMP

Kidney preservation, as currently performed in the transplantation clinic, is based on reversible inhibition of the isolated organ's metabolism by hypothermia. Cooling is induced by a brief flush with a chilled electrolyte solution immediately after the organ is removed from the donor, and as the degree of metabolic inhibition is dependent on tissue temperature[1], rapid cooling would be expected to minimize preservation injury. We have, however, previously reported a highly deleterious effect on post-transplant function of rapid cooling of rabbit kidneys before a brief storage[2,3].

The aim of the present study was to examine the effect of cooling rate during flushing of kidneys before prolonged storage, imitating the clinical situation.

METHODS

Rabbit kidneys were used for the experiments. Donor animals were anesthetized with fentanyl citrate, fluanisone and pentobarbitone as described earlier[4]. The animals were pretreated with i.v. furosemide (5 mg), mannitol (1 g), chlorpromazine (4 mg/kg body weight) and heparin (500 units) before removal of left kidneys for preservation. The kidneys were flushed from a hanging bottle with 5 ml/g kidney weight of hypertonic citrate solution[5], and subsequently stored at $+2\,°C$ for 24 h before auto-transplantation[4], after which a contralateral nephrectomy was performed. Graft function was measured by daily serum creatinine determinations and creatinine clearance over 24 h, 2 weeks post-transplant[4].

Two groups of experiments were carried out. *Group I:* Twenty-two kidneys were flushed at ambient room temperature with the solution pre-cooled to $+2\,°C$ and from a height of 115 cm. This produced an average cooling rate of $3.7\,°C/min$ measured with a thermocouple 5 mm below the renal capsule. In *group 2* twenty-two kidneys were flushed with the same precooled solution, from a height of 135 cm to compensate for the increased viscosity of the fluid and at an ambient temperature of $+2\,°C$

producing an average cooling rate of 7.2 °C/min. Two kidneys in each group were removed 24 h post-transplant, and fixed by perfusion with 2.5% glutaraldehyde for histological examination after post-fixation with osmium tetraoxide. A further two grafts in each group surviving 2 weeks post-transplant were processed for histology.

RESULTS AND DISCUSSION

Perfusate flow rate during washout was not different in the two groups (Table 23.1), and as perfusion height was increased in group 2 proportionally to the increased perfusate viscosity at the lower temperature, this means that vascular resistance to flow was similar during flush at the two temperatures.

Table 23.1 Cooling rate and post-transplant function after 24 hours of cold storage

Cooling rate (°C/min)	Perfusate flow rate (ml/g kidney/min)	Mean S-creatinine (μmol/l)	Survival ratio
3.7	2.1 ± 0.5	298 ± 137	20/20
7.2	2.0 ± 0.5	412 ± 200	14/20
Level of significance for differences	ns	$p < 0.05$	$p < 0.05$

Mean ± SD

Immediate post-transplant function, measured as a mean of serum creatinine levels on the first three postoperative days, was significantly lower in the rapidly cooled group than in the slowly cooled, and only 14 of 20 grafts cooled at the higher rate before cold storage permitted survival of the recipient animals. All of 20 kidneys cooled at the lower rate had sufficient post-transplant function for survival of the animals during the experimental period of 2 weeks (Table 23.1). However, the function of surviving grafts in the two groups was not different when measured as peak creatinine levels and endogenous creatinine clearance 2 weeks post-transplant (Table 23.2).

Histological examination of two grafts cooled as in group 1 and removed 24 h post-transplant revealed normal morphology (Figure 23.1), whereas similar grafts of group 2 showed patchy necrosis of proximal tubular cells

Table 23.2 Cooling rate and post-transplant function of surviving grafts

Cooling rate (°C/min)	Peak creatinine (μmol/l)	Creatinine clearance (ml/min)
3.7	356 ± 167	5.5 ± 2.5
7.2	330 ± 117	6.1 ± 2.6
Level of significance for differences	ns	ns

Mean ± SD

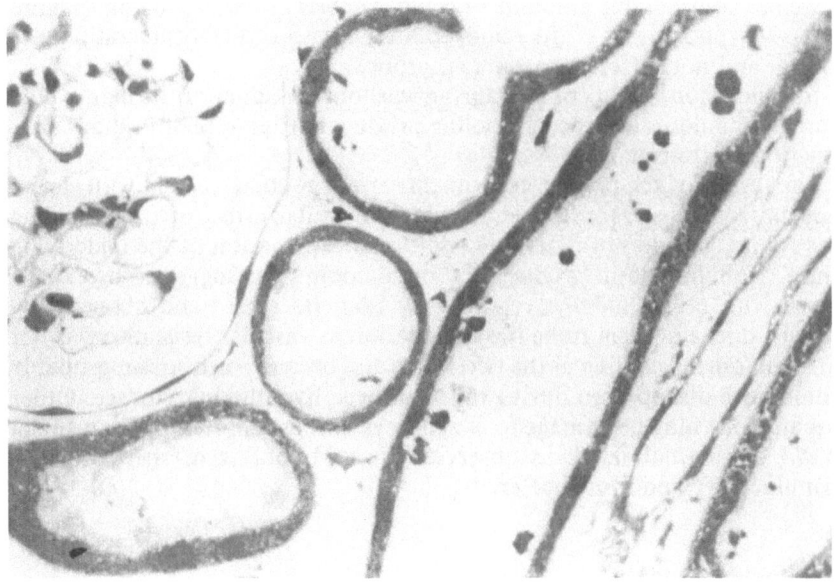

Figure 23.1 Graft cooled as in group 1 and removed 24 h post-transplant. Normal morphology. (Magnification ×512)

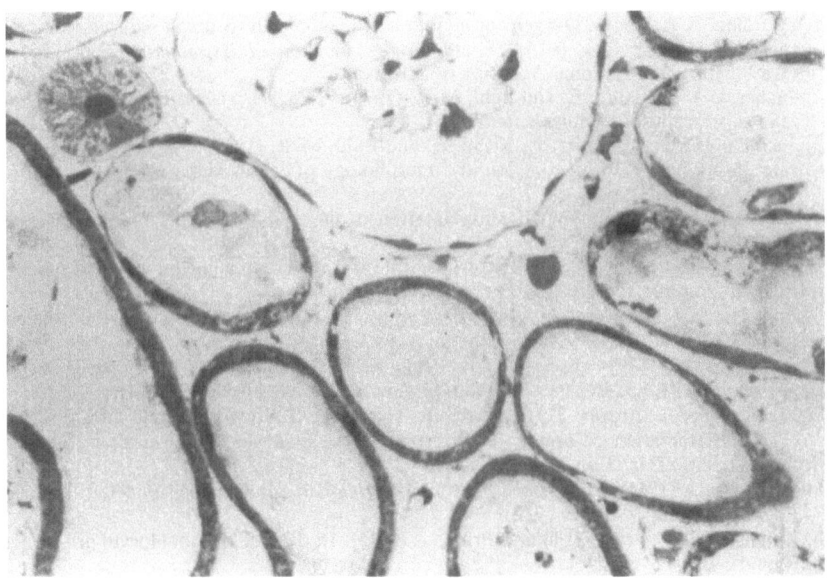

Figure 23.2 Graft cooled as in group 2 and removed 24 h post-transplant. Proximal tubular epithelium shows patchy necrosis, and cellular debris is seen in tubular lumina. (Magnification ×512)

as well as considerable amounts of cellular debris in tubular lumina (Figure 23.2). Morphology of grafts removed after 2 weeks of transplantation was normal and not different in the two groups.

In conclusion, rapid cooling during washout of kidney grafts before cold storage is undesirable as such cooling produces a high rate of primary non-functioning transplants.

The results of the present experiments are in good agreement with earlier reports from this laboratory[2,3], in which a similar effect of rapid cooling was found, but do not offer any additional explanation of the underlying cause. Vascular spasm produced by rapid cooling, as suggested by experiments with rabbit kidneys reported by Fonteles et al.[6] and observed by Belzer[7], does not seem to be the explanation as vascular resistance was not different during cooling at the two rates, and because such spasm probably would have disappeared during the prolonged hypothermic storage. Other explanations may be damage to enzyme systems as reported by Francavilla et al.[8] or thermal shock as observed in rapid cooling of spermatozoa[9], granulocytes[10] and some bacteria[11].

Acknowledgement

This work was supported by The Danish Medical Research Council.

References

1. Fuhrman, F. A. (1956). Oxygen consumption of mammalian tissues at reduced temperatures. In Dripps, R. D. (ed.), *The Physiology of Induced Hypothermia*, pp. 50–51. (Washington DC: National Academy of Sciences)
2. Jacobsen, I. A., Kemp, E. and Buhl, M. R. (1979). An adverse effect of rapid cooling in kidney preservation. *Transplantation*, **27**, 135
3. Jacobsen, I. A., Chemnitz, J., Kemp, E. and Buhl, M. R. (1980). The effect of cooling rate during perfusion on function and morphology of rabbit kidney grafts. *Scand. J. Urol. Nephrol.*, **54**, 90
4. Jacobsen, I. A. (1978). Renal transplantation in the rabbit: a model for preservation studies. *Lab. Anim.*, **12**, 63
5. Ross, H., Marshall, V. C. and Escott, M. L. (1976). 72 hour canine kidney preservation without continuous perfusion. *Transplantation*, **21**, 498
6. Fonteles, M. C. and Karow, A. M. (1976). An alpha-adrenotropic study of the isolated rabbit kidney at normo- and hypothermia. *Arch. Int. Pharmacodyn. Ther.*, **223**, 196
7. Belzer, F. O. (1979). Discussion, in Pegg, D. E. and Jacobsen, I. A. (eds.) *Organ Preservation II*, pp. 255–256. (Edinburgh: Churchill Livingstone)
8. Francavilla, A., Brown, T. H., Fiore, R., Cascardo, S., Taylor, P. and Groth, C. G. (1973). Preservation of organs for transplantation. Evidence of detrimental effect of rapid cooling. *Eur. Surg. Res.*, **5**, 384
9. Smith, A. U. (1961). *Biological Effects of Freezing and Supercooling*, p. 440. (London: Edward Arnold)
10. Knight, S. C., Farrant, J. and O'Brien, J. (1975). In defence of granulocyte preservers (Letter). *Lancet*, **1**, 929
11. Meynell, G. G. (1958). The effect of sudden chilling on *Escherichia coli*. *J. Gen. Microbiol.*, **19**, 380

24
Washout of red blood cells from kidneys damaged by warm ischaemia

J. FOREMAN, M. C. WUSTEMAN and D. E. PEGG

It is generally accepted that the vasculature of kidneys to be transplanted should first be cleared of donor blood: this is particularly important, and also more difficult, when there has been a significant period of warm ischaemia[1]. We have previously shown that the composition of the perfusate affects both the vascular resistance and the completeness of red cell removal from ischaemic rabbit kidneys[2]. Enquiries have revealed considerable variation in the composition of flush perfusates in clinical use in the United Kingdom at the present time, and the situation is further complicated by the use of common eponyms to describe dissimilar formulations. This study was designed to compare some of the solutions in use today with the WF5PD solution previously described by us[2], using rabbit kidneys subjected to 60 min of warm ischaemia as the model.

The composition of each of the solutions tested is shown in Table 24.1.

Table 24.1 Composition of flush perfusates

Constituent (per litre)	WF5PD	Hypertonic citrate	Cambridge flush solution	Cardiff flush solution	Collins* C_2 solution
Na^+ (mmol)	70.2	83.7	83.7	11.5	10.0
K^+ (mmol)	4.0	79.5	79.5	158.0	115.0
Mg^{2+} (mmol)	36.0	40.6	34.9	–	30.0
Citrate (mmol)	–	54.4	54.4	–	–
SO_4^{2-} (mmol)	1.0	40.6	34.9	–	30.0
$H_2PO_4^-$ (mmol)	0.8	–	–	17.0	15.0
HPO_4^{2-} (mmol)	1.2	–	–	62.0	42.5
Cl^- (mmol)	116.0	–	–	17.0	15.0
HCO_3^- (mmol)	25.0	–	–	11.0	10.0
EDTA (mmol)	–	–	–	0.25	–
Mannitol (mmol)	–	185.5	92.8	–	–
Glucose (mmol)	167.0	–	–	167.0	140
Dextran 40 (g)	50.0	–	–	–	–
Papaverine (mg)	30.0	–	–	–	–
HEPES (mmol)	10.0	–	–	–	–
Osmolality (mosmol/kg)	400	400	280	380	360

* Not studied in these experiments – included for comparison

Hypertonic citrate solution was prepared from analytical grade reagents according to the data of Ross, Marshall and Escott[3]. Cambridge flush solution is the local variant of that solution and is prepared by the New Addenbrooke's Hospital Pharmacy: it contains somewhat less magnesium sulphate and only half the amount of mannitol; it is slightly hypotonic. The Cardiff flush solution is a variant of the so-called Euro-Collins formulation (Rijksen, J. F. W. B., personal communication), itself a variant of Collins' C2 solution[4]. This solution is commonly referred to as Collins' solution, but in our view should not be, since the differences are substantial, see Table 24.1. This is the solution currently prepared by the University Hospital of Wales Pharmacy and provided by the UK Transplant Service.

The animals used in this study were New Zealand White rabbits, anaesthetized, hydrated and heparinized as previously described[2]. Each kidney was excised, incubated in 100 ml of 0.9% sodium chloride solution at 37°C for 1 h, and then perfused at a measured renal artery pressure of 60 mmHg with 100 ml of the appropriate solution that had been precooled to 4°C. Six kidneys were used for each perfusate. The venous effluent was collected in a fraction collector and the haemoglobin content of each fraction, and of the kidney after 100 ml had been perfused, was measured. All the techniques used have been fully described[2].

The results obtained with the four solutions studied are illustrated in Figure 24.1 and Table 24.2. It is apparent that there are considerable differences between the solutions, both in respect of mean flow rate and of efficiency of removal of red cells. The dextran 40-containing WF5PD solution gave the most rapid flush but shared with the Cardiff solution the property of leaving the largest amounts of residual red cells. The two citrate-containing solutions gave the lowest levels of retained haemoglobin but the 100 ml flush took much longer. The Ross and Marshall formulation of hypertonic citrate offered the best compromise: although the final residual red cell content was similar to that achieved with the Cambridge solution, the mean flow rate was higher, and already by 4 min the bulk of the contained blood had been removed.

We draw several conclusions from this study. First, there are significant differences between solutions in current use in their efficiency for removing red blood cells from ischaemic kidneys. Secondly, it may be necessary to perfuse for much longer times than is often done, in order to remove blood efficiently; apparent clarity of the effluent perfusate does not necessarily indicate completion of the flush. Thirdly, those perfusates that give the lowest vascular resistance may not give the most complete blood removal.

Table 24.2 Effect of perfusate on the removal of red cells from rabbit kidneys

Washout solution	Mean flow rate (ml/min/g kidney) (n = 6)	Residual haemoglobin (mg/g kidney) (n = 6)
WF5 PD	1.3 ± 0.1	0.70 ± 0.09
Hypertonic citrate	0.5 ± 0.1	0.29 ± 0.02
Cardiff flush solution	1.1 ± 0.2	0.72 ± 0.19
Cambridge flush solution	0.3 ± 0.0	0.26 ± 0.06

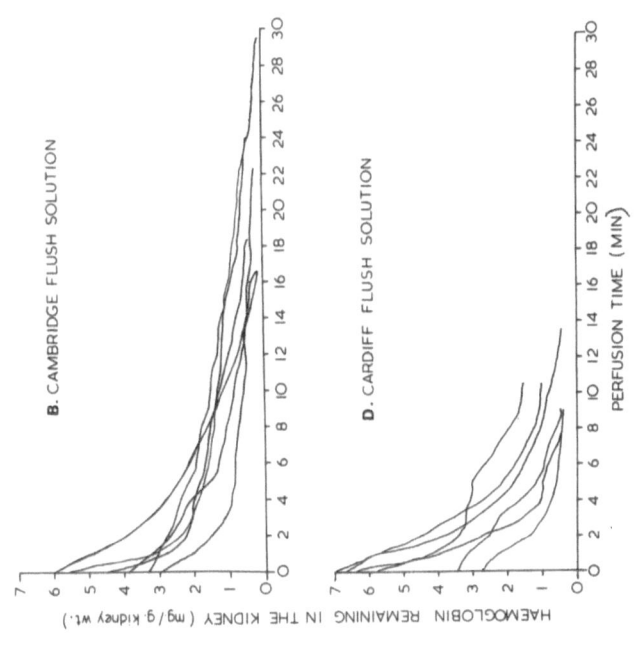

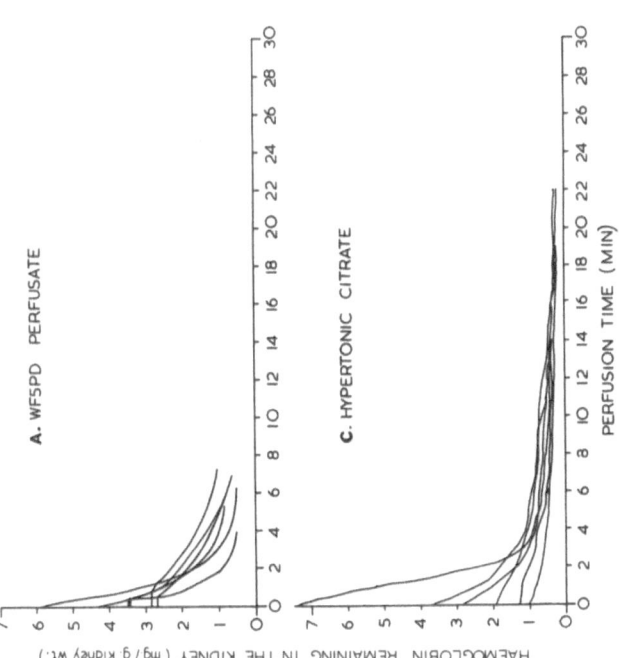

Figure 24.1 Haemoglobin washout curves for rabbit kidneys subjected to 60 min of warm ischaemia prior to perfusion with 100 ml of the indicated solution

These findings emphasize the need for proper control of washout solution formulations.

References

1. Pegg, D. E. (1978). An approach to hypothermic renal preservation. *Cryobiology,* **15,** 1
2. Wusteman, M. C., Jacobsen, I. A. and Pegg, D. E. (1978). A new solution for initial perfusion of transplant kidneys. *Scand. J. Urol. Nephrol.,* **12,** 281
3. Ross, H., Marshall, V. C. and Escott, M. L. (1976). 72-hour canine kidney preservation without continuous perfusion. *Transplantation,* **21,** 498
4. Collins, G. M., Bravo-Shugarman, M. and Terasaki, P. (1969). Kidney preservation for transportation. *Lancet,* **2,** 1219

25
Comparative evaluation of a new low ionic strength, hyperkalaemic flush solution

G. M. COLLINS, N. A. HALASZ and G. M. FAHY

The majority of flush solutions utilized for hypothermic kidney storage have been hypertonic and contained high concentrations of potassium ions[1-5]. Recently Fahy *et al.* reported that a new flush solution 'RPS-2'[6] was superior to Collins' solution for maintaining tissue slice K/Na ratios following hypothermic storage. The unique features of this new solution are that it is isotonic, has a low ionic strength, and [K$^+$] is only 42 mmol/l.

This report describes evaluation of the new solution by comparison with continuous albumin perfusion and hypothermic storage using C2 and some low ionic strength isotonic solutions. The experiments were conducted in the rabbit using a test model, which we have described previously, for measuring renal function after storage[7]. Kidneys were preserved on ice by an initial 30 ml cold flush at 100 mmHg with one of the solutions shown in Table 25.1 or by continuous hypothermic albumin perfusion on a Waters (MOX 100) perfusion machine. Following 24 h storage, kidneys were

Table 25.1 Flush solution composition (mmol/l)

Constituent	Solution			
	C2	*RPS-0*	*RPS-2*	*LIC*
K	115	42	42	42
Na	10	10	10	10
Mg	28	2	2	2
Cl	15	34	34	4
HCO$_3$	10	10	10	10
HPO$_4$	57.5	7	7	24
SO$_4$	30	–	–	–
Glucose	139	180	180	233
Osmolarity	320	285	290	290
Ca	–	–	1	–
Glutathione	–	–	5	–
Adenine	–	–	1	–

187

connected by a silastic shunt to the aorta and vena cava of a host perfusor rabbit. Thirty minutes were allowed for recovery and then urine was collected for 1 h to measure endogenous creatinine clearance.

The results are shown in Table 25.2. All methods of preservation produced a significant impairment of function by comparison with the unpreserved controls. The RPS-2 solution was significantly superior to C2 ($p < 0.05$), confirming Fahy's observations. It was possible, however, to further improve upon the basic electrolyte composition of the Fahy solution, RPS-0, by substitution of phosphate for chloride ions ($p < 0.05$). This low ionic strength intracellular type flush solution (LIC) yielded the best function of all of the methods tested (compared with RPS-2, $0.05 < p < 0.1$).

Table 25.2 24 hour rabbit kidney preservation: function on a shunt

Treatment	Number of experiments	Creatinine clearance (ml/h)	
		Mean	SD
Control	15	291	145
Perfusion	16	140	45
C2	15	69	33
RPS-2	10	121	58
RPS-0	10	92	54
LIC	50	161	61

Further work is needed to determine whether the mode of action of LIC is similar to that of other well-established flush solutions and whether its superiority can be demonstrated when tested in a transplant model and in species other than the rabbit. Preliminary data from our laboratory (to be published) suggest that the results in the dog may be different. This raises the interesting question as to which species of lower animal should be used to predict the utility in man of experimentally derived preservation solutions.

Acknowledgement

Supported by the Veterans Administration Medical Research Service and the PHSAM 20193 and 26324.

References

1. Collins, G. M., Bravo-Shugarman, M. B. and Terasaki, P. I. (1969). Kidney preservation for transportation. 3. Initial perfusion and 30-hour ice storage. *Lancet,* 2, 1219
2. Sacks, S. A., Petritsch, P. H. and Kaufman, J. J. (1973). Canine kidney preservation using a new perfusate. *Lancet,* 1, 1024
3. Ross, H., Marshall, V. C. and Escott, M. L. (1976). 72-hour canine kidney preservation without continuous perfusion. *Transplantation,* 21, 498

4. Acquatella, H., Gonzalez, M. P., Morales, J. M. *et al.* (1972). Ionic and histologic changes in the kidney after perfusion and storage for transplantation. *Transplantation,* **14,** 480

5. Vij, D., Chee, M. and Toledo-Pereyra, L. G. (1980). Failure of hypertonic citrate solution to preserve canine renal transplants after 24 hours of hypothermic storage. *Transplantation,* **29,** 90

6. Fahy, G. M., Hornblower, M. and Williams, H. (1979). An improved perfusate for hypothermic renal preservation. I. Initial *in vitro* optimization based on tissue electrolyte transport. *Cryobiology,* **16,** 618

7. Carter, J. N., Green, R. D., Halasz, N. A. *et al.* (1981). Ex-vivo perfusion: a renal preservation model. *J. Surg. Res.,* **31,** 55

26
Hypothermic preservation of the rat pancreas

J. KLEMPNAUER, D. E. PEGG, M. J. TAYLOR and M. J. DIAPER

A number of papers report varying degrees of success in short-term preservation of the pancreas: techniques studied include hypothermia after initial perfusion, continuous hypothermic perfusion, hypothermia combined with hyperbaric oxygen and cryopreservation. The simplest approach, initial perfusion followed by storage at 0–4 °C, has proved effective for 24 h using a 'protide gel' solution[1], fructose-bicarbonate solution[2], modified cryoprecipitated plasma[3], Collins' C3 solution[4] or Sacks' solution[5]. The only report of effective 48 h preservation used a preliminary perfusion with plasma supplemented by potassium, glucose and albumin to produce a total osmolality of 450 mosmol/kg[5]. Similarly, continuous perfusion using cryoprecipitated plasma[4,6,7] or purified human albumin solution[2] has been effective for 24 h storage, some investigators stressing the need for a low perfusion pressure[7,8] and the inclusion of methylprednisolone[9]. However, direct comparisons of initial perfusion with continuous perfusion have failed to show any benefit from the more complex continuous perfusion method[2–4]. The use of hyperbaric oxygen likewise confers no apparent advantage[10], and cryopreservation of the whole pancreas is clearly inferior[11]. Thus, the available evidence suggests that the simplest approach, that of initial perfusion with a chilled solution, followed by storage at 0–4 °C gives results at 24 h that are as good as any more complicated method.

The above studies were all carried out in the dog using allografts, and assessment of preservation was inevitably complicated by graft rejection or immunosuppression. Moreover, the selection of perfusate formulations has been haphazard, and it is impossible to deduce which of the many formulations might be best. For these reasons we decided to study the preservation of the isolated rat pancreas, where isologous transplantation is possible, and to examine 24 and 48 h preservation using flush solutions that were modified in a stepwise manner similar to that used in studies of renal preservation[12,13]. Function was assessed by isografting into streptozotocin-diabetic rats: a parallel study, using *in vitro* assessment in a normothermic perfusion assay, will be reported separately[14].

METHODS

Inbred WAG rats were used in all experiments. Donors were of either sex weighing 130–170 g; 220–270 g males served as recipients. A single i.v. injection of 65 mg/kg streptozotocin was given to induce diabetes, which was confirmed by blood glucose measurements above 22 mmol/l and a substantial weight loss 2–3 weeks later.

After entering the abdomen through a long midline incision the common bile duct was ligated at the liver hilum and at its entrance into the duodenum, resulting in a duct-ligated pancreas. After transection of the hepatic artery and dissection from the greater omentum, the right gastroepiploic artery and vein were ligated. Then the pancreas was dissected from the duodenum, preserving the pancreaticoduodenal arcade and ligating all communicating vessels. The superior mesenteric artery and vein were ligated at the level of their first jejunal branches. The transverse colon was removed by blunt dissection and the middle colic artery and the inferior mesenteric vein were transected. After splenectomy the short gastric vessels and the left gastric artery and vein were ligated and cut. An aortic segment giving off the coeliac axis and the superior mesenteric artery was then isolated and the right renal artery was ligated. The aorta was cannulated below the superior mesenteric artery and clamped just above the coeliac axis. Perfusion was commenced immediately. The portal vein was cut at the start of the perfusion to provide venous outflow. Removal of the pancreas took 35 ± 5 min.

The composition of the perfusates was varied in such a manner that factors contributing to good preservation could be identified; see Table 26.1. Twenty ml of the appropriate solution was delivered to the arterial cannula at a pressure of 80 mmHg and a temperature of ~10 °C using the technique previously described for rabbit kidneys[15]. The perfusion lasted 4–5 min for solutions PP1–4 and 7–8 min for solutions PP5–7. Each pancreas was then stored in a glass beaker containing 20 ml of the same solution, surrounded by melting ice, for 24 or 48 h.

Transplantation was by end-to-side anastomoses between donor aorta

Table 26.1 Composition of perfusates (mmol/l)

	PP1	PP2	PP3	PP4	PP5	PP6	PP7
Na$^+$	140	140	70	70	70	70	70
K$^+$	5	5	5	5	75	75	75
Mg^{2+}	1	1	51	51	1	1	1
Cl$^-$	140	140	170	70	140	70	140
HCO$_3$$^-$	5	5	5	5	5	5	5
SO$_4^{2-}$	1	1	1	–	1	–	1
Glycerophosphate	–	–	–	51	–	36	–
HEPES*	20	20	20	20	20	20	20
Mannitol	–	50	50	105	50	75	50
Heparin (IU)	5000	5000	5000	5000	5000	5000	5000
pH	7.0	7.0	7.0	7.0	7.0	7.0	7.6
Osmolality (mosmol/kg)	315	365	365	360	370	360	370

* HEPES = N-2-hydroxyethylpiperazine-N'-2-ethanesulphonate

192

and recipient infrarenal aorta and between donor portal vein and recipient inferior vena cava using continuous overrunning 8–O Ethilon® sutures. The time between removal of the pancreas from cold storage and re-establishing the blood supply was approximately 20 min.

Non-fasting blood glucose levels and body weight of the rats were monitored on days 1, 2, 3, 5, 7 and 10 after transplantation, then at weekly intervals for 3 months, and thereafter at monthly intervals for at least 6 months. About 3 weeks after transplantation an intravenous glucose tolerance test (IVGTT) was performed under fentanyl–fluanisone anaesthesia. Glucose (1 g/kg i.v.) was administered, and blood samples were taken 10 and 5 min prior to glucose injection and 2, 5, 10, 20, 40 and 60 min thereafter. Glucose disappearance rates or k-values were calculated; k-values above 1.5 are considered normal, 1.0–1.5 indicates latent diabetes, and k-values below 1.0 are considered frankly diabetic.

RESULTS AND DISCUSSION

When unpreserved transplanted pancreases were revascularized, they flushed immediately and gained a homogeneous pink colour. Normo-glycaemia was established within 24 h – see Figure 26.1. The non-fasting blood glucose levels did not differ from those prior to induction of diabetes. After streptozotocin treatment the animals lost 16.5% of their body weight, but within 10 days after transplantation they regained 15.8%.

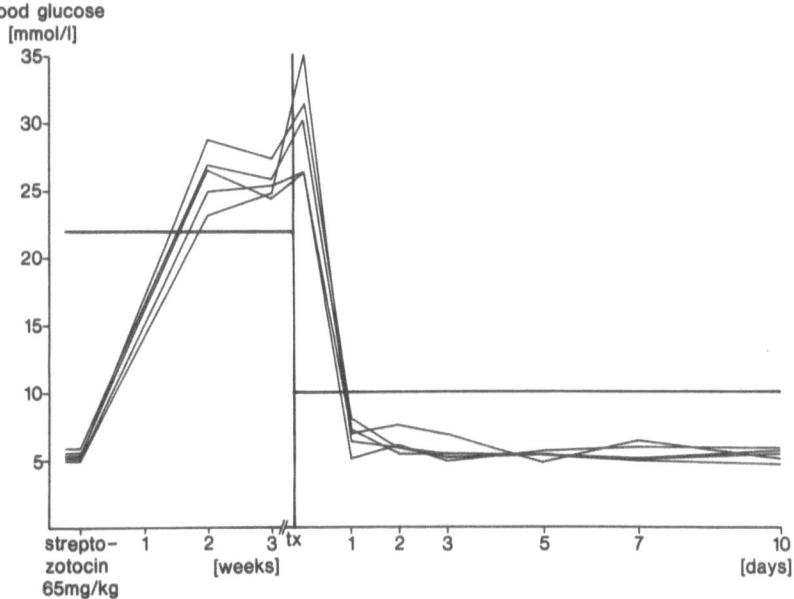

Figure 26.1 Blood glucose levels in WAG rats following streptozotocin treatment and isologous pancreas transplantation using freshly isolated, unpreserved pancreases

The k-value 3 weeks after transplantation was 3.00, which is not significantly different from healthy untreated controls (2.77) and well above the value for diabetics (0.01). All five animals in this group are alive, well and normoglycaemic 6 months later. The results with preserved pancreases were:

PP1

The appearance of the pancreases after preservation in this simple balanced salt solution and immediately after revascularization was excellent. All animals became normoglycaemic after transplantation. Two pancreases ceased to function on day 2 and 3 respectively and 10 days after transplantation these two rats increased their body weight only by 6%; k-values were only ~0.30. The remaining three animals gained 18% in body weight and had normal k-values (2.77); they are still alive and normoglycaemic.

PP2

The osmolality of this solution was increased to 365 mosmol/kg by the addition of 50 mmol/l of the slowly permeating neutral solute mannitol. The preserved pancreases had an excellent appearance immediately after transplantation. Blood glucose levels dropped to normal within 24 h, but on day 1 two animals were found in hypoglycaemic coma with blood glucose levels of 0.9 and 1.2 mmol/l respectively. One recovered after the intravenous administration of glucose, but the other died 2 h later. The surviving five animals had a good endocrine function with a weight gain of 17% and a mean k-value of 3.75. One animal became diabetic again 120 days after transplantation, but the remaining four rats are still alive and normoglycaemic.

PP3

Half of the Na^+ was replaced by Mg^{2+} in this solution while retaining the same total osmolality. As Mg^{2+} is divalent, this resulted in a simultaneous increase in Cl^- concentration: it was found that the replacement of 70 mmol/l NaCl by 50 mmol/l Mg Cl_2 gave the same total osmolality. The preserved organs were all slow to perfuse with blood and retained a mottled appearance. Four of five animals died from pancreatitis, one within 2 h of transplantation, another on day 1 after the blood glucose had returned to normal, and the other two on days 8 and 10 respectively. The surviving animal had a normal blood glucose level after transplantation, but it lost weight and was latently diabetic ($k = 1.3$): 45 days after transplantation it died, being frankly diabetic.

PP4

In this solution half of the original Cl$^-$ concentration was replaced by glycerophosphate: since glycerophosphate is divalent it was necessary to increase the mannitol concentration to keep the osmolality constant. These pancreases also had a mottled appearance after revascularization, though not as bad as with PP3. One animal died from pancreatitis 3 h after transplantation and another from hypoglycaemia on day 2. The remaining three animals had normal glucose levels and showed a weight gain of 14.4%. However, one was frankly diabetic ($k = 0.02$), one was latently diabetic ($k = 1.0$) and only one was normal ($k = 2.9$). The frankly diabetic animal died 140 days after transplantation, but the two remaining animals are still alive and normoglycaemic.

PP5

This perfusate contained Cl$^-$ as the major anion, but half of the Na$^+$ was replaced by K$^+$. Each of the five pancreases had an oedematous appearance, but assumed a normal pink colour gradually after revascularization. Endocrine function was excellent – see Figure 26.2: normoglycaemia was established within 24 h and maintained for more than 6 months. The weight gain of 10.4% was a little low, but the mean k-value of 2.65 was almost identical to the normal controls. All five animals are still alive and normoglycaemic.

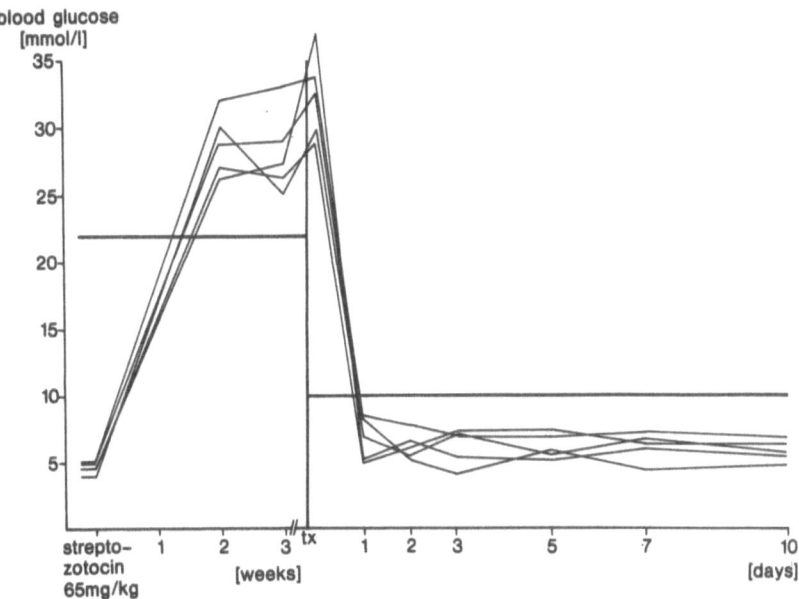

Figure 26.2 Blood glucose levels in WAG rats following streptozotocin treatment and isologous transplantation of pancreases preserved at 0 °C for 24 h after perfusion with solution PP5

195

PP6

Half of the original Cl^- was replaced by glycerophosphate in this solution while maintaining the approximately equimolar balance of Na^+ and K^+. As with PP4, it was necessary to adjust the mannitol concentration to maintain constant osmolality. The pancreases preserved with PP6 were also slow to reperfuse but they were less oedematous than those preserved with PP5. They all showed excellent endocrine function ($k = 2.59$) and the weight gain of 15.7% was virtually identical to that of freshly transplanted organs. All animals are still alive and normoglycaemic.

PP7

This solution had the same composition as PP5, but the pH was increased from 7.0 to 7.6. All the five pancreases preserved with PP7 were slow to reperfuse with blood, but the animals had good endocrine function with normal blood glucose levels and a weight gain of 18.5%. (Due to a technical mishap unfortunately no IVGTT data are available.) One animal relapsed into a fully diabetic state 30 days after transplantation, but the remaining animals are still alive and normoglycaemic.

PP5: 48 hours

The five pancreases preserved for 48 h with PP5 were oedematous and soft. They were slow to reperfuse with blood and retained a mottled appearance. Three animals died from pancreatitis, one 2 h after transplantation and one 11 h after transplantation (blood glucose level 6.8 mmol/l). The third animal died 26 h after transplantation with no evidence of endocrine function. Two animals were normoglycaemic within 24 h, but one developed hypoglycaemic attacks on days 2 and 5, and in spite of repeated oral and i.v. glucose one animal died on day 5: the remaining rat returned to stable blood glucose levels, showed a weight gain of 10.4% and a k-value of 2.13. This animal is still alive and normoglycaemic.

These results show that the two most significant factors in the design of a preservation solution for the rat pancreas are the inclusion of an impermeant neutral solute and replacement of some Na^+ by K^+. This is consistent with evidence from renal preservation studies[12,13,16,17]: 50 mmol/l of mannitol should be adequate to balance impermeant intracellular solutes[18]. The evidence concerning Mg^{2+} in renal preservation is inconclusive[12,13,19-21], but in these studies the addition of Mg^{2+} was detrimental, leading to a high incidence of pancreatitis. The addition of glycerophosphate to the Mg^{2+}-rich solution may have reduced this effect (the groups are too small for reliable statistical analysis) but the addition of glycerophosphate to the K^+-rich solution had no detectable effect on pancreases preserved for 24 h. Glycerophosphate, with a molecular weight of 171 daltons, has been beneficial in maintaining lysosomal integrity[22], in improving the viability of smooth muscle stored at subzero temperatures[23] and in preventing swelling of renal cortical slices stored at $4\,°C^{24}$. It is possible that the optimal pH may be higher at $0\,°C$ than at $37\,°C^{25}$, but raising the perfusate pH to 7.6 had no effect. Only solution PP5 (K+-rich, high osmolality) was studied at 48h, and this failed to give adequate preservation.

We conclude that preservation of the rat pancreas for 24h is possible, using the simple technique of initial perfusion followed by storage on ice: such pancreases were indistinguishable from grafts transplanted without storage when pancreas perfusate 5 (PP5) was used, but reliable preservation for 48h was not possible.

Acknowledgement

J. Klempnauer was in receipt of a NATO Research Scholarship provided by the German Academic Exchange Service.

References

1. Solassol, C., Serrou, B. C., Gelis, C., Michel, H., Cabasson, J., Averous, M., Paren, M. and Romieu, C. (1971). 8 and 24 hours of canine pancreas preservation by a simple cooling technique using a gel. *Proc. Eur. Exp. Surg. 6th Congress*, p. 272
2. Brynger, H. (1975). Twenty-four hour preservation of the duct-ligated canine pancreatic allograft. *Eur. Surg. Res.*, **7**, 341
3. Toledo-Pereyra, L. H., Valjee, K. D. and Chee, M. (1979). Preservation of the pancreas for transplantation. *Surg. Gynecol. Obstet.*, **148**, 57
4. De Gruyl, J., Westbroek, D. L., MacDicken, I., Ridderhof, E., Verschoor, L. and Van Strik, R. (1977). Cryoprecipitated plasma perfusion preservation and cold storage preservation of duct-ligated pancreatic allografts. *Br. J. Surg.*, **64**, 490
5. Toledo-Pereyra, L. H., Chee, M., Condie, R. M., Najarian, J. S. and Lillehei, R. C. (1979). Forty-eight hours hypothermic storage of whole canine pancreas allografts. Improved preservation with a colloid hyperosmolar solution. *Cryobiology*, **16**, 221
6. Dijkhuis, C. M., Westbroek, D. L., De Gruyl, J., Oldenhof, J. and Drop, A. (1972). 24-hour isolated canine pancreas preservation on the Belzer machine. *Proc. Eur. Soc. Exp. Surg. 7th Congress*, p. 270
7. Tersigni, R., Toledo-Pereyra, L. H., Pinkham, J. and Najarian, J. S. (1975). Pancreaticoduodenal preservation by hypothermic pulsatile perfusion for 24 hours. *Ann. Surg.*, **182**, 743
8. De Gruyl, J., Westbroek, D. L., Dijkhuis, C. M., Vriesendorp, H. M., MacDicken I., Elion-Gerritsen, W., Verschoor, L., Hulsmans, H. A. M. and Horchner, P. (1973). Influence of DL-A matching, ALS and 24 hour preservation on isolated pancreas allograft survival. *Transplant. Proc.*, **V**, 755
9. Tersigni, R., Toledo-Pereyra, L. H. and Najarian, J. S. (1975). Effects of methylprednisolone, glucagon, and allopurinol in the protection of pancreatic duodenal allografts perfused for 24 hours. *Surgery*, **78**, 599
10. Idezuki, Y., Goetz, F. C. and Lillehei, R. C. (1969). Experimental allotransplantation of the preserved pancreas and duodenum. *Surgery*, **65**, 485
11. Zimmerman, G., Tennyson, C. and Drapanas, T. (1971). Studies of preservation of liver and pancreas by freezing techniques. *Transplant. Proc.*, **III**, 657
12. Fuller, B. J. and Pegg, D. E. (1976). Assessment of renal preservation by normothermic bloodless perfusion. *Cryobiology*, **13**, 177
13. Green, C. J. and Pegg, D. E. (1979). The mechanism of action of intracellular renal preservation solutions. *World J. Surg.*, **3**, 115

14. Pegg, D. E., Klempnauer, J., Diaper, M. P. and Taylor, M. J. (1982). Assessment of hypothermic preservation of the pancreas in the rat by a normothermic perfusion assay. *J. Surg. Res.* (In press)
15. Wusteman, M. C., Jacobsen, I. A. and Pegg, D. E. (1978). A new solution for initial perfusion of transplant kidneys. *Scand. J. Urol. Nephrol.,* **12,** 281
16. Acquatella, H., Perez-Gonzales, M., Morales, J. M. and Whittembury, G. (1972). Ionic and histologic changes in the kidney after perfusion and storage for transplantation. *Transplantation,* **14,** 480
17. Downes, G., Hoffmann, R., Huang, J. and Belzer, F. O. (1973). Mechanism of action of washout solutions for kidney preservation. *Transplantation,* **16,** 46
18. Robinson, J. R. (1971). Control of water content of non-metabolizing kidney slices by sodium chloride and polyethylene glycol (PEG 6000). *J. Physiol.,* **213,** 227
19. Collins, G. M., Bravo-Shugarman, M. and Terasaki, P. I. (1969). Kidney preservation for transportation. *Lancet,* **2,** 1219
20. Collins, G. M. and Halasz, N. A. (1976). Forty-eight hour ice storage of kidneys: importance of cation content. *Surgery,* **79,** 432
21. Sacks, S. A., Woo, Y. C., Smith, R. B., Ehrlich, R. M. and Kaufman, J. J. (1978). Magnesium: not essential for renal preservation by initial perfusion and hypothermic storage. *Transplant. Proc.,* **10,** 287
22. Lee, D. (1972). The effect of glycerol, ethanol and dimethylsulphoxide on rat liver lysosomes. *Biochim. Biophys. Acta,* **266,** 50
23. Elford, B. C. and Walter, C. A. (1972). Effects of electrolyte composition and pH on the structure and function of smooth muscle cooled to $-79\,°C$ in unfrozen media. *Cryobiology,* **9,** 82
24. Karow, A. M, Jr and Fahy, G. M. (1979). Inhibition of colloid cell swelling in rabbit kidney cortex by disodium glycerophosphate. *Cryobiology,* **16,** 35
25. Halasz, N. A., Collins, G. M. and White, F. M. (1979). The right pH for preservation? In Pegg, D. E. and Jacobsen, I. A. (eds.) *Organ Preservation II,* p. 259. (Edinburgh: Churchill Livingstone)

27
Deuterium oxide (D₂O) for organ preservation

J. H. FISCHER, G. REIFFERSCHEIDT, M. FUHS, M. WENZEL and
W. ISSELHARD

Organ preservation nowadays is limited by the development of cellular damage which is mainly damage to cellular membranes. The course of damage can be slowed down by oxygenated preservation, i.e. continuous perfusion or retrograde oxygen persufflation, but it cannot be prevented. Many efforts have been made to reduce the damaging effects by use of special flush solutions which reduce oedema formation and electrolyte redistribution but a real protection of membranes has not yet been achieved.

Therefore we tried to utilize the effect of deuterium oxide (the oxide of the non-radioactive stable isotope of hydrogen) which is known to replace H- by D-linkages in biological macromolecules and thus to stabilize their structure[1]. It has been shown previously[2] that erythrocytes are more resistant to thermic or osmotic damage in the presence of D_2O. Moreover we could demonstrate[3] that in asphyxia the maintenance of blood pressure and thereby survival and revivability can be prolonged significantly by D_2O.

In experiments on kidney, heart or liver preservation we used flush solutions containing 99% D_2O instead of H_2O. We determined the changes in metabolic parameters of these organs as well as the degree of fluid accumulation indicating cellular swelling, and in some preliminary experiments we tested post-transplant functional recovery.

For ischaemic kidneys at hypothermia or normothermia, the inhibition of oedema formation is of central importance for post-transplant function. Moreover the cellular content of energy-rich substances reflects renal viability provided the metabolic state has been normal before the onset of ischaemia[4]. Also in liver preservation, oedema formation and cellular energy are central parameters for organ viability[5]. In hearts the tolerance to ischaemic damage is also related to the maintenance of ATP or the total nucleotide content as shown by several authors[6].

Kidney preservation

Rat kidneys were stored by hypothermic ischaemia (HIS) at 6 °C for 48 h or by normothermic ischaemia (NI) at 37 °C for 60 min following flush perfusion with Ringer's solution containing glucose and mannitol (400 mosmol/kg). In both experiments the maintenance of the sum of adenine nucleotides (SAN = ATP + ADP + AMP) per g dry weight was significantly better ($p < 0.02$) when D_2O-flush solutions were used. Moreover in HIS, the oedema formation (as indicated by changes in the dry weight/wet weight ratio) could be significantly reduced ($p < 0.001$) by D_2O. The D_2O content of kidneys at the end of NI was $46 \pm 4\%$ (mean $\pm$ SD) of the total tissue water, while it amounted to $92 \pm 3\%$ after 48 h HIS in the flush solution. (Determination of D_2O contents was by NMR-spectrometry.)

In preliminary experiments, dog kidneys demonstrated life-supporting function following 48 h HIS or after 30 min NI and 24 h HIS and autotransplantation with contralateral nephrectomy using D_2O–Collins solution for flush and storage.

Heart preservation

Rat hearts were stored at different temperatures (7 °C, 17 °C, 27 °C) following a flush with Ringer's solution on the basis of H_2O or 99% D_2O for 160 min (7 °C), 80 min (17 °C) or 40 min (27 °C). The D_2O content

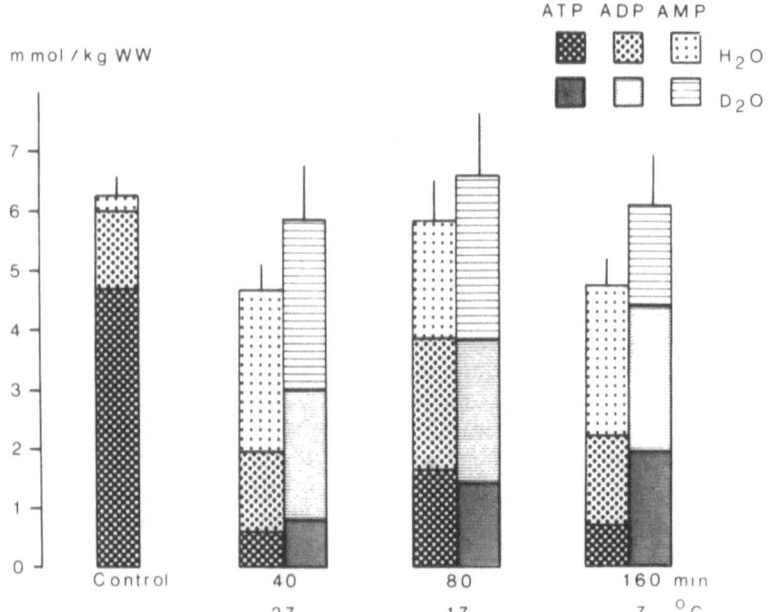

Figure 27.1 Adenine nucleotide levels in hearts after hypothermic ischaemic storage in D_2O- and H_2O-based solutions (mmol/kg wet weight, mean $\pm$ SD, $n = 5$–10 per group)

amounted to $71 \pm 14\%$ of total tissue water, resulting in a better maintenance of adenine nucleotides (SAN) at all temperatures (Figure 27.1). D$_2$O was found to be most effective in hypothermia at 7 °C, with significantly better maintenance of SAN, energy charge potential (ECP) and creatine phosphate (CrP). In rats with 25% D$_2$O in the total body water after infusion of D$_2$O–Ringer's solution, the SAN of the heart was significantly increased before and after a 20 min period of normothermic ischaemia (37 °C), compared to controls without D$_2$O.

Liver preservation

Rat livers were flushed *in situ* with cold solutions of different types (Ringer–glucose–mannitol (RGM), Collins' solution C2[7], Lambotte's solution KMgS[5] and our own solution C2-S), which were composed on the basis of H$_2$O or 99% D$_2$O (see Table 27.1). The livers were stored in the flush solution at 6 °C for 24 h (HIS). Oedema formation was reduced by D$_2$O but also by sucrose. The maintenance of cellular adenine nucleotides (calculated per g dry weight) differed in the four groups with respect to the action of D$_2$O. The values were lowered in RGM perfusate while they were stabilized significantly in C2-S (Figure 27.2).

Table 27.1 Composition of flush solutions (mmol/l)

	RGM	C2	KMgS	C2-S
Na$^+$	147	10	–	110
K$^+$	4	115	95	115
Ca^{2+}	2	–	–	–
Mg^{2+}	–	30	80	30
Cl$^-$	155	15	–	15
HCO$_3^-$	–	10	15	10
SO$_4^{2-}$	–	30	120	80
HPO$_4^{2-}$, H$_2$PO$_4^-$	–	57.5	–	57.5
Glucose	33.3	138.8	50	–
Mannitol	197.6	–	–	–
Sucrose	–	–	99.3	99.3
HEPES buffer	–	–	–	10
mosmol/kg	500	320	405	400

In experiments using the three-cuff technique for rat liver transplantation – a technique which has recently been developed in our laboratory[8] – preliminary results indicate life-supporting function of livers preserved in D$_2$O–C2-S for 18 h by hypothermic ischaemic storage.

Thus our experiments show that D$_2$O significantly influences metabolism and membrane processes. It reduces cellular oedema formation in the liver similarly to a high sucrose content of the flush solution, but while sucrose acts by its osmotic effect, and cellular oedema can occur during its removal in the course of organ reperfusion, D$_2$O influences the cellular membranes directly. The D$_2$O effect on cellular metabolism is dependent on the ionic composition of the tissue fluid, as shown in Figure 27.2, and therefore it

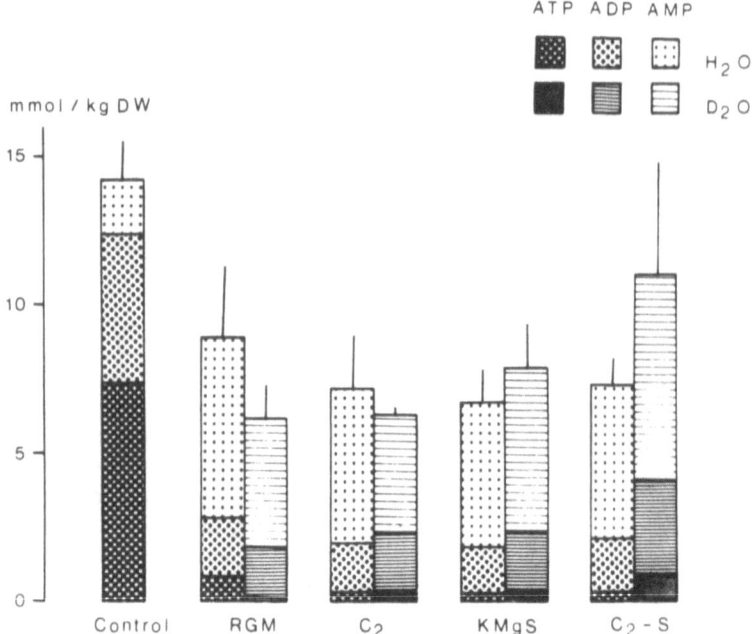

Figure 27.2 Adenine nucleotide levels in livers after 24 h of hypothermic ischaemic storage (mmol/kg dry weight, mean ± SD, $n = 5$-10 per group)

cannot be predicted for different tissues or new preservation solutions.

In transplantation experiments there is no danger of noxious effects of D_2O on the recipient because a D_2O content in the total body water up to 25% can be tolerated for long periods[9]. After transplantation of D_2O-preserved organs (kidney, liver or heart) the D_2O is immediately distributed over the whole body resulting in D_2O contents of whole body water below 5% – a value which is further reduced continuously by normal water excretion and replacement by H_2O.

Acknowledgement

This work was supported by a grant from the Deutsche Forschungs-gemeinschaft, SFB68.

References

1. Wenzel, M. and Lemm, U. (1980). Stabilization of enzymes and antisera in heavy water (D_2O). *J. Clin. Chem. Clin. Biochem.*, **18**, 684
2. Wenzel, M. (1976). Schutzeffekt von Schwerem Wasser (D_2O) bei der Schädigung von Human-Erythrocyten durch thermische und osmotische Einflüsse. *J. Clin. Chem. Clin. Biochem.*, **14**, 185

3. Fischer, J. H., Asmuth, C. and Wenzel, M. (1981). Asphyxie-Schutz durch Schweres Wasser (D$_2$O). *Experientia,* **37**, 263
4. Fischer, J. H., Kulus, D., Hansen-Schmidt, I. and Isselhard, W. (1981). Adenine nucleotide levels of canine kidneys during hypothermic aerobic or anaerobic storage in Collins' solution. *Eur. Surg. Res.,* **13**, 181
5. Lambotte, L. and Wojcik, S. (1978). Measurement of cellular oedema in anoxia and its prevention by hyperosmolar solutions. *Surgery,* **83**, 94
6. Bretschneider, H. J. (1980). Myocardial protection. *Thorac. Cardiovasc. Surg.,* **28**, 295
7. Collins, G. M., Bravo-Shugarman, M. and Terasaki, P. J. (1969). Kidney preservation for transportation. *Lancet,* **2**, 1219
8. Miyata, M., Fischer, J. H., Fuhs, M., Isselhard, W. and Kasai, Y. (1980). A simple method for orthotopic liver transplantation in the rat. *Transplantation,* **30**, 335
9. Thompson, J. F. (1963). *Biological Effects of Deuterium.* (Oxford: Pergamon Press)

28
Retrograde oxygen persufflation – a technique for preservation of ischaemically damaged organs

J. H. FISCHER and W. ISSELHARD

Hypothermic ischaemic storage (HIS) of kidneys after flush perfusion with special solutions is an effective and sufficient preservation technique for periods up to 24 h. It is widely used in transplant centres, and exclusively in Eurotransplant. But there is a problem: after periods of normothermic ischaemia only the administration of oxygen allows preservation with sufficient maintenance of viability. However, continuous perfusion techniques are not available in many transplant centres and for sufficient surface oxygenation of the whole kidney gas pressures of 7–10 atmospheres would be necessary.

Our technique – called retrograde oxygen persufflation (ROP) – achieves good oxygenation of the whole kidney without perfusion or elevated gas pressures by using a part of the vascular system for gaseous oxygen: the veins. Thus it does not contact arteries or capillaries but reaches the whole organ by diffusion from the venous system.

In canine experiments we used cold Collins' solution C2[1] for flush perfusion from a height of 100 cm. During hypothermic storage at 6 °C, gaseous oxygen was administered through the renal vein at a pressure of 50–60 mmHg (6.7–8.0 kPa). The gas escaped from capsular veins which were opened by multiple pricks with a thin needle[2] reaching a maximal depth of 1–2 mm. Measurements of renal adenine nucleotides or lactate levels demonstrate an optimal oxygenation of the whole kidney by oxygen diffusion from the persufflated veins (Figure 28.1). The energy charge potential (ECP)[3], which is significantly reduced even by the 2 min period of ischaemia necessary for cannulation of the renal vessels, is quite normal after a 24 h period of ROP preservation. The ECP is similar to the values found during continuous oxygenated perfusion and even after 24 h ROP following a 30 min period of normothermic ischaemia (NI) nearly normal ECP values are found (Figure 28.1). The maintenance of the total adenine nucleotide content (SAN = ATP + ADP + AMP) is even better in ROP than in continuous perfusion because no washout of nucleotides or their

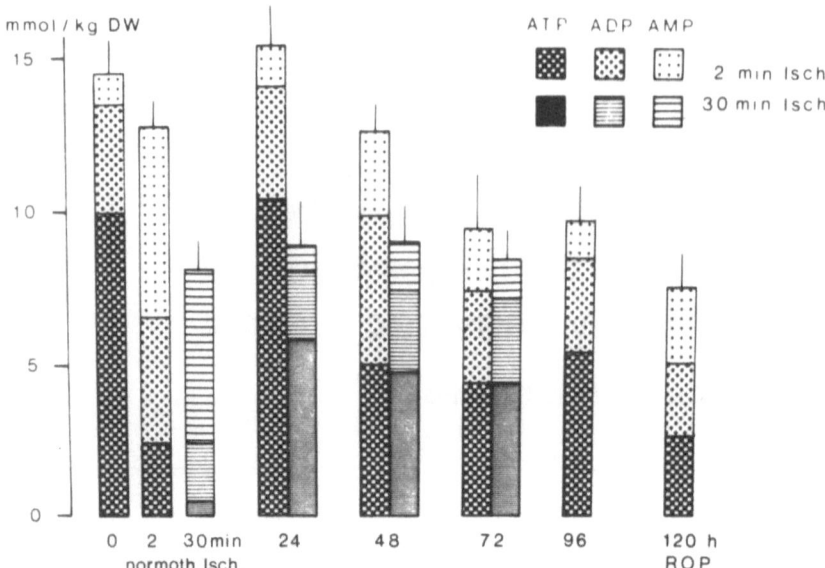

Figure 28.1 Nucleotide content of canine renal cortical tissue during ROP in Collins' C2 solution at 6 °C following initial periods of 2 or 30 min normothermic ischaemia (mean ± SD, calculated per kilogram tissue dry weight). For method, see reference no. 5. (Number of kidneys in each group: 5–11)

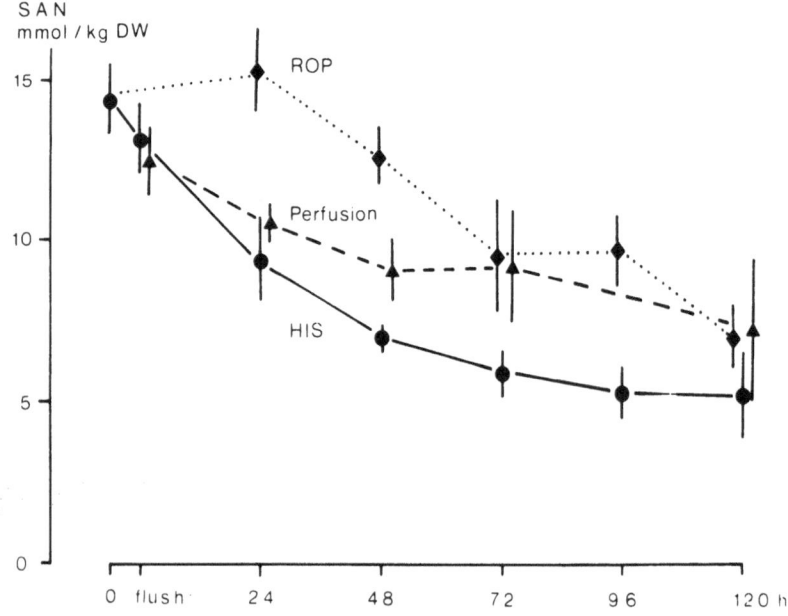

Figure 28.2 Total adenine nucleotide content (SAN = ATP + ADP + AMP) of canine renal cortex during hypothermic (6 °C) preservation (without NI) in HIS or ROP in Collins' C2 solution or continuous perfusion[4,5] (mean ± SD, number of kidneys in each group: control: 8, ROP: 5, HIS: 5, perfusion: 4)

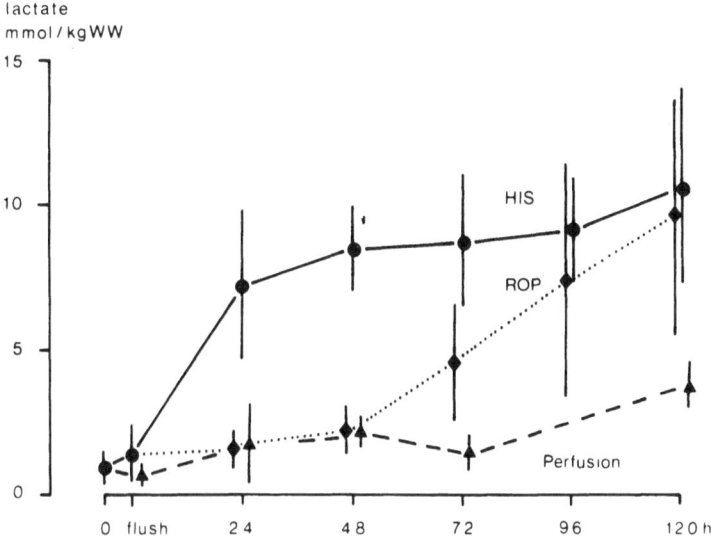

Figure 28.3 Lactate contents in canine renal cortical tissue during hypothermic preservation. Mean ± SD calculated per kilogram tissue wet weight. (The wet weight basis is chosen because lactate is dissolved in intra- and extracellular water)

metabolites occurs (Figure 28.2). During the 2nd and 3rd day of ROP preservation nucleotide levels decrease, probably because of the shortage of adequate cellular substrates for aerobic metabolism, an explanation which is supported by the increase in lactate levels after 48 h in contrast to the lack of lactate accumulation in continuously perfused kidneys[4,5] (Figure 28.3). We saw a similar effect in our continuous perfusion experiments at 6 °C[4,6]: up to 48 h oxygenated perfusion without any exogenous substrate was sufficient for renal energy production as shown by stable ECP values; thereafter only with a supply of exogenous substrate could a decrease of ECP be prevented. Even with ROP, the hypothermically (6 °C) preserved kidney is not able to restore tissue adenine nucleotides after 30 min NI. ECP and SAN values, as well as lactate levels, indicate the sufficiency of aerobic metabolism and substrate supply. But for viability testing these parameters are of limited value because a near-normal ECP can be obtained by sufficient tissue oxygenation even in severely damaged organs, and normal SAN values reflect good viability (if there is no structural damage in addition) but low SAN values can be found in viable as well as in non-viable kidneys damaged by NI. Also, an increase of lactate levels indicates problems in aerobic pathways only if glycolysis itself is not damaged by initial NI[5].

Therefore we tested the functional recovery of canine kidneys after transplantation following ROP preservation. We determined the immediate functional recovery for 3 h after transplantation of the preserved organ to the neck of the donor animal in comparison to the function of the normal contralateral kidney which remained untouched *in situ*. Constant plasma levels of 15–20 mg/100 ml inulin and 1–2 mg/100 ml PAH were produced by continuous infusion of these substances and the clearances determined for both kidneys. Figure 28.4 shows the results of these clearance tests as percentages of the function of the normal contralateral kidney (mean ± SD). 'Control transplants' were kidneys flushed with cold Ringer's solution and immediately retransplanted. '24 h perfusion' indicates a continuous oxygenated perfusion using a total volume of 200 ml of perfusate containing albumin and glucose in an extracellular type solution[4,6]. All preservations using 'storage' (HIS) or ROP were performed using Collins' C2 solution. All types of HIS and ROP experiments were performed on kidneys without NI (only 2 min NI for cannulation of the vessels) or after 30 min NI. In combinations of HIS and ROP, the storage period always preceded ROP. For 30 min NI the kidneys were totally excised, weighed and placed in the open abdomen with the temperature ranging from 31 to 33 °C. In the 24 h storage and in the 24 h ROP groups the kidneys were additionally flush-perfused with Ringer's solution at 37 °C before beginning the 30 min NI period, but the functional outcome was not different from control experiments without this additional measure[2,7].

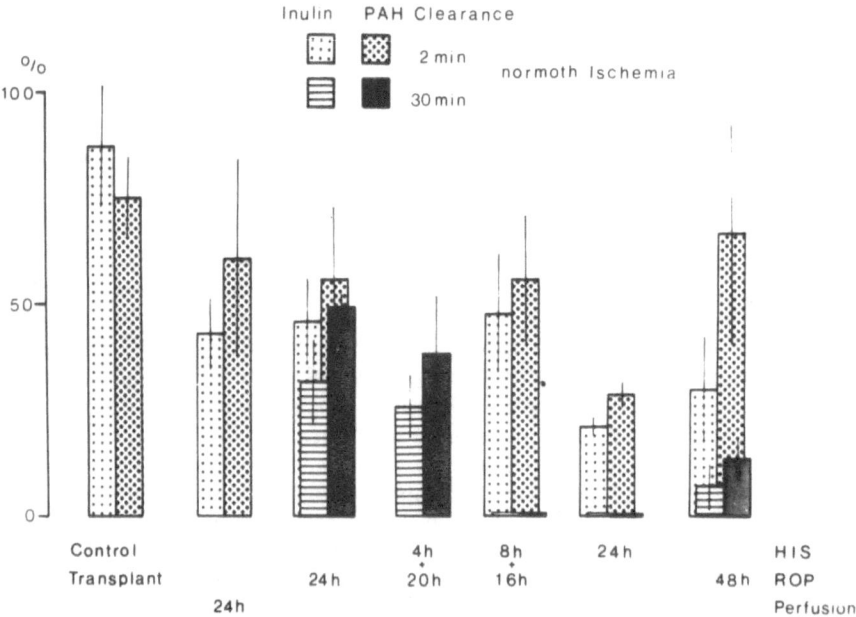

Figure 28.4 Immediate function of canine kidneys after preservation at 6 °C and autotransplantation (mean ± SD, number of kidneys in each group: 4–6)

The quality of immediate function shown in Figure 28.4 indicates that:

(1) 24 h ROP preservation results in a functional recovery similar to 24 h continuous perfusion and significantly higher than after 24 h HIS.

(2) After 30 min NI, 24 h ROP guarantees sufficient immediate function, while after 30 min NI and 24 h HIS in our experiments no
immediate functional recovery occurred.

(3) The start of ROP preservation in initially HIS-preserved kidneys can
be delayed 8 h if there is no pre-damage but for only 4 h if 30 min NI
preceded the HIS period.

(4) ROP preservation for 48 h is possible in kidneys without pre-damage
– function being especially reduced in inulin clearance (glomerular
damage or proximal tubular obstruction), while in organs damaged
by 30 min NI insufficient immediate recovery can be expected after a
2-day preservation period.

One day after the transplantation the clearance values had further
increased in the 24 h ROP-preserved (with and without NI), in the 4 h HIS
and 20 h ROP preserved organs, and also after 24 h of HIS without NI, the
increase amounting to an additional 20%. In the other groups no
significant increase was found during the first post-transplant day.

Experiments using other flush solutions with the same experimental
protocol resulted in insufficient function in most instances after 30 min NI
and 24 h ROP using gas pressures of 50–60 mmHg (6.7–8.0 kPa) (Figure
28.5 and Table 28.1). The damage in these kidneys correlates with
increasing gas flow rates, while during ROP in C2 solution a spontaneous
reduction of gas flow rates occurs[2,8]. A reduction of the gas pressure allows
ROP preservation also in these solutions, as shown by the experiment of
Ross and Escott[9]. These authors found significantly better function in
canine kidneys preserved for 24 h in hypertonic citrate solution[9,10] after
30 min NI if the organs were ROP-preserved using a gas pressure of
10–12 mmHg (1.3–1.6 kPa). It is important to realize that such a low gas
pressure results in partial oxygenation of the kidney. In our control experiments using C2 and a gas pressure of 30 mmHg (4 kPa) SAN decreased by

Table 28.1 Composition of the flush solutions. Collins' C2 solution, Sacks' solution II[11], Lambotte's solution KMgS[12], Ross' hypertonic citrate solution[10] (mmol/l)

	Collins C2	Sacks II	Lambotte KMgS	Ross Citrate	Ringer +G +M
Na$^+$	10	14	—	80	147
K$^+$	115	126	95	80	4
Ca^{++}	—	—	—	—	2
Mg^{++}	30	8	80	35	—
Cl$^-$	15	16	—	—	155
HCO$_3^-$	10	20	15	—	—
SO$_4^{2-}$	30	—	120	35	—
H$_2$PO$_4^-$, HPO$_4^{2-}$	57.5	77.5	—	—	—
Citrate	—	—	—	55	—
Glucose	138.8	—	50	—	33.3
Mannitol	—	205.9	—	186.6	98.8
Sucrose	—	—	99.3	—	—
mosmol/l	320	430	405	400	400

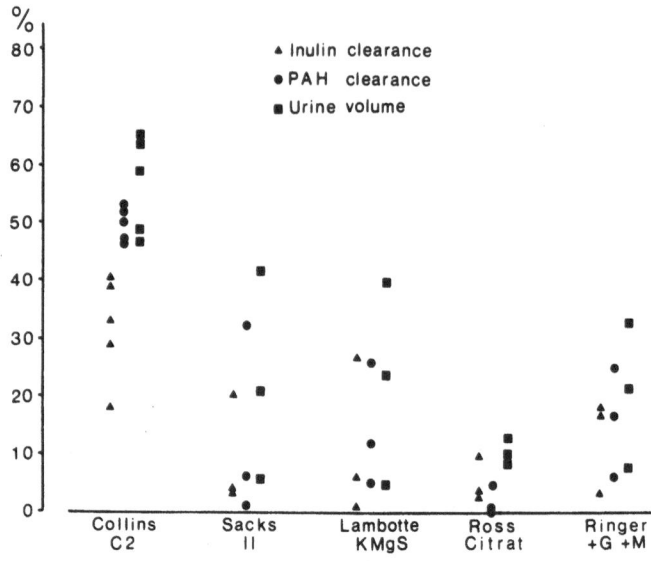

Figure 28.5 Inulin and PAH clearances and urine output of canine kidneys after autotransplantation following 30 min normothermic ischaemia and 24 h ROP preservation (6 °C, 50–60 mmHg gas pressure) using different flush solutions

27% on average in 24 h with ECP values around 0.65 and some lactate production indicating moderate hypoxia.

Thus the ROP preservation technique allows sufficient oxygenation of the whole kidney if gas pressures of 50–60 mmHg (6.7–8.0 kPa) are applied and it results in sufficient aerobic energy production from endogenous substrates for 24–48 h. ROP guarantees immediate functional recovery of kidneys pre-damaged by up to 30 min NI after a 24 h preservation period if Collins' C2 solution is used, and it is also effective after short initial periods of HIS preservation. Even reduced oxygen gas pressures – necessary for ROP with other flush solutions – seem to be effective and to result in some improvement of renal functional recovery.

Acknowledgement

This work was supported by a grant from the Deutsche Forschungs-gemeinschaft, SFB68.

References

1. Collins, G. M., Bravo-Shugarman, M. and Terasaki, P. I. (1969). Kidney preservation for transportation. Initial perfusion and 30-hour ice storage. *Lancet*, **2**, 1219
2. Fischer, J. H., Czerniak, A., Hauer, U. and Isselhard, W. (1978). A new simple method for optimal storage of ischaemically damaged kidneys. *Transplantation*, **25**, 43
3. Atkinson, D. E. (1968). The energy charge of the adenylate pool as a regulatory parameter. Interaction with feedback modifiers. *Biochemistry NY*, **7**, 4030

4. Fischer, J. H., Armbruster, D., Grebe, W., Czerniak, A. and Isselhard, W. (1980). Effects of differences in substrate supply on the energy metabolism of hypothermically perfused canine kidneys. *Cryobiology,* **17,** 135

5. Fischer, J. H., Kulus, D., Hansen-Schmidt, I. and Isselhard, W. (1981). Adenine nucleotide levels of canine kidneys during hypothermic aerobic or anaerobic storage in Collins' solution. *Eur. Surg. Res.,* **13,** 181

6. Fischer, J. H., Isselhard, W., Hauer, U. and Menge, M. (1979). Free fatty acid and glucose metabolism during hypothermic perfusion of canine kidneys. *Eur. Surg. Res.,* **11,** 107

7. Fischer, J. H., Czerniak, A., Kulus, D., Hansen-Schmidt, I. and Isselhard, W. (1979). Persufflations-Konservierung von Nieren in intrazellulären Lösungen über 48 und 72 Stunden. In Schellerer, W. and Schildberg, F. W. (eds.) *Chirurgie aktuell. Vol. 5: Aktuelles aus der Abdominal- und Unfallchirurgie,* pp. 257–259. (Erlangen: Peri'med)

8. Fischer, J. H., Miyata, M., Isselhard, W. and Casser, H. R. (1979). Hypotherme Lagerung unter aeroben Bedingungen – Einfluss unterschiedlicher Freispüllösungen auf die Funktionserhaltung der Niere. *Arch. Klin. Chir., Suppl. Chir. Forum,* p. 307

9. Ross, H. and Escott, M. L. (1979). Gaseous oxygen perfusion of the renal vessels as an adjunct in kidney preservation. *Transplantation,* **28,** 362

10. Ross, H., Marshall, V. C. and Escott, M. L. (1976). 72 hr canine kidney preservation without continuous perfusion. *Transplantation,* **21,** 498

11. Sacks, S. A., Petritsch, P. H. and Kaufman, J. J. (1973). Canine kidney preservation using a new perfusate. *Lancet,* **1,** 1024

12. Lambotte, L. and Wojcik, S. (1978). Measurement of cellular edema in anoxia and its prevention by hyperosmolar solutions. *Surgery,* **83,** 94

PART V
PRESERVATION BY CONTINUOUS PERFUSION

29
Kidney preservation by continuous perfusion

R. W. G. JOHNSON

Artificial perfusion has been a tool of physiological research for more than 100 years; over the last 20 years these techniques have been applied to the objective of organ preservation for transplantation and what started as an empirical art form allowing inconsistent 10–24 h storage has improved to an unsophisticated science in which 24 h storage is a fact and 8-day storage an occasional possibility.

Isolated warm perfusions of the kidney with a study of urine production were first reported by Richards and Plant in 1922[1] and similar investigations have since been described by other authors[2,3]. Carrel[4] tried to perfuse individual organs by combining previous techniques with the antiseptic methods developed during the First World War and a sterilizable perfusion apparatus; this failed entirely. Following Lindbergh's design of a coil apparatus which could be kept sterile, and a pump whereby pulsatile circulation of fluid could be maintained and properly oxygenated, Carrel was able to perfuse a cat's thyroid for 18 days. The perfusing fluid was cat serum in Tyrode solution. The gas mixture was carbon dioxide, 3%; oxygen 21%; and nitrogen 76%. Kidneys, he found, were more refractory and degenerated rapidly.

From his extensive experience of organ perfusion Carrel was able in a few sentences to set down requirements for artificial perfusions that still stand today:

> The life of the perfused tissue depends on many factors. The fluid must be free from floating particles that may act as emboli. If blood is used there should be no agglutinated corpuscles. The temperature, the osmotic pressure, pH of the fluid, the pulse rate, the maximum pressure and the minimum pressure have to be exactly adjusted. The chemical composition of the nutrient medium and its oxygenation are of capital importance. Moreover it is imperative that the organ be free from all bacteria. Even if all conditions save one are satisfactory the result of the experiment is utter failure.

It only needs to be added that perfusate distribution needs to be uniform within the vascular compartment for adequate tissue nourishment. The problems which affect organ perfusion are in essence supply and distribution.

What then are the minimum requirements merely to sustain life? How do these requirements vary with temperature, duration of perfusion and the specific identity of the organ?

Adequate answers require a precise biochemical definition of life itself. Current preservation experiments, however empirical, show that kidneys may be kept alive for periods of up to 8 days if they are offered oxygen, an energy-rich substrate such as glucose, and electrolyte and colloid concentrations appropriate for the maintenance of reasonable oncotic and ionic balance across capillary and cellular membranes. There remains the unsettled possibility that hormones, vitamins, amino acids, polypeptides and lipids may singly or severally be necessary for the subtler demands of long-term perfusion. Carrel and Lindbergh more than any other authors made it clear that even relatively crude synthetic media may nourish some organs for days or weeks. Thus, however incomplete and imprecise our fundamental knowledge of baseline metabolic requirements, the devising of satisfactory perfusates has not proved impossible.

The limiting factors in contemporary preservation experiments in so far as they have been identified have centred on technical problems with the perfusion apparatus and vascular events in the organ being perfused. Both phenomena mainly affect the second requirement for preservation by perfusion; *viz.*: uniform distribution to all cells. Distribution of the perfusate throughout the organ presents the greatest difficulty in precisely those organs with which clinical transplantation is concerned: the kidney and the liver.

Early perfusion experiments concentrated on the use of whole or diluted blood at room temperature or at 37 °C. Perfusions with blood commonly met with a marked increase in renal vascular resistance within a few minutes of starting: the so-called 'outflow block'. Animal experiments implicated multiple contributing factors including microvascular blockage by cellular aggregates and vascular responses consequent upon neural, humoral and intrinsic effects. Noradrenalin was found[1] to cause swelling and a rise in perfusion pressure. Trueta[5] described a renal response to trauma in which cortical blood flow was differentially abolished and the arterial blood was shunted through juxtamedullary arteriovenous connections. This phenomenon has been demonstrated in dogs[6]: both kidneys exhibited absence of cortical staining and increased amounts of Indian ink were found in the corticomedullary junction as a response to simple mobilization of one kidney. In arteriographic studies in dogs[7] perfused with Ringer lactate and low molecular weight dextran at 10 °C, cortical perfusion was better when vascular collapse was prevented by maintaining a venous pressure of about $10 \text{ cmH}_2\text{O}$. Infiltration of the renal pedicle with procaine or incorporation of procaine in the perfusate has been used in canine and porcine renal perfusion by many authors[8,9].

The phenomenon of outflow block could also be minimized by

maintaining oxygen and CO_2 at near normal levels and hypothermia seemed to delay the onset of the block[10,11]. Austen and McLoughlin[12] compared pulsatile against steady pressure and found much better flow and sustenance of tissues with pulsatile flow. Any artificial perfusion of necessity introduces interfaces, solid or gaseous, which by their very nature are not physiological and have been found to induce changes in blood that are inimical to the conduct of perfusion. Whole blood seems relatively unaltered by the surfaces of modern plastics such as PVC and silicone rubber, and there is reason to believe that oxygenators are the principal culprits in inducing erythrocyte and platelet aggregation[13,14], denaturation of proteins[15] and release of histamine and serotonin[16]. The polarizing forces which exist at any liquid–gas interface are very effective in denaturing proteins. Glass wool filtration is an effective method of removing microemboli[13]. When hypothermia is combined with perfusion, blood becomes a less suitable perfusate for two reasons: the oxygen dissociation curve with haemoglobin shifts to the right and there is avid uptake of oxygen but no release at $10\,°C$[17]. Secondly, the viscosity of blood increases markedly[18]. Humphries[9] used blood diluted with a balanced salt solution and then serum and plasma to perfuse dogs' kidneys at $10\,°C$ with a pulsatile pressure of $40–110\,mmHg$ in a circuit that included a membrane oxygenator and a glasswool filter; although he obtained $24–48\,h$ of preservation and was even able to perfuse viable kidneys for $72\,h$ on occasion his results were very inconsistent.

Problems continued to exist with prolonged perfusions using acellular fluids at low temperatures. The kidneys became oedematous and developed increasing vascular resistance. The oedema was reduced if albumin, or to some extent if dextran, was added to the perfusate. Two factors contributed to the renal vascular resistance: spasm, which could be reduced with procaine or papaverine, and the presence of a particulate material in the perfusate. Conventional microscopic studies showed no evidence of thrombi; however, when frozen sections were taken fat stains revealed multiple small emboli in renal arterioles and fat droplets in the tubules and intratubular cells. Rapid thawing of freeze-dried plasma causes lipoproteins to flocculate. The flocculation could be removed by passing the plasma under pressure through banks of micropore filters of pore diameter 1.2, 0.45 and $0.22\,\mu m$. Perfusion of the kidney with this filtered plasma completely eliminated rise in perfusion pressure. After $72\,h$ of perfusion kidney function was proven by reimplantation with immediate contralateral nephrectomy[19].

Cryoprecipitated plasma as described by Belzer, however, was rather difficult and time-consuming to prepare. Its composition was also variable, especially in terms of its fat content. The low density lipoproteins present in plasma, even after microfiltration, remain unstable and continue to precipitate in the presence of extremes of temperature, pH and ionic strength of upon exposure to interfaces such as gas–liquid. The clear plasma which Belzer obtained after preliminary denaturation and subsequent microfiltration becomes layered and cloudy if allowed to stand[20]. Belzer overcame this problem by making up his perfusate fresh and avoiding gas–liquid interfaces by introducing a sophisticated silicone rubber oxygenator and using scrupulous adjustment of pH. These developments, together with the initial microfiltration, resulted in an escalation both of cost and complexity.

Albumen-based perfusates eliminate the need for microfiltration and provide a stable perfusate of predictable composition. The first of these was modified plasma protein fraction (PPF) introduced by Johnson in 1971[21,22]. The perfusate was human albumen (4.5 g%) dissolved in saline. It contained no unstable lipoproteins, no fibrinogen and no gamma-globulin, it was hepatitis-free and contained no blood group antibodies. PPF required the addition of sugar, potassium and a bicarbonate buffer[23]. Using PPF, dog kidneys were stored for 24 h after up to 60 min of warm ischaemia[24] on a much simplified apparatus and for 72 h[23] in the absence of warm ischaemia. A second solution based on Kabi albumen but of essentially the same composition was introduced by Claes and Blohmé[25] and they were able to achieve 96 h storage on a much simplified Gambro machine. Cryoprecipitated plasma and the albumen-based perfusates have now been in use in clinical practice for 10 years. They have been used on a wide variety of machines with equally satisfactory results. More recently plasma treated with silica gel has been introduced as a perfusate[26,27]. Silica gel removes fibrinogen, cholesterol and lipoproteins.

In the laboratory attempts to increase storage times have continued. Storage times have been progressively extended from 4 days[25] through 5 days[28,23,29]; 7 days[30,23,29] to 8 days[29]. With extension of time the method has become progressively less predictable and much effort has been expended in trying to determine the factors which limit machine storage[23,31].

Perfusate volume has been considered by some authors to be critical[32,33,31]. 800 ml was thought to be the minimum volume required to prevent trace substrate exhaustion and to dilute accumulating ammonia. In fact, perfusate volume is not as critical as has been suggested. Kidneys have been successfully stored for up to 8 days[34,29] with a perfusate volume of only 400 ml and without perfusate exchange. No benefit has ever been established for perfusate exchange; on the contrary it has been shown that a fresh kidney can be successfully stored for 24 h in perfusate that has previously been used for 3-day storage[35]. This experiment is not conclusive since a fresh kidney can easily be stored under anaerobic conditions for 24 h and it may be that the organ's intrinsic stores are sufficient for 24 h.

Accumulation of ammonia is not a consistent feature of long-term kidney perfusion although rising pH is a problem. Cohen[29] was unable to demonstrate ammonia in the perfusate during 5- and 8-day storage but there was a continuous release of bicarbonate, produced presumably from aerobic glycolysis.

Oxygen consumption and glucose utilization are well-established features of continuous hypothermic pefusion. It is most unlikely that shortage of oxygen is a critical feature as the volume consumed is so small: 0.0012 ml/g/min at 10 °C after equilibration. Substrate exhaustion is also unlikely in quantity although it may be deficient in quality. The kidney is able to utilize a wide range of substrate even at 10 °C. Huang and her colleagues[36] first demonstrated the utilization of oleate and this was confirmed by Petterson[37] who in a comprehensive study demonstrated that the kidney has a preference for short-chain fatty acids which are utilized for energy production to the same extent as glucose. It has further been shown that ischaemically injured kidneys can replace their depleted ATP stores during continuous hypothermic perfusion in the presence of oxygen, glucose and hypoxanthine[38].

Physical factors have been implicated in limiting perfusion storage. Endothelial injury is a fact and it has always seemed likely that indifferent pumping techniques might be responsible. No-one has yet been able to show a significant difference between pulsatile and non-pulsatile perfusion[39,40] but these experiments have all been confined to storage intervals of less than 48 h. All of the very long perfusion successes have been with pulsatile flow and low perfusion pressures, < 40 mmHg. Despite the steady extension of storage time, little is known about the metabolic needs of the kidney during prolonged storage. Enzyme studies indicate that the kidney starts to decline from the start of cold storage and that continuous perfusion merely slows the rate[23]. Van der Wijk et al.[41] have shown that the kidney can be 'recharged' by removing it from the machine and allowing 2 h of warm circulation with a host dog's blood. The kidney then tolerates a further 3 days of storage with excellent preservation producing a total of 6 days of storage with low serum creatinines in the recipient. Whether this benefit is from rewarming or from provision of missing nutrients remains to be seen.

PRESERVATION OF ISCHAEMICALLY INJURED KIDNEYS

Twenty-four and 48-h preservation have been achieved by simple hypothermia, using intracellular electrolyte solutions, hypertonic solutions, and hypertonic citrate; by a combination of hypothermia and hyperbaria, and by continuous hypothermic perfusion. It is important to test these methods in circumstances resembling the clinical situation and to determine their safety margins. Since cadaver kidneys have most often been exposed to ischaemic injury prior to preservation it is important to evaluate storage methods with ischaemically injured kidneys. Frost[42] was the first to point out that kidneys subjected to 15 min warm ischaemia failed to function after 24 h of storage using Collins' solution. This finding was independently confirmed by Johnson[24] who also showed that kidneys subjected to up to 45 min of warm ischaemia functioned immediately after 24 h of machine preservation. Johnson et al.[23] have also reported successful 48 h machine storage after 30 min of warm ischaemia. Both Toledo-Pereyra et al.[43] and Ross and Escott[44] have shown that kidneys do not function well after warm ischaemic injury when stored by simple hypothermia with either Sacks' solution or hypertonic citrate. Ross has shown that this problem can be resolved by bubbling oxygen into the renal vein during storage, suggesting that it is the oxygen debt that is the problem and this is made worse in an anaerobic environment. When the pathogenesis of cold injury and ischaemic injury is considered it is not surprising that a kidney that has already acquired an oxygen debt as a result of ischaemic injury will indeed be made worse when placed in a situation where its oxygen debt cannot be corrected.

In organ preservation two factors operate which interfere with cell volume regulation: one is cooling itself, which effectively turns off the sodium pump by its effect on chemical reaction rates. The other is anoxia which reduces the synthesis of the ATP necessary to run the sodium pump. Cooling at present is unavoidable and its effects appear to be readily and completely reversible on rewarming as long as sufficient ATP is available.

The effect of anoxia is more serious because it appears to be less readily recoverable. Anoxic injury is characteristically associated with a mottled, cyanosed, vasospastic kidney. The failure of blood flow to return to a kidney that has suffered a period of warm injury was first described by Sheehan and Davis[45] and is known as the 'no-reflow' phenomenon. There is no doubt that this is a very important factor in determining the success of kidneys preserved after warm injury.

A number of authors[5,6,31] have demonstrated changes in distribution of the kidney microcirculation in response to handling, hypovolaemic shock and warm ischaemia. Ischaemia increases renal vascular resistance[46] but this is not due to intravascular coagulation since it is not improved by heparinization. Prevention of vascular collapse by simultaneous clamping of artery and vein was beneficial[46] and in Johnson's study[47] of continuous perfusion it was found that vascular resistance of ischaemically damaged kidneys decreased during perfusion until after 12 h it was similar to undamaged kidneys. This finding has been confirmed in rabbit kidneys[31]. Pretreatment with chlorpromazine also prevents the no-reflow phenomenon[46,48]. High vascular resistance is therefore at least partly responsible for the difficulty in preserving ischaemically injured kidneys.

Flores et al.[49] have suggested that pretreatment with mannitol prevents swelling of the endothelium and blockage of the vessels. However, after anoxic injury mannitol alone does not improve renal blood flow whereas administration of Dextran 40 to prevent cell sludging does. This finding fits into Pegg's hypothesis[31] that it is blockage of the microcirculation by rigid anoxic red cells that causes the no-reflow phenomenon. Anoxic red cells rapidly become depleted of ATP and under these circumstances Ca^{2+}, which would normally be chelated by ATP, binds with cell membrane rendering it more rigid[50].

Direct experimental evidence for the importance of adenine nucleotide reserves and particularly ATP in warm ischaemia is strong; the adenine nucleotide content of kidneys subjected to warm ischaemia correlates with their ability to support life[51,52]. Bergstrom and his colleagues[53] showed how rapidly ATP levels declined; they also provided important evidence that the maintenance of high ATP reserves correlated with the effectiveness of different preservation methods. ATP levels were best maintained by continuous perfusion; indeed it has recently been shown that ischaemically injured kidneys can resynthesize ATP during continuous hypothermic perfusion in the presence of oxygen, glucose and hypoxanthine[38].

Continuous perfusion has been in use since 1967 and is the method of choice in 82% of American centres[54].

Machine preservation is expensive and, despite considerable modification in design and in perfusate composition, it is a much more complex technique. Transportation on a machine is altogether more difficult. The advantages are very much prolonged safe storage time and the safe preservation of ischaemic kidneys. The continuous washout of metabolic by-products, with buffering and provision of an aerobic milieu, means that oxygen debt is rapidly corrected and that energy stores are conserved. In addition patency of the microcirculation is maintained. The merits of machine storage must not be exaggerated; bad technique with machine storage is disastrous and leads to unnecessary wastage. Some centres have reserved machine storage for testing doubtful kidneys. This creates two problems: firstly, through lack of practice they are unlikely to be able to make a realistic judgement; and secondly, through inferior technique they are likely to damage the organ further. It is true that machine preservation provides an opportunity for continuous monitoring of the kidney during storage; there are, however, no reliable tests of deterioration during storage. The only tests that have been shown to be beneficial are those that indicate probability of immediate function rather than likelihood of primary non-function.

It has also been suggested that continuous perfusion with cryo-precipitated homologous plasma is associated with an increased rate of early graft loss[55]. This has been attributed to an immunological injury caused by cytotoxic IgM present in homologous plasma[56].

Albumin-based perfusates have also been widely used in clinical practice. These perfusates contain no immunoglobulins and no blood-group antibodies. There has never been any association between them and early graft failure. Excellent immediate function has been reported for human kidneys after up to 45 h of machine storage[57] with plasma protein fraction. Continuous perfusion is not for the occasional user. In practised hands it provides the highest quality of preservation for the longest period of time.

References

1. Richards, A. N. and Plant, O. H. (1922). Urine formation in the perfused kidney. *Am. J. Physiol.,* **59**, 184
2. Bayliss, L. E. and Ogden, E. (1932). 'Vasotonins' and the pump-oxygenator kidney preparation. *J. Physiol.,* **77**, 34
3. Hemingway, A. (1931). Some observations on the perfusion of the isolated kidney by a pump. *J. Physiol. (Lond.),* **7**, 201
4. Carrel, A. and Lindbergh, C. A. (1938). *The Culture of Organs.* (New York: Paul B. Hoeber Inc.)
5. Trueta, J. (1947). *Studies of the Renal Circulation.* (Oxford: Blackwell Scientific Publications)
6. Hardaway, R. M., McKay, D. G. and Hollowell, O. W. (1961). Vascular spasm and disseminated intravascular coagulation. *Arch. Surg.,* **83**, 31
7. Defalco, A. J., Mundth, E. D., Brettschneider, L., Jacobsen, Y. G. and McClenathan, J. E. (1965). A possible explanation for transplant anuria. *Surg. Gynecol. Obstet.,* **121**, 748

8. Telander, R. L. (1962). Prolonged normothermic perfusion of the isolated baboon and sheep kidney with maintenance of function. *Surg. Forum,* **13**

9. Humphries, A. L., Moretz, W. H. and Converse-Pierce, E (1964). 24 hour kidney storage with report of a successful canine autotransplant after total nephrectomy. *Surgery,* **55,** 524

10. Kestens, P. J., Austen, W. G. and McDermott, W. V. (1959). Biochemical and physiological studies on the viable extracorporeal liver. *Surg. Forum,* **10,** 225

11. Kestens, P. J. and McDermott, W. V. (1961). Perfusion and replacement of the canine liver. *Surgery,* **50,** 196

12. Austen, W. G. and McLoughlin, E. D. (1965). In vitro small bowel perfusion. *Surg. Forum,* **16,** 359

13. Belzer, F. O., Hatsumi, Y., Park, B. S. and Vetto, R. M. (1964). Factors influencing renal blood flow during isolated perfusion. *Surg. Forum,* **15,** 222

14. Swank, R. L., Fellman, J. H. and Hissen, W. W. (1963). Aggregation of RBCs by 5-hydroxytryptamine. *Circulat. Res.,* **13,** 392

15. Lee, W. H., Krumhaar, D., Fonkalsrud, E. W., Schjeide, O. A. and Maloney, J. V. (1961). Denaturation of plasma proteins as a cause of morbidity and death after cardiac operations. *Surgery,* **50,** 29

16. Huggins, C. E. (1961). Survival of hamsters after 4 hours of cardiac arrest at 0°C. *Surg. Forum,* **12,** 413

17. Callaghan, P. B., Lider, J., Paton, B. C. and Swan, H. (1961). Effect of varying carbon dioxide tensions on. the oxy-haemoglobin association curves under hypothermic conditions. *Ann. Surg.,* **154,** 903

18. Humphries, A. L. (1967). Problems of organ preservation. *Transplantation,* **5,** 1138

19. Belzer, F. O., Ashby, B. S. and Dunphy, J. E. (1967). 24 and 72 hour preservation of canine kidneys. *Lancet,* **2,** 536

20. Belzer, F. O., Ashby, B. S., Huang, J. S. and Dunphy, J. E. (1968). Aetiology of rising perfusion pressure in isolated organ perfusion. *Ann. Surg.,* **168,** 382

21. Johnson, R. W. G., Anderson, M., Flear, C. T. G., Murray, S., Swinney, J. and Taylor, R. M. R. (1971). Evaluation of a new perfusate for kidney preservation. *Eur. Surg. Res.,* **3,** 215

22. Johnson, R. W. G., Anderson, M., Flear, C. T. G., Murray, S., Swinney, J. and Taylor, R. M. R. (1972). Evaluation of a new perfusate for kidney preservation. *Transplantation,* **13,** 270

23. Johnson, R. W. G., Cohen, G. L. and Ballardie, F. W. (1979). The limitations of continuous perfusion with plasma protein fraction. In Pegg, D. E. and Jacobsen, I. A. (eds.) *Organ Preservation II,* p. 18. (Edinburgh: Churchill-Livingstone)

24. Johnson, R. W. G., Anderson, M., Morley, A. R., Taylor, R. M. R. and Swinney, J. (1972). Twenty four hour preservation of kidneys injured by prolonged warm ischaemia. *Transplantation,* **13,** 174

25. Claes, G. and Blohmé, I. (1971). Klinisk användning av kontinverlig perfusion för njurpreservation. *Nord. Med.,* **86,** 881

26. Toledo-Pereyra, L. H., Condie, R. M., Callender, C. O., Mozes, M. F., Moberg, A. W., Santiago-Delphin, E. A., Simmons, R. L. and Najarian, J. S. (1974). Hypothermic pulsatile kidney preservation. *Arch. Surg.,* **109,** 816

27. Toledo-Pereyra, L. H., Condie, R. M., Malmberg, R., Simmons, R. L. and Najarian, J. S. (1974). A fibrinogen free perfusate for preservation of kidneys for 120 hours. *Surg. Gynaecol. Obstet.,* **138,** 901

28. Woods, J. E. (1971). Successful three- to seven-day preservation of canine kidneys. *Arch. Surg.,* **102,** 614

29. Cohen, G. L. and Johnson, R. W. G. (1978). Optimum perfusate pH for 5- and 7-day canine kidney preservation. *Br. J. Surg.,* **65,** 823

30. Liu, W. P., Humphries, A. L., Russell, R., Stoddard, L. D., Garcia, L. A. and Serkes, K. D. (1973). 3- and 7-day perfusion of dog kidneys with human plasma protein fraction IV-4. *Surg. Forum,* **24,** 316

31. Pegg, D. E. (1978). An approach to hypothermic renal preservation. *Cryobiology,* **15,** 1

32. Abouna, G. M., Lim, F., Cook, J. S., Grubb, W., Craig, S. S., Seibel, H. R. and Hume, D. M. (1972). 3-day canine kidney preservation. *Surgery,* **71,** 436

33. Grundman, R., Berr, F., Pitschi, H., Kirchloff, R. and Pichlmaier, H. (1974). 96-hour preservation of canine kidneys. *Transplantation,* **17,** 299
34. Cohen, G. L. and Johnson, R. W. G. (1980). Perfusate buffering for 8-day canine kidney storage. *Proc. Eur. Soc. Artif. Org.,* **7,** 235
35. Williams, J. T., Hoffman, R. and Belzer, F. O. (1973). Lack of correlation between periodic perfusate changes and subsequent renal function. *Transplantation,* **15,** 629
36. Huang, J. S., Downes, G. L. and Belzer, F. O. (1971). Utilization of fatty acids in perfused hypothermic dog kidneys. *J. Lipid Res.,* **12,** 622
37. Petterson, S., Claes, G. and Schersten, T. (1974). Fatty acid and glucose utilization during continuous hypothermic perfusion of dog kidney. *Eur. Surg. Res.,* **6,** 79
38. Pegg, D. E., Wusteman, M. C. and Foreman, J. (1981). Metabolism of normal and ischaemically injured rabbit kidneys during perfusion for 48 hours at 10 °C. *Transplantation,* **32,** 437
39. Pegg, D. E. and Green, C. J. (1973). Renal preservation by hypothermic perfusion. The importance of pressure control. *Cryobiology,* **10,** 56
40. Pegg, D. E. and Green, C. J. (1976). Renal preservation by hypothermic perfusion. The lack of influence of pulsatile flow. *Cryobiology,* **13,** 161
41. Van der Wijk, J., Sloof, M. J. H., Rijkmans, B. G. and Kootstra, G. (1980). Successful 96 and 144 hour experimental kidney preservation. *Cryobiology,* **17,** 473
42. Frost, A. B., Ackerman, J., Finch, W. T. and Manlove, A. (1970). Kidney preservation for transportation. *Lancet,* **1,** 620
43. Toledo-Pereyra, L. H. and Condie, R. M. (1978). Comparison of Sacks solution and a new colloid hyperosmolar solution for hypothermic renal storage. *Transplantation,* **26,** 166
44. Ross, H. and Escott, M. L. (1979). Gaseous oxygen perfusion of the renal vessels as an adjunct to kidney preservation. *Transplantation,* **28,** 362
45. Sheehan, H. L. and Davis, J. C. (1959). Renal ischaemia with failed reflow. *J. Pathol. Bacteriol.,* **78,** 105
46. Løkkegaard, H. and Bilde, T. (1972). Vascular resistance in hypothermically perfused kidneys following 1 hour of warm ischaemia. *Acta. Med. Scand.,* **191,** 429
47. Johnson, R. W. G. (1972). The effect of ischaemic injury on kidneys preserved for 24 hours before transplantation. *Br. J. Surg.,* **59,** 10
48. Løkkegaard, H., Bilde, T., Gyrde-Hansen, N., Jaglicic, D., Jensen, E., Nerstrom, B. and Rasmussen, F. (1973). The effect of chlorpromazine on preservation of kidneys with one hour's warm ischaemia. Renal clearance in pigs with autotransplanted 24-hour preserved kidneys. *Acta Med. Scand.,* **189,** 243
49. Flores, J., Di Bona, D. R., Frega, N. and Leaf, A. (1972). Cell volume regulation and ischaemic tissue damage. *J. Membrane Biol.,* **10,** 331
50. Weed, R. I., La Celle, P. I. and Merrill, E. W. (1969). Metabolic dependence of red cell deformability. *J. Clin. Invest.,* **48,** 795
51. Calman, K. C. (1974). The prediction of organ viability. *Cryobiology,* **11,** 1
52. Calman, K. C. (1974). The prediction of organ viability. Testing the hypothesis. *Cryobiology,* **11,** 7
53. Bergstrom, J., Collste, H., Groth, C. G., Hultman, E. and Melia, B. (1971). Water, electrolyte and metabolite content of cortical tissue from dog kidneys preserved by hypothermia. *Proc. Eur. Dialysis Transplant Assoc.,* **8,** 313
54. Belzer, F. O. and Southard, J. H. (1980). The future of kidney preservation. *Transplantation,* **30,** 161
55. Clarke, E. A., Terasaki, P. I., Opelz, G. and Mickey, M. R. (1974). Cadaver kidney transplant failures at 1 month. *N. Engl. J. Med.,* **291,** 1099
56. Light, J. A., Annable, C., Perloff, L. J., Sulkin, M. D., Hill, G. S., Etheredge, E. E. and Spees, E. K. (1975). Immune injury from organ preservation. *Transplantation,* **19,** 511
57. Johnson, R. W. G., Cohen, G. L., Mallick, N. P. and Orr, W. McN. (1979). Renal function and early cadaver graft survival after continuous hypothermic perfusion with plasma protein fraction (PPF). *Transplant. Proc.,* **11,** 1476

30
Continuous perfusion and transplantation of rat kidneys

T. ANDRÉEN, L. FRÖDIN and B. HARVIG

The advantages of hypothermic storage have lately been discussed by Marshall[1] and Collins[2], and continuous perfusion by Belzer[3]. Both methods are excellent for clinical use but further research is necessary to explain what happens in the kidney during the hypothermic state and what changes are of importance for functional restitution after transplantation.

In our laboratories morphology, circulation and function in the rat kidney have been studied after hypothermic storage and transplantation[4-7]. The present work was necessitated by the need of a model for studies of continuous perfusion of rat kidneys to compare this method of preservation with hypothermic storage.

METHODS

Sixty-six male Sprague–Dawley rats (250–400 g) were used for the experiments. The donor rats were anaesthetized by intraperitoneal Inactin® 120 mg/kg and the recipients by ether. The operations were performed under controlled temperature conditions. Donor rats were pretreated with phenoxybenzamine 1.3 mg/kg and heparin 100 IU. Initial perfusion and operative procedures, donor-operation and transplantation were performed according to Harvig and Norlén[8].

Warm ischaemia was 5 min. Continuous perfusion was started without interruption of the flow immediately after initial perfusion in a lucite micropuncture cup. The temperature was kept constant by an ice-bath at +6 to +8 °C. The perfusion was performed by a roller-pump (LKB 2115) and constant flow was used with continuous registration of perfusion pressures by a pressure transducer (Statham P37). Oxygen was not actively added but the surface of the perfusate was open to air. Temperature was registered continuously by a needle thermistor inserted into the renal parenchyma. After an initial perfusion of 20 min the perfusate was recirculated through the kidney (Figure 30.1).

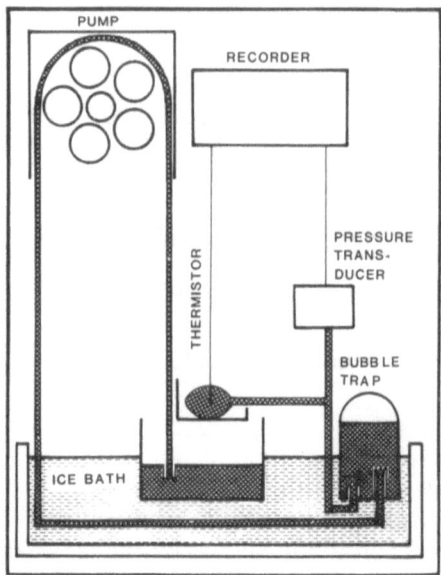

Figure 30.1 Perfusion model

The following perfusates were used: Perfudex® (Pharmacia), a modified Collins solution with 5% albumin added and an extracellular electrolyte solution with 6% albumin. The compositions of the perfusates are listed in Table 30.1.

Table 30.1 Composition of perfusates

	A Perfudex	B Modified Collins solution + 5% albumin	C Extracellular + 6% albumin
Cl⁻ (mmol/l)	142.0	15.2	83.10
Na⁺ (mmol/l)	138.0	9.3	87.76
K⁺ (mmol/l)	6.0	118.0	4.10
PO_4^{2-} (mmol/l)		57.6	
HCO_3 (mmol/l)	1.0	12.0	8.76
Mg^{2+} (mmol/l)			5.13
SO_4^{2-} (mmol/l)	0.8		5.13
$H_2PO_4^- HPO_4^{2-}$ (mmol/l)	0.8		
Dextran 40 (g/l)	50.0		58.39
Glucose (g/l)		50.0	11.24
Albumin (g/l)		50.0	58.39

Cold ischaemia was 6, 12 and 16 h. Transplantation was performed in 37 recipients. Flow of perfusate during the initial perfusion was 1.3 or 0.9 ml/min and during continuous perfusion 1.3, 0.5 or 0.3 ml/min. In groups 1 and 2 perfusion was performed without transplantation, whereas in groups 3, 4, 5, 6 and 7 transplantation was done. The experimental groups are characterized in Table 30.2.

All recipients were followed postoperatively with regard to survival and body weight. In groups 5, 6 and 7 plasma creatinine and haematocrits were followed. In four cases in groups 6 and 7 the kidney wet weight before and after continuous perfusion was registered.

Table 30.2 Characteristics of the experimental groups

			Group				
	1	*2*	*3*	*4*	*5*	*6*	*7*
Number of kidneys	4	4	8	10	6	8	5
Cold ischaemia (hours)	20	8	16	12	6	12	6
Perfusate	A	B	C	C	C	C	C
Flow rate (ml/min) — Initial perfusion	1.3	1.3	1.3	1.3	1.3	0.9	0.9
Flow rate (ml/min) — Continuous perfusion	1.3	0.5	0.5	0.5	0.5	0.3	0.3
Transplantation	No	No	Yes	Yes	Yes	Yes	Yes

RESULTS

Except for group 7 the pressure increased during perfusion. The pressure recordings are summarized in Figure 30.2.

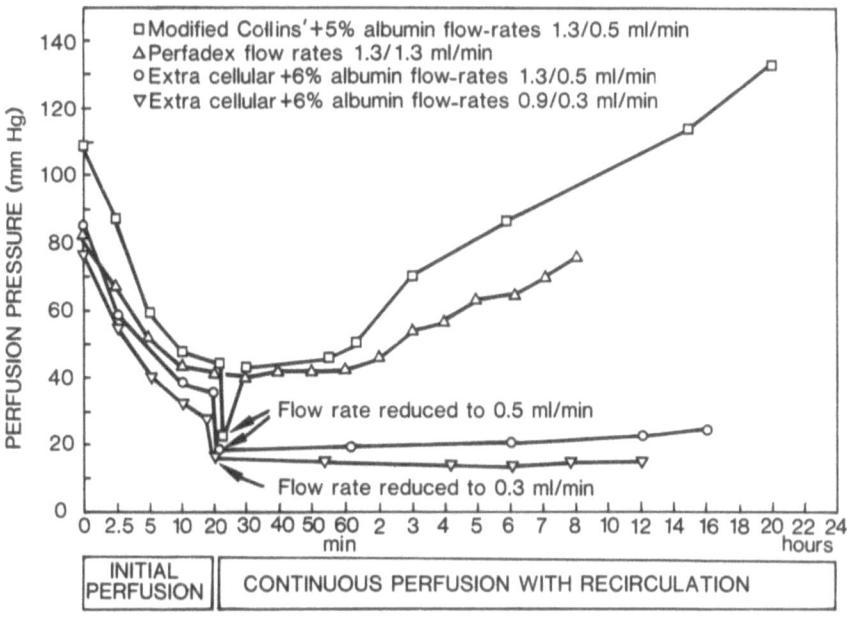

Figure 30.2 Perfusion pressure recordings. Curve o contains groups 3, 4 and 5; curve ∇ contains groups 6 and 7

In the recipients, survival was achieved in groups 4, 5, 6 and 7. Body weight decreased in survivors for 4–7 days. Loss of weight was accentuated in rats with long cold ischaemia and high creatinine values. Plasma creatinine values for survivors increased more in groups with prolonged cold ischaemia and in groups with higher flow rates and increasing pressure during continuous perfusion. Survival and body weight changes 5 days after transplantation for survivors are shown in Table 30.3 together with cold ischaemia time, flow rates (initial perfusion/continuous perfusion), and changes in perfusion pressure during the continuous perfusion. Figure

Table 30.3 Survival and body weight change 5 days post-transplant

| | Group | | | |
	4	5	6	7
Survival	1/10	3/6	6/8	5/5
Body weight changes (as percentages of initial body weight)	−16	−8	−13	−1.4
Cold ischaemia (hours)	12	6	12	6
Flow rate (ml/min) Initial perfusion	1.3	1.3	0.9	0.9
Flow rate (ml/min) Continuous perfusion	0.5	0.5	0.3	0.3
Mean perfusion pressure changes from start to end of continuous perfusion (mmHg)	+3.7	+2.3	+2.5	−1.6

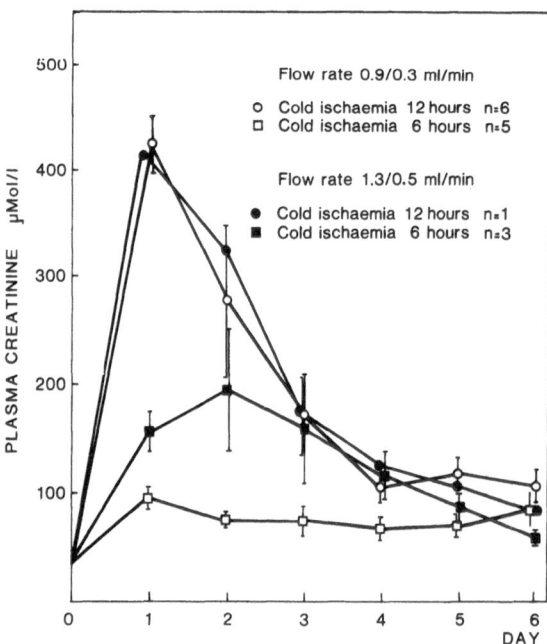

Figure 30.3 Plasma creatinine for survivors

30.3 shows plasma creatinine values for the survivors in the different groups.

Haematocrits in the postoperative course had no predictive value as to survival; although there was a tendency for survivors in group 7 to have more normal values with less pronounced daily variations than survivors in group 4, 5 and 6. No animal with a plasma creatinine level above 507 mmol/l during the first two postoperative days survived. Wet weight of kidneys after continuous perfusion in groups 6 and 7 showed a mean increase of 30% and 45% respectively.

DISCUSSION

It was possible to design a simple model for continuous perfusion of rat kidneys and achieve survivors after 12 h of cold ischaemia for more than 50% of the rats when the perfusate flow was diminished to 0.9 for initial perfusion and 0.3 ml/min for continuous perfusion. These results are similar to those obtained in rat kidneys after initial perfusion 1.3 ml/min and hypothermic storage for 12 h, using the same strain of rats[8]. The better results with flow rates of 0.9 and 0.3 ml/min (group 6 and 7 compared to group 4 and 5) emphasizes the importance of flow-pressure relations used during initial perfusion and continuous perfusion. This is in accordance with the results of Frödin et al.[9], pointing out different functional results according to the method used for initial perfusion. The relatively low flow of 0.3 ml/min, corresponding to about 0.2 ml/min/g gave better results than perfusing with 0.5 ml/min (0.4 ml/min/g). This should be compared to about 1.7 ml/min/g used for human kidneys. This could indicate a weakness in our model but could also suggest a difference between species. The rat kidney could be more susceptible to ischaemic trauma and perfusion, which in some respects may make this model more sensitive. It also indicates that results from animal models must be interpreted with caution.

The increase of pressure during perfusion, and the heavy oedema found in some cases, emphasizes the statement above. Bearing these considerations in mind we conclude that continuous perfusion of rat kidneys can be performed and that studies of the kidneys after transplantation may add further information on preservation.

References

1. Marshall, V. C. (1980). Renal preservation prior to transplantation. *Transplantation,* **30,** 165

2. Collins, G. M. and Halasz, N. A. (1979). Experimental and clinical results with intracellular washout solutions. In Pegg, D. E. and Jacobsen, I. A. (eds.) *Organ Preservation II,* pp. 68-85. (Edinburgh: Churchill-Livingstone)

3. Belzer, F. D. and Southard, J. H. (1981). The future of kidney preservation. *Transplantation,* **30,** 161

4. Harvig, B., Engberg, A. and Ericsson, J. L. E. (1980). Effects of cold ischaemia on the preserved and transplanted rat kidney. *Virch. Arch. Cell Pathol.,* **34,** 173

5. Frödin, L. (1975). Renal transplantation in the rat. The effect of colloidal and non-colloidal perfusates on the clearing of blood from the *in vitro* perfused rat kidney. *Scand. J. Urol. Nephrol.*, **9**, 75
6. Norlén, B. J., Engberg, A., Källskog, Ö. and Wolgast, M. (1978). Intrarenal hemodynamics in the transplanted rat kidney. *Kidney Int.*, **14**, 1
7. Norlén, B. J., Engberg, A., Källskog, Ö. and Wolgast, M. (1978). Nephron function of the transplanted rat kidney. *Kidney Int.*, **14**, 10
8. Harvig, B. and Norlén, B. J. (1980). A technique for studies *in vivo* and *in vitro* on the preserved and transplanted rat kidney. *Urol. Res.*, **8**, 107
9. Frödin, L., Engberg, A., Källskog, Ö. and Wolgast, M. (1975). Cortical pressure gradients measured *in vivo* and during isolated perfusion with reference to renal function after transplantation. *J. Clin. Lab. Invest.*, **35**, 463

31
Cold storage and machine preservation of kidney: studies with the isolated rat kidney

V. MARSHALL, P. JABLONSKI, B. HOWDEN, E. LESLIE, D. RAE and
D. F. SCOTT

Recently the isolated normothermically perfused rat kidney has been used as a test system of kidney preservation[1-3]. Kidneys flushed with hypertonic citrate solution before ice-storage functioned better than others flushed with Collins', Sacks' or Perfudex solutions[1]. The citrate flushing solution required both citrate and magnesium for efficacy but tricarballyate, a non-metabolizable analogue, could replace citrate if suitably buffered[3]. Hyper-osmolality did not enhance the efficacy of the solution; an isosmolar solution was more effective[3]. Subsequent studies have shown that replacing part or all of the mannitol with glucose further enhanced the efficacy of the isosmolar citrate solution.

In this study the isolated perfused rat kidney has been used to examine the effect of storage conditions (intermittent flushing, single-pass perfusion and perfusion with a recycling volume during 24 h storage). The effects of added albumin, oxygenation, pH and temperature on the efficacy of storage were also tested.

METHODS

The operative procedure was essentially as outlined by Jablonski et al.[3]. Male Sprague–Dawley rats were used, and the right kidney was cannulated. All kidneys were immediately flushed with 10 ml of cold isosmolar citrate solution containing glucose (Na 78 mmol/l, K 84 mmol/l, Mg 40 mmol/l, citrate 54 mmol/l, sulphate 40 mmol/l, glucose 100 mmol/l; 300 mosmol/kg). Bovine serum albumin (5%) was added to this solution in some experiments. The temperature of the flushing solution was 0–2 °C and the pH was 7.1 at these temperatures unless otherwise stated. In some studies the flushing solutions were oxygenated (P_{O_2} 650 mmHg) prior to flushing, by passing the solution through an oxygenator gassed with oxygen. Solutions of the same composition as the flushing solutions were used for intermittent flushing or continuous perfusion. Kidneys were perfused continuously at 0–4 °C either by single pass infusion or by recycling of the perfusate using a roller pump.

At the end of the 24 h storage period preservation was tested by normothermic *ex vivo* perfusion. The kidney was perfused normothermically for 60 min via the renal artery with 80 ml of 6.5–6.7% dialysed bovine serum albumin/Krebs Henseleit buffer with 10 mmol/l glucose[3]. Glomerular filtration rate (GFR), urinary:plasma (U/P) inulin ratio, total sodium reabsorption (T_{Na}) and percentage sodium reabsorption (%Na) were assessed at intervals over the test period. Tissue adenine nucleotides were measured before and at the end of the test perfusion. Results are presented graphically, GFR and T_{Na} ($\pm$ SEM) are plotted at each 10 min time interval during the test perfusion period and data are compared statistically at each time interval.

RESULTS

Cold storage after a single flush

The addition of albumin to the flushing solution improved GFR and T_{Na} but not to a significant level; oxygenation of the basic solution (Figure 31.1) also improved function, but not significantly. Renal ATP was significantly elevated by oxygenation (no oxygen 0.95 ± 0.15 versus oxygen $1.83 \pm 0.25\,\mu$mol/g dry weight, $p < 0.02$). Total adenine nucleotides were unchanged.

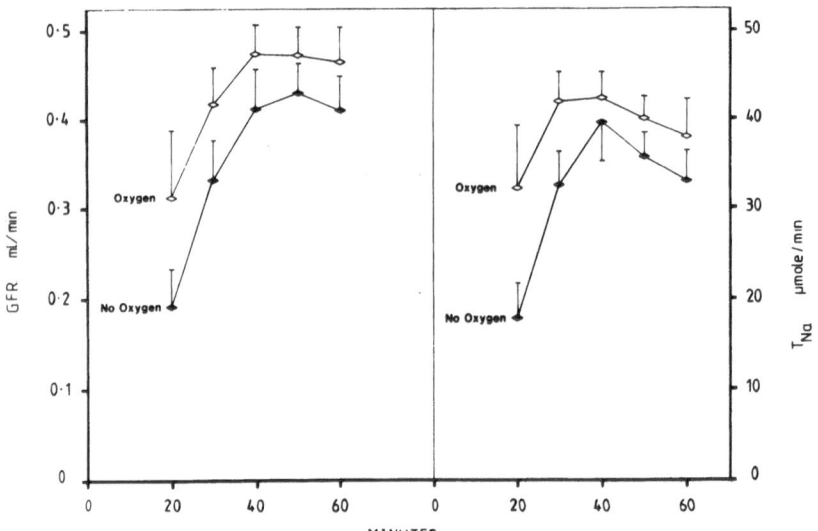

Figure 31.1 Effect of oxygenation on renal function after single flush and 24 h ice-storage. ◇, Oxygen; ◆, no oxygen

Increasing the temperature of flushing and storage from 0 to 5 °C significantly ($p < 0.002$) worsened subsequent function (Figure 31.2). Reducing the pH to 6.6 resulted in lower T_{Na} ($p < 0.02$) but GFR was not significantly lowered. Increasing pH to 7.6 had no significant effect (Figure 31.3).

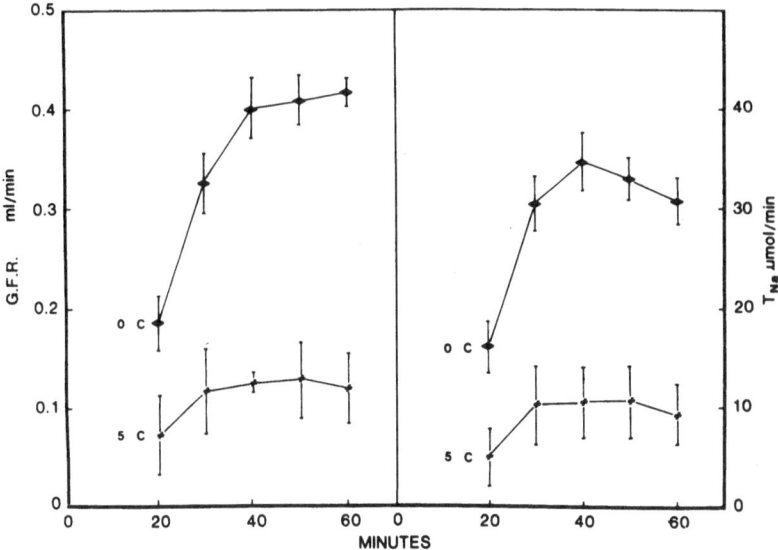

Figure 31.2 Effect of temperature on renal function after single flush and 24 h ice-storage. #, 5 °C; ♦, 0 °C

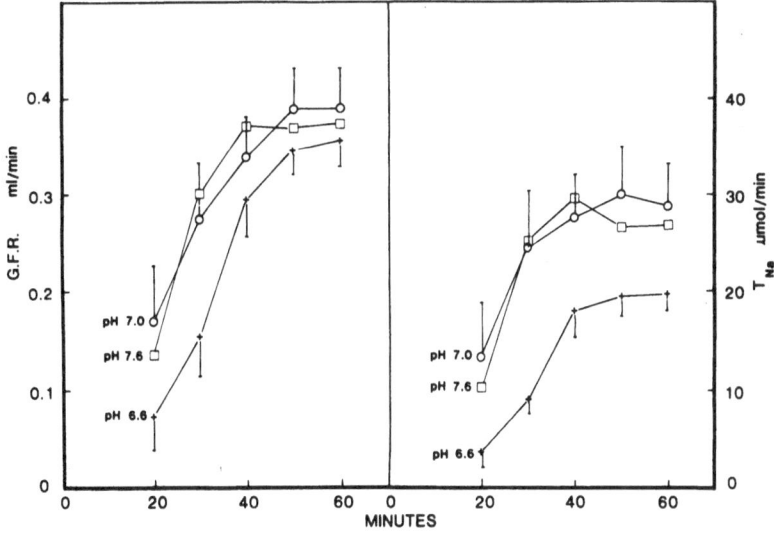

Figure 31.3 Effect of pH on renal function after single flush and 24 h ice-storage. +, pH 6.6; o, pH 7.0; □, pH 7.6

233

Intermittent flushing and continuous perfusion

Flushing the kidneys at 4 h intervals during the period of cold storage was detrimental (Figure 31.4) and oxygenation of the flushing solution did not abolish this effect.

Continuous slow perfusion of the kidneys during storage (5 ml/h) by single pass, or by recycling 20 ml of perfusate was also deleterious (Figure 31.4). The kidneys were oedematous (percentage dry weight: single flush = 17.3 ± 0.3, perfused = 14.0 ± 0.1, $p < 0.02$), suggesting the requirement of an oncotic agent such as albumin during continuous perfusion.

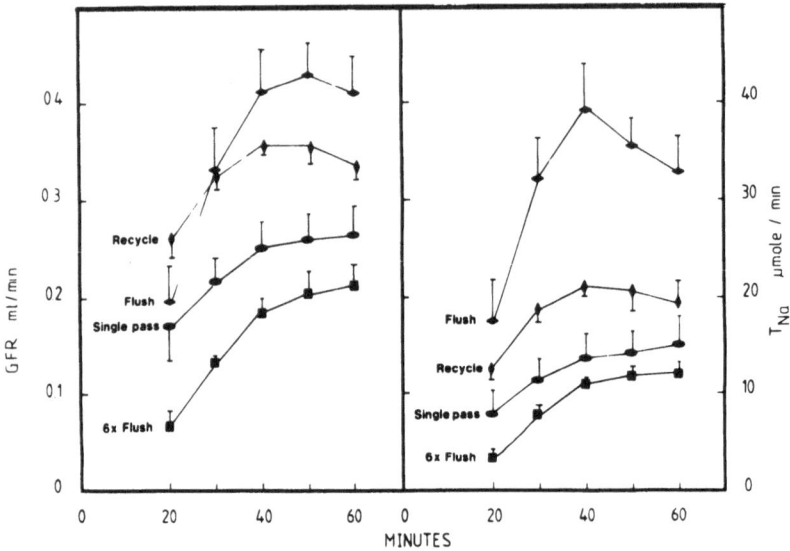

Figure 31.4 Effect of storage conditions on renal function – 24 h storage – solutions not containing albumin. ◆ , Single flush and 24 h ice-storage; ■, intermittent flush every 4 h during 24 h ice-storage; ● , continuous single-pass perfusion (5 ml/h) at 0–4 °C for 24 h; ◆, continuous perfusion (5 ml/h) with recycling 20 ml perfusate at 0–4 °C for 24 h

The addition of albumin abolished the detrimental effect of storage by continuous perfusion. In kidneys perfused with an albumin-containing solution immediate function after storage was improved, but not ultimate function.

Oxygenation of the albumin-containing perfusate improved T_{Na} still further (Figure 31.5). Continuous perfusion with recycling of a 20 ml perfusate was more effective than single-pass perfusion (Figure 31.6), improving both GFR and T_{Na}.

Increasing the rate of perfusion from 5 ml/h to 2 ml/min marginally improved GFR ($p < 0.02$) but T_{Na} was not significantly increased.

Best function after 24 h of storage was obtained by continuous cold perfusion with recycling of the oxygenated perfusate containing albumin.

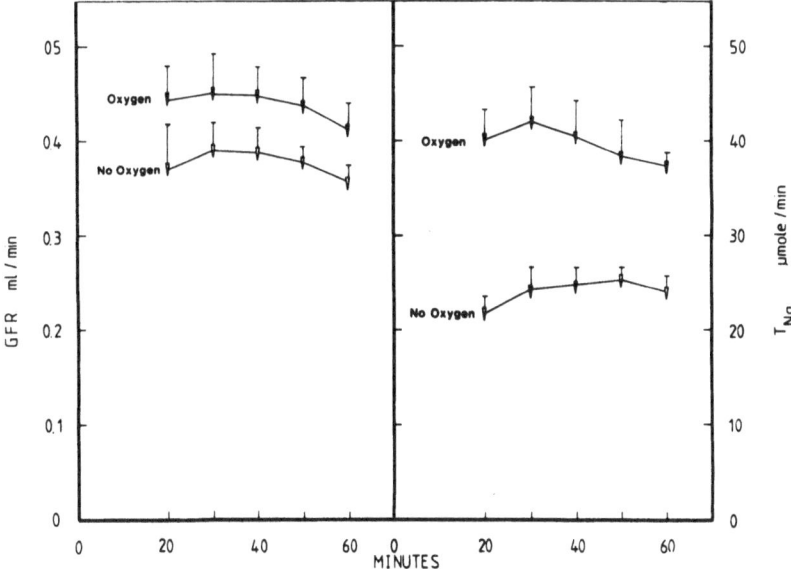

Figure 31.5 Effect of oxygenation of perfusate on renal function after continuous perfusion (5 ml/h) with albumin-containing solution for 24 h at 0–4 °C. ▼ Oxygen; ▽ no oxygen

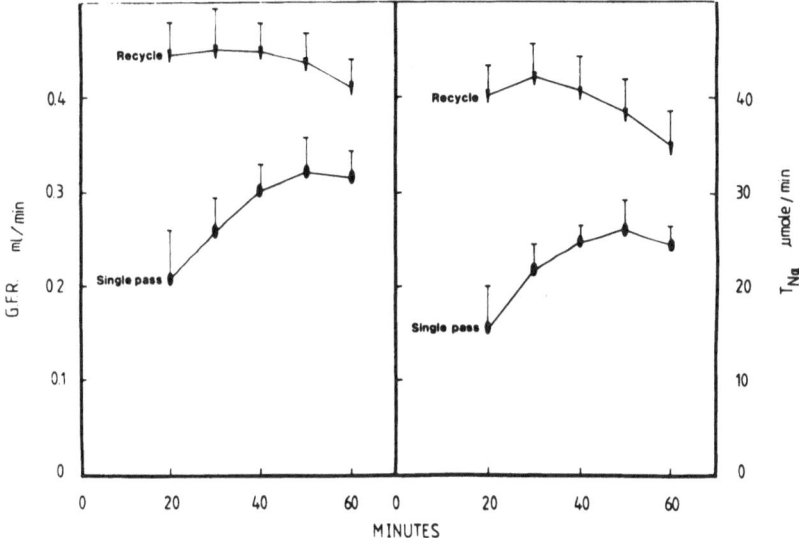

Figure 31.6 Effect of method of continuous perfusion on renal function – perfusion (5 ml/h) with oxygenated, albumin-containing solution for 24 h at 0–4 °C. ▼, Recycling 20 ml perfusate; ●, single-pass perfusion

DISCUSSION

The use of the isolated perfused rat kidney model as a screening test enables rapid investigations of multiple variables. Validation of its application to

235

preservation is, as yet, incomplete. The test measures initial renal function immediately after storage and this may not reflect ultimate function, although in the dog model with reimplantation of the stored kidney early function has been shown to correlate with later function[4]. Use of the test immediately after progressively increasing periods of warm or cold ischaemic storage shows functional deterioration directly proportional to the increasing ischaemia[2]. Ultimate validation by a transplantation model remains necessary.

The results of this study confirm and extend results obtained experimentally and clinically[6], that machine-preserved kidneys function only marginally better than kidneys which are simply flushed once and stored at 0 °C when there is no period of warm ischaemia and storage is only for 24 h.

In the present test system, using the basic flushing solution, intermittent flushing during cold storage was clearly detrimental. Energy stores after a single flush and cold storage could, however, be significantly improved by oxygenation of the flushing solution. Additive benefits of oxygenation during cold storage have also been suggested by retrograde oxygen persufflation[4,5]. During continuous perfusion storage the necessity for albumin and the benefits of perfusate oxygenation shown in the present system have also been demonstrated in larger animal models[7,8].

Optimal temperatures of flushing, storage and of perfusion are clearly important. These experiments suggest that flushing and cold storage are more effective at 0 °C than at 5 °C. Continuing metabolism occurs during hypothermia with gradual depletion of energy stores, and this effect would be greater at the higher temperature. Rate of cooling is also likely to be important. Kidneys preserved by continuous perfusion are usually perfused at somewhat higher temperatures (5–10 °C) than kidneys stored by simple hypothermia. It is technically difficult to maintain temperatures at 0 °C in a perfusion circuit, and it has been suggested that preservation of mitochondrial function is better at higher temperatures[9]. In our experiments kidneys were continuously perfused at 0–4 °C – further studies are required to determine the effects of varying perfusate temperatures.

The deleterious effect of single-pass perfusion may have been due to a leaching out of essential metabolites from the kidney and this may be more pronounced when relatively small kidneys (such as rat) are perfused. Potentially beneficial effects of such perfusion (removal of toxic waste products, continuous supply of nutrients and oxygen) may thus be negated.

No comparisons have yet been made with the perfusates used in clinical practice, which have generally extracellular electrolyte composition and which do not contain citrate, or such high concentrations of $MgSO_4$. It is thus not yet possible to determine whether citrate and magnesium have any specifically beneficial effect in continuous perfusion.

In summary, optimum maintenance of renal function and energy stores during 24 h storage was obtained by continuous perfusion at 0–4 °C with a recycled volume of oxygenated citrate solution containing both albumin and glucose.

Acknowledgement

This work was supported in part by a grant from the National Health and Medical Research Council.

References

1. Bishop, M. C. and Ross, B. D. (1978). Evaluation of hypertonic citrate flushing solution for kidney preservation using the isolated perfused rat kidney. *Transplantation*, **25**, 235
2. Marshall, V., Ross, B., Bishop, M. and Morris, P. (1978). Evaluation of renal preservation using the isolated perfused rat kidney. *Transplantation*, **26**, 315
3. Jablonski, P., Howden, B., Marshall, V. and Scott, D. F. (1980). Evaluation of citrate flushing solution using the isolated perfused rat kidney. *Transplantation*, **30**, 239
4. Fischer, J. H., Czerniak, A., Hauer, U. *et al.* (1978). A new simple method for optimal storage of ischemically damaged kidneys. *Transplantation*, **25**, 43
5. Ross, H. and Escott, M. L. (1979). Gaseous oxygen perfusion of the renal vessels as an adjunct in kidney preservation. *Transplantation*, **28**, 362
6. Marshall, V. C., Ross, H., Scott, D. F. *et al.* (1977). Preservation of cadaver renal allografts: Comparison of ice storage and machine perfusion. *Med. J. Austr.*, **2**, 353
7. Pegg, D. E. and Farrant, J. (1967). *In vitro* perfusion of the rabbit kidney. *Cryobiology*, **3**, 373
8. Belzer, F. O., Ashby, B. S. and Dunphy, J. E. (1967). 24 h and 72 h preservation of canine kidneys. *Lancet*, **2**, 536
9. Belzer, F. O. and Southard, J. H. (1980). The future of kidney preservation. *Transplantation*, **30**, 161

32
Light microscopy findings in intermediate term kidney preservation

J. VAN DER WIJK, C. VOORDES, B. G. RIJKMANS and
G. KOOTSTRA

In machine preservation of kidneys histological changes may occur, which do not exist after simple cooling[1,2]. The graft survival after 1 year may also be lower in machine preservation[3]. However, other authors describe good results of machine preservation[4]. Experimental studies show that high perfusion pressure and hypotonic perfusates are coupled with morphological disorders[5]. In this study the function and biopsies of kidneys which were machine perfused for 96 and 144 h at low pressure and with a hypertonic perfusate are studied.

METHODS

Mongrel dogs with a mean weight of 22 kg and normal renal function were divided into two groups. Nephrectomy, preservation, autotransplantation and contralateral nephrectomy were performed as described previously[6].

Group 1

Ten kidneys were machine perfused for 96 h. After 96 h, autotransplantation and contralateral nephrectomy was done. Thirty minutes later a surgical biopsy was done in four cases. The biopsies were fixed in formalin and processed for light microscopy. Four-micron sections were stained with haematoxylin and eosin. The function of the preserved kidneys was determined by daily serum creatinine measurements. After 14 days the dogs were sacrificed, an autopsy was performed, and the kidneys were examined macroscopically and microscopically.

Group 2

In six kidneys the procedure was similar to the kidneys of group 1. In this group however the perfusion lasted for 144 h. Biopsies from kidneys were studied after 14 days if the animal survived, but if it died (mean = 4 days) the kidney tissue was studied at autopsy.

RESULTS

The biopsies taken before machine preservation but after Euro-Collins flushing showed only slight changes. These changes consisted of tubular damage and some kidneys showed focal interstitial nephritis. During perfusion of the kidneys of group 1 with constant pressure, the perfusion flow increased. The end flow (mean 113 ml/min) was in all cases higher than the initial flow (mean 67 ml/min) (Table 32.1).

Table 32.1 Perfusate flow rate in kidneys perfused for 96 h

Kidney no.	Flow	
	Initial (ml/min)	Final (ml/min)
1	80	120
2	60	120
3	50	100
4	90	120
5	70	110
6	80	120
7	30	90
8	60	110
9	80	120
10	70	120

The perfusion of the kidneys of group 2 showed the same perfusion characteristics. The initial flow (mean 65 ml/min) increased in this group to 108 ml/min (Table 32.2).

The results of light microscopic investigation of the biopsies, taken 30 min after recirculation of the kidneys of group 1, are reported in Table 32.3; those of group 2 in Table 32.4. In the biopsies from group 1, minimal tubular damage and minimal interstitial oedema were seen. Fibrin deposits, casts or disorders in glomeruli and vessels were not seen. In the biopsies

Table 32.2 Perfusion flow rates in kidneys perfused for 144 h

Kidney no.	Flow	
	Initial (ml/min)	Final (ml/min)
11	80	100
12	50	100
13	60	110
14	70	110
15	70	115
16	60	120

from group 2, with one exception, the tubular damage was moderate to severe, and it is remarkable that all biopsies contained neutrophils. In group 1 all kidneys had life-sustaining function; however, the serum creatinine did not reach the preoperative level. In group 2, only one kidney had life-sustaining function. Remarkably this was the kidney which showed no further damage (K14) in the 30 min biopsy. After 14 days one kidney of group 1 showed multiple abscesses (K10). Histologically these proved to be a purulent interstitial nephritis. In the other kidneys of group 1 and group 2 no macroscopic changes were found.

Table 32.3 Morphological characteristics after 30 min of recirculation of kidneys perfused for 96 h

Kidney no.	Fibrin	Neutrophils	Tubular degeneration	Casts	Oedema
7	0	0	+	0	+
8	0	+ +	+ + +	0	+
9	0	0	0	0	+ +
10	0	+ +	+	0	0

Table 32.4 Morphological characteristics after 30 min of recirculation of kidneys perfused for 144 h

Kidney no.	Fibrin	Neutrophils	Tubular degeneration	Casts	Oedema
11	0	+ +	+ + +	0	0
12	0	+ +	+ +	0	0
13	0	+	+ +	0	0
14	0	+	0	0	0
15	0	+	+ +	0	0
16	0	+	+ +	0	0

The light microscopic findings at autopsy of group 1 and group 2 are listed in Tables 32.5 and 32.6. All biopsies contain neutrophils, and the biopsies of group 2 also contain casts and tubular damage. Damage to glomeruli and vessels is not seen.

During perfusion for 96 and 144 h with a hypertonic perfusate (albumin Kabi® 4.5 g/100 ml), the flow increased with a constant low perfusion

Table 32.5 Morphological characteristics at autopsy of kidneys perfused for 96 h

Kidney no.	Fibrin	Neutrophils	Tubular degeneration	Casts	Oedema
1	0	+ +	+	+	+
2	0	+	0	0	+
3	0	+	0	0	+
4	0	+ +	0	0	0
5	0	+ +	0	0	0
6	0	+	0	0	0
7	0	+	0	+	0
8	+	+ + +	+ + +	0	+ + +
9	0	+ +	0	0	0
10	abscess	—	—	—	—

Table 32.6 Morphological characteristics at autopsy of kidneys perfused for 144 h

Kidney no.	Fibrin	Neutrophils	Tubular degeneration	Casts	Oedema
11	0	+ +	+ +	+ + +	+
12	0	+ +	+ +	+ + +	+
13	0	+	+	+ +	0
14	0	+	0	0	0
15	0	+	0	+ + +	0
16	0	+ +	+	+ +	0

pressure. Possibly vasoconstriction played some part in causing the initially lower flow. Damage to the endothelia might be caused by attempting to increase the flow by raising the perfusion pressure. Others have also mentioned damage due to high perfusion pressures[7].

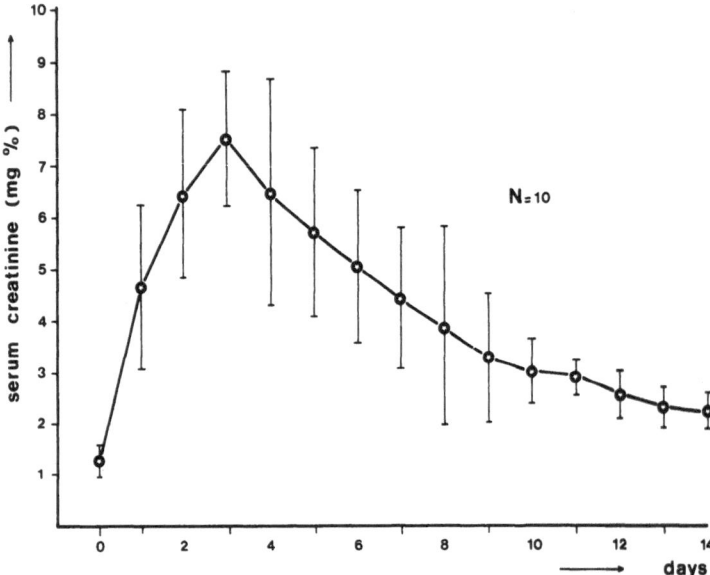

Figure 32.1 Mean serum creatinines after 96 h preservation, autotransplantation and contralateral nephrectomy

DISCUSSION

In our study the perfusion characteristics had no prognostic value for kidney function after autotransplantation. Light microscopic findings in our study were not specific. After 96 h machine preservation, only a small amount of tubular damage and interstitial oedema was found after grafting. In biopsies taken after 144 h machine preservation and recirculation of the kidney, tubular damage had increased in comparison with the biopsies of the 96 h preservation. Biopsies after 144 h machine preservation also contained more neutrophils. In the 144h perfused kidneys, as in the 96h perfused kidneys, neutrophils were found in the interstitium, but most neutrophils were found in the biopsies of the 144h perfused kidneys. The ureterocutaneostomy is partially responsible for this[8], but the biopsies taken after 144h machine preservation and 30min after autotransplantation also showed neutrophils. A long exposure in the organ container, and perfusion with a perfusate that did not contain antibiotics, could be responsible. By increasing the preservation time to 144h the amount of tubular damage increased, and after autotransplantation of these 144h-preserved kidneys, many casts were seen in the biopsies. These changes have also been seen in biopsies of kidneys which had an ischaemic period[9]. One cause of the tubular damage with increasing preservation time could be a lack of nutrients, or bad perfusion of the renal cortex during the preservation. Casts could consist of necrotic remnants of tubular cells which have been passed into the tubular lumen. The changes that have been described as perfusion nephropathy[1] did not occur. We did, however, find a correlation between the presence of tubular damage in the biopsy taken after recirculation and post-transplantation function.

References

1. Spector, D., Limas, C., Frost, J.L. *et al.* (1976). Perfusion nephropathy in human transplants. *N. Engl. J. Med.,* **295**, 1217
2. Hill, G.S., Light, J.A. and Perloff, L.J. (1976). Perfusion related injury in renal transplantation. *Surgery,* **79**, 440
3. Clark, E.A., Mickey, M.R., Opelz, G. *et al.* (1973). Evaluation of Belzer and Collins kidney preservation methods. *Lancet,* **1**, 361
4. Burleson, R.L., Jones, D.B., Yenikomshian, A.M. *et al.* (1978). Clinical renal preservation by cryoperfusion with an albumin perfusate. *Arch. Surg.,* **113**. 688
5. Whittier, F.C., Cross, D.E. and Pierce, G.E. (1975). The influence of protein concentration of the perfusate on weight gain and kidney transplant outcome. *Proc. Dialysis Transplant Forum,* **36**
6. Wijk, J. van der, Slooff, M.J.H., Rijkmans, B.G. and Koostra, G. (1980). Successful 96- and 144 hour experimental kidney preservation: a combination of standard machine preservation and newly developed normothermic *ex vivo* perfusion. *Cryobiology,* **17**, 473
7. Cerra, F.B., Raza, S., Andres, G.A. *et al.* (1977). The endothelial damage of pulsatile renal preservation and its relationship to perfusion pressure and colloid osmotic pressure. *Surgery,* **81**, 534
8. Herrman, Th.J. and Turcotte, J.G. (1969). Preservation of canine kidneys by hypothermia and low flow perfusion with bloodless perfusate. *Arch. Surg.,* **98**, 121
9. Fin, W.F. (1980). Postischemic acute renal failure initiation, maintenance and recovery. *Invest. Urol.,* **17**, 427

33
Five days preservation of canine kidneys using a preservation machine

A. OZAKI, K. FUKAO, M. SANO, T. OKAMURA and Y. IWASAKI

Four-day preservation of the canine kidney has been successful using Belzer's plasma[1] and a perfusion machine[2]. However, 5 days preservation was unsuccessful with the same method and the same perfusate. In search of a better method of preserving canine kidneys, further experiment has been attempted.

METHODS

Mongrel dogs weighing 15–25 kg were anaesthetized; one kidney was removed and flushed with 100 ml of electrolyte solution containing procaine 200 mg/l, and heparin 5000 units/l, at 4 °C. During preservation the perfusate was not changed and the circulating temperature was 6 °C. After preservation kidneys were transplanted and a contralateral nephrectomy was done.

Group 1

Five kidneys were preserved on the circuit for 120 h using Belzer's cryo-precipitated plasma (CPP).

Group 2

Four kidneys were preserved on the circuit for 120 h using modified Belzer's plasma (MB plasma). This perfusate contained 50 ml of an amino acid solution (12% Ispol, Diago-Eiyo Chemical Inc., Japan) instead of 25% mannitol, and distilled water is increased to yield an osmolality of around 320 mosmol/kg.

Group 3

Four kidneys were preserved on the circuit for 168 h using MB plasma. Samples of the perfusate were taken every 24 h and lactate dehydrogenase (LDH), electrolytes, GOT, and GPT, were measured.

The circuit was composed of a non-pulsatile roller pump, a membrane oxygenator, a refrigerator and heat exchanger, a pH controller, and a pressure controller (Senko Medical Instrument Inc., Tokyo). The pH was set to 7.75 at 6 °C, and the pressure was set at 40–60 mmHg.

RESULTS AND DISCUSSION

Group 1

All five dogs were dead within 8 days and the transplanted kidneys secreted no urine.

Group 2

Two dogs died, 6 and 10 days after retransplantation, and the other two dogs lived more than 60 days with normal serum creatinines.

Group 3

All four dogs were dead within 6 days after retransplantation because of uraemia (Table 33.1).

Table 33.1 Five- to seven-day canine kidney preservation

Perfusate	Success at	
	5 days	7 days
Belzer's CPP	0/5	—
Modified Belzer perfusate	2/4	0/4

The LDH change in the perfusate was prominent among the parameters examined (Figure 33.1). In group 1 LDH increased to more than 800 units on the fifth day, whereas in group 2 it was 208 ± 142 units on the same day. In group 3, LDH was 465 ± 35 units on the 7th day. Electrolyte, GOT and GPT changes were not notable.

Since 96 h preservation of canine kidneys was successful, 120 h preservation has been attempted with the same method. However, no kidneys functioned. To investigate the histological changes, one kidney was preserved on the perfusing machine and biopsied periodically. The substance which is stained by PAS increased in the lumina of glomerular capillaries after 96 h, and capillary obstruction with this substance seemed to be the cause of the failure of 120 h preservation[3]. This substance was thought to be the necrotizing endothelium of capillaries. Thinking that amino acids may have protective effects on endothelium during low-temperature preservation, the amino acid solution, Ispol, was added to the perfusate. Since the osmolality of Ispol is about 1200 mosmol/kg, mannitol was excluded from the perfusate to maintain the appropriate osmolality. Using this perfusate, two out of four canine kidneys functioned after 120 h

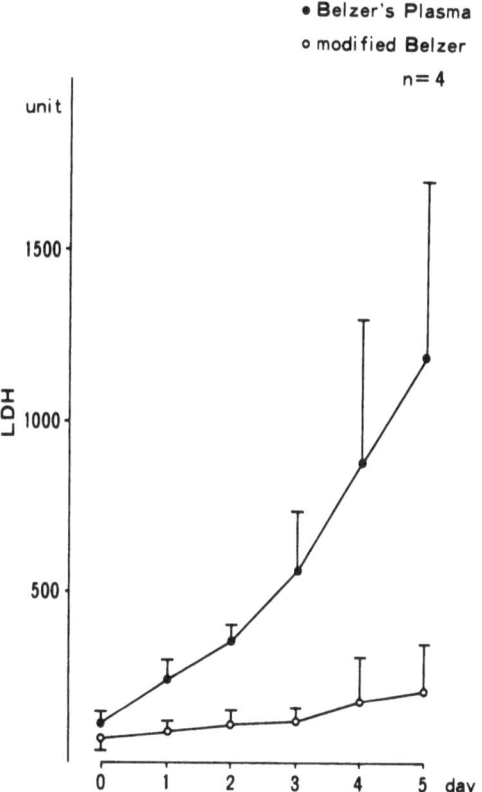

Figure 33.1 LDH release during preservation of canine kidneys

preservation; the other two died of uraemia, although their kidneys excreted some urine. MB plasma seems to be superior to CPP in low-temperature perfusion preservation. It might be speculated that some kinds of amino acid may be effective as membrane stabilizers or they may protect preserved tissues from damage in some other way.

Amino acids in the perfusate were analysed periodically. Most of them increased gradually, glutamine being an exception. This means that amino acids are not used during preservation, but are exuded from the preserved tissues. Therefore it is merely speculation that amino acids work as membrane stabilizers or protective factors in preserved organs. Seven days preservation was unsuccessful with MB plasma.

As parameters for viability of preserved kidneys, LDH, GOT, GPT, Na, K, and Cl were analysed but only LDH seemed to indicate viability to some extent. The rate of increase of LDH was less in MB plasma than Belzer's plasma during 5 days of preservation.

Temperature was set at 6 °C in our experiment, and pH was set at 7.75 ± 0.05 at this temperature. This pH will become about 7.40 at 37 °C[4]. We used this pH because of previous experience, but some workers prefer a lower pH at low temperatures. The optimum pH and temperature for perfusion preservation is not yet clear.

Toledo-Pereyra succeeded in 5-day preservation of canine kidneys using fibrinogen-free plasma[5], and Humphries, Woods, and Johnson succeeded in 7-day preservation of canine kidneys[6-8]. Johnson further succeeded in 8-day preservation using plasma protein fraction (PPF) and he stressed the importance of pretreatment of the dog before nephrectomy[9]. Since PPF is expensive we have been using CPP for our experiments. It is not yet clear why PPF is better than CPP; since proteinase is supposed to be one of the factors to damage the cell membrane, PPF, in which proteinase is inactivated, should be a better perfusate than CPP, in which proteinase is still active.

References

1. Belzer, F.O. and Kountz, S.L. (1970). Preservation and transplantation of human cadaver kidneys: a two-year experience. *Ann. Surg.*, **172**, 394
2. Ozaki, A., Asano, T., Amemiya, H., Ochiai, T., Sato, H., Iwasaki, Y., Okamura, T., Fukao, K. and Yokoyama, T. (1977). Successful 96-hour preservation of canine kidneys using a new machine. *Transplant. Proc.*, **9**, 247
3. Ozaki, A., Sano, M., Fukao, K. and Iwasaki, Y. (1980). The horizon of canine kidney preservation using a perfusing machine. *Low Temp. Med.*, **6**, 7
4. Halasz, N.A., Collins, G.M. and White, F.M. (1979). The right pH for preservation? In Pegg, D.E. and Jacobsen, I.A. (eds.) *Organ Preservation II,* pp. 259-266. (London: Churchill-Livingstone)
5. Toledo-Pereyra, L.H., Condie, R.M., Malmberg, R., Simmons, R.L. and Najarian, J.S. (1974). A fibrinogen-free plasma perfusate for preservation of kidneys for one hundred and twenty hours. *Surg. Gynecol. Obstet.*, **138**, 901
6. Humphries, A.L., Carcia, L.A. and Serkes, K.D. (1974). Perfusates for long-term preservation by continuous perfusion. *Transplant. Proc.*, **6**, 249
7. Woods, J.E. (1971). Successful three to seven day preservation of canine kidneys. *Arch. Surg.*, **102**, 614
8. Johnson, R.W.G., Cohen, G.L. and Ballardie, F.D. (1979). The limitation of continuous perfusion with plasma protein fraction. In Pegg, D.E. and Jacobsen, I.A. (eds.) *Organ Preservation II,* pp. 18-32. (London: Churchill-Livingstone)
9. Johnson, R.W.G. (1980). In Workshop: Organ Preservation. 8th Congress of Society for Organ Transplantation. 30 June-4 July, Boston

34
Lysosomal enzyme release during successful 5-, 7- and 8-day canine kidney storage

G. L. COHEN, F. W. BALLARDIE, A. MAINWARING and R. W. G. JOHNSON

The maintenance of lysosomal integrity is thought to be vital for successful organ storage. Lysosomal enzyme release during storage should therefore correlate significantly with loss in viability or function after re-implantation. To test this hypothesis we investigated the release of the kidney proximal tubular lysosomal enzyme N-acetyl-β-D-glucosaminidase (NAG) during prolonged hypothermic canine kidney storage and attempted to relate this to the function of the reimplanted kidney.

METHODS

We used 39 beagle dogs of between 10 and 17 kg body weight. The dogs were anaesthetized with thiopentone and then breathed spontaneously a halothane–N_2O–O_2 anaesthetic. All but two of the dogs received frusemide pre-treatment prior to nephrectomy. The kidneys were flushed cold with a mannitol-based solution within 3 min of division of the renal artery and then transferred to a modified Belzer pulsatile perfusion apparatus kept in a cold room at 8 °C. The perfusate was based on plasma protein fraction; samples of perfusate were removed at frequent intervals throughout the period of storage and deep frozen for later estimation of their NAG content. After 5, 7 or 8 days storage the kidneys were reimplanted as autografts and an immediate contralateral nephrectomy performed. During the reimplantation operation the kidneys were kept at 8 °C within a cooler coil to minimize any injury occurring after the end of perfusion. Postoperatively serum creatinine was measured daily for 1 week and then every 2 days in the survivors.

NAG was estimated by the method of Leabeck and Walker[1] using a 2.6 millimolar substrate. The NAG results were expressed as milli-International Units per gram of the pre-perfusion kidney weight and were corrected for loss of perfusate by sampling and evaporation (1 IU of NAG = amount of NAG hydrolysing 1 μmol of substrate in 1 min at 37 °C).

RESULTS AND DISCUSSION

The rate of NAG loss during storage was almost constant. There was no significant correlation between peak post-reimplantation serum creatinine and the total NAG released by each viable kidney (Table 34.1). There was also no significant difference between the total amount of NAG released by the non-viable and viable kidneys after each period of perfusion (Table 34.2). Histology of the best-preserved viable 5-day stored kidney at the end of perfusion showed mitochondrial swelling and vacuolation of the endoplasmic reticulum but no glomerular injury. However, 20 of the 22 non-

Table 34.1 Correlation between NAG release and function of viable kidneys

Dog no.	Frusemide (mg)	Perfusion time (h)	Peak creatinine (mmol/l)	Total NAG released (mIU/g)
36	40	120.7	0.29	16.7
75	40	119.5	0.34	23.3
57	40	118.2	0.36	12.4
94	0	120	0.37	23.3
79	120	118.3	0.44	16.7
59	40	119.6	0.45	15.0
49	40	119	0.46	12.1
65	40	119.7	0.52	18.3
61	80	119.9	0.56	12.0
54	40	119.8	0.58	15.3
50	40	119.7	0.74	14.0
45	20	120.1	0.81	15.1
78	0	119	0.94	23.4
80	100	167.5	0.52	12.5
81	100	167.3	0.63	22
92	180	193.1	0.92	21.5
95	180	192.7	0.74	18.3

$r = 0.2$

Table 34.2 Correlation between NAG release and viability

Storage time (days)	Viable kidneys	Non-viable kidneys	Peak creatinine (mmol/l) mean ± SD	Total NAG released (mIU/g) mean ± SD	
5	13		0.53 ± 0.2	16.7 ± 4.2	n.s.
5		14	1.1 ± 0.5	20.4 ± 11.8	
7	2		0.58 ± 0.08	17.3 ± 6.7	n.s.
7		3	0.99 ± 0.19	16.2 ± 7.1	
8	2		0.83 ± 0.13	19.9 ± 2.3	n.s.
8		5	1.04 ± 0.53	28.7 ± 4.8	

viable kidneys showed a picture similar to Figure 34.1 with a non-specific 'glomerulitis' in which there was minimal occlusion of glomerular vessels. Immunohistology showed no evidence of an active immunological process.

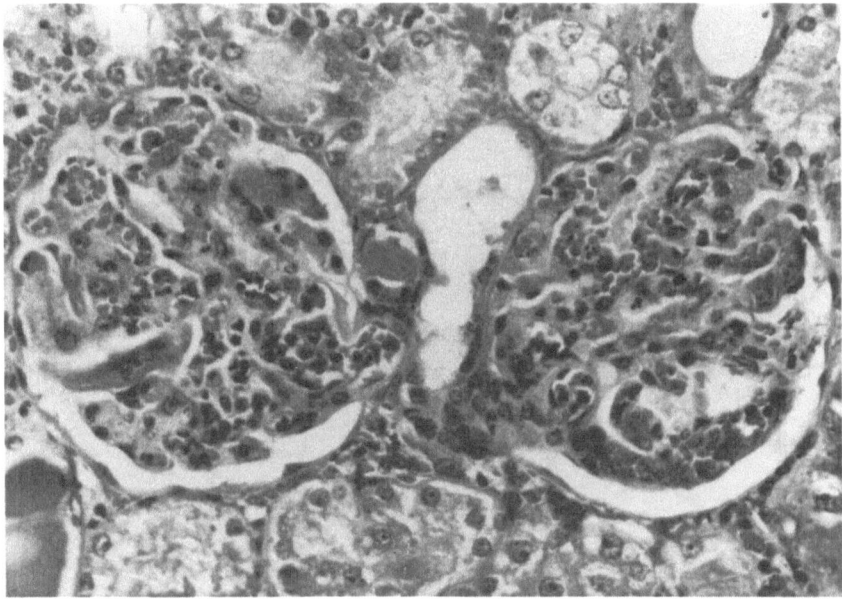

Figure 34.1   Glomerulus of a typical non-viable kidney 2 days after reimplantation. (× 280)

These results show that if a sensitive assay technique is used lysosomal enzyme release can be demonstrated during hypothermic kidney storage even in the absence of pre-existing warm injury; they also show that kidneys can remain viable after up to 8 days storage despite lysosomal enzyme release. The development of glomerular pathology after re-implantation may be the explanation for our failure to find significant correlation between NAG release and function.

Reference

1. Leabeck, D. H. and Walker, P. G. (1961). Studies on glucosaminidase. The fluorimetric assay of N-acetyl-β-glucosaminidase. *Biochem. J.,* **78,** 151

35
Aerobic and anaerobic perfusion of canine kidneys with a new perfusate

F. O. BELZER, R. M. HOFFMANN and J. H. SOUTHARD

Perfusion preservation was introduced in clinical transplantation in 1967[1] and simple cold storage in 1969[2]. Since then many articles have appeared in the literature suggesting superiority of one method over the other[3-5]. In general, however, it has been accepted that continuous hypothermic perfusion preservation is superior for kidneys subjected to periods of warm ischaemia and also allows preservation for up to 72 h. Simple hypothermic storage appears to be safe for up to 48 h in kidneys not subjected to warm ischaemia and up to 24 h in kidneys with warm ischaemia. The better results with perfusion preservation have been thought to be due to continued aerobic metabolism.

In our laboratory we have become interested in the idea that O_2 toxicity may limit long-term preservation[6]. The presence of high levels of O_2 induces the formation of lipid peroxides which are toxic to cells and organelles such as mitochondria[7,8]. To investigate this problem we have studied the effects of perfusion preservation under N_2 on renal viability and certain biochemical parameters and compared these results to perfusion in the presence of O_2. To effectively carry out anaerobic perfusion we developed a new perfusate containing gluconate in place of Cl^-.

METHODS

The dogs used in these experiments were adult mongrels weighing an average of 20 kg. Under general anaesthesia a unilateral nephrectomy was performed, the kidney was flushed with saline solution at 4 °C and placed on a mini-Belzer perfusion circuit. Perfusion pressure was adjusted to 60/20 mmHg which usually settled around 50/20 mmHg during the 3-day perfusion. After 72 h the kidney was autotransplanted, and the contralateral kidney was removed and placed on the perfusion circuit for 3 days for biochemical and physiological determinations. Kidneys were randomized into three groups. In *group I* oxygenation was provided by a membrane oxygenator using room air. In *group II* nitrogen was passed through the oxygenator, and suction was applied to the cassette to remove any air. The perfusate pH in both groups remained approximately 7.5 ± 0.2 during the preservation. In group I the average perfusate Po_2 was 200 mmHg, corrected for room temperature. In the nitrogen experiments the Po_2 was 10 mmHg, also corrected. The composition of the perfusate is shown in Table 35.1. A large proportion of Cl^- was replaced by the impermeant or slowly permeable anions, gluconate and phosphate. The perfusate also contained 1.5 g/l of inulin plus [^{3}H]inulin (20 μCi/l). In *group III* the kidneys were flushed out with the same perfusate without albumin, stored at 6–8 °C for 72 h and then autotransplanted. The level of Na^+ in the washout solution was adjusted to 140 mmol/l by the addition of NaCl. Postoperatively daily serum creatinine determinations were made.

Table 35.1 Composition of perfusate

Substance	Amount
Na gluconate	80 mmol/l
K_2HPO_4, KH_2PO_4	25 mmol/l
Glucose	10 mmol/l
Glutathione	3 mmol/l
Mg gluconate	5 mmol/l
Human serum albumin (HSA)	3.75 g/l
Penicillin	6×10^5 U/l
Dexamethasone	12 mg/l
Penosulphathelien	12 mg/l
NaOH	–*
NaCl	~35–45 mmol/l
Final values	
Na$^+$	140–145 mmol/l
K$^+$	25 mmol/l
Gluconate	80 mmol/l
pH (room temp.)	7.5

The perfusate is made in distilled, deionized water. The level of Na^+ in the HSA varies between 19 and 24 mmol per 37.5 g HSA. The amount of NaCl is dependent upon the amount of Na^+ added with the HSA.

* NaOH is added to raise the pH to the desired level.

Biochemical determinations

Following the preservation period the non-transplanted kidney was processed immediately. Methods for total tissue water[9], electrolyte levels[9], adenine nucleotides[10] and inulin permeable space[11] determinations have been reported. Malondialdehyde was determined on homogenates of cortex tissue (in KCl: 1.15%) by the thiobarbiturate method of Ohkawa *et al.*[12] except that in place of the extraction of the reaction products by organic solvents, millipore filtration (0.22 μm filter) was used to remove the turbidity. The optical density of the solution was determined at 532 nm and the nmol malondialdehyde was calculated using an extinction coefficient of 1.56×10^5. Respiration rates were determined polarographically on homogenates of kidney cortex tissue (see Chapter 16).

Table 35.2 Post-transplant renal function (serum creatinine) of kidneys preserved under N_2, air, or cold-stored for 3 days

Group	Serum creatinine (mg/dl) on indicated post-transplant day									
	1	*2*	*3*	*4*	*5*	*6*	*7*	*8*	*9*	*10*
Perfused N_2	3.4±.5	4.0±.6	4.2±1.3	4.1±.3	3.0±1.2	2.3±1.1	1.7±.8	1.3±.4	1.8±.4	1.2±.4
Perfused air	3.2±.6	4.4±.4	3.9±.8	3.3±.9	2.8±.9	1.7±.3	1.4±.2	1.3±.1	–	–
Cold stored	3.7±.9	6.7±1.3	7.5±.8	>8	>8	Died				

Dog kidneys were perfused for 3 days at 6–8 °C under N_2 (six kidneys), room air (six kidneys) or by simple washout and cold storage (three kidneys). The perfusate and washout solutions were similar and contained HSA-gluconate as described in Methods. Results are expressed as the mean ± SEM

RESULTS

Postoperative renal function is shown in Table 35.2. Most of the dogs receiving perfused kidneys had normal renal function by the seventh day. In some dogs normal function was present by day four to five. In both perfusion preservation groups all dogs survived and the degree of damage which occurred during preservation appeared to be about equal in both the air and nitrogen groups. All dogs receiving kidneys preserved by simple cold storage alone died in uraemia.

Some of the physiological and biochemical parameters are shown in Table 35.3 and compared to control kidneys. During perfusion the kidneys became oedematous due to an expansion of the inulin permeable space. Total adenine nucleotides after 3 days of preservation were about half of normal in the perfused kidneys and 20% of normal in the cold-stored kidneys. Cation determinations showed that after 3 days of preservation there was an increase in intracellular sodium and a decrease of intracellular potassium, suggesting that the sodium pump is only partially effective.

The formation of malondialdehyde was used as a measure of the degree of lipid peroxidation. At the end of 3 days of preservation with air there was approximately a 3-fold increase in lipid peroxide end products in the

Table 35.3 Biochemical effects of preservation by perfusion under N_2 or air and cold storage for 3 days

Determination	Preservation conditions			
	None	Perfusion – N_2	Perfusion – air	Cold store
Total tissue H_2O (kg/kg dry wt)	3.45 ± 0.2	3.98 ± 0.2	4.35 ± 0.23	3.88 ± 0.13
Inulin permeable space (%)	40 ± 5	57 ± 7	57 ± 4	—
Na^+ intracellular (mmol/l)	54 ± 10	73 ± 8	65 ± 5	62 ± 14
K^+ intracellular (mmol/l)	121 ± 15	96 ± 4	93 ± 7	105 ± 10
ATP (μmol/g wet wt)	1.25 ± 0.15	0.56 ± 0.1	0.59 ± 0.1	0.24 ± 0.05
ADP (μmol/g wet wt)	0.38 ± 0.05	$0.35 \pm .04$	0.23 ± 0.08	0.41 ± 0.06
AMP (μmol/g wet wt)	0.29 ± 0.05	$0.25 \pm .05$	$0.16 \pm .06$	$0.23 \pm .07$
TAN	2.12 ± 0.15	1.16 ± 0.14	0.92 ± 0.14	0.88 ± 0.18
Peroxide value	253 ± 100	319 ± 104	847 ± 292	250 ± 58
Pyruvate + ADP	$3.18 \pm 0.12*$	1.40 ± 0.14	1.59 ± 0.27	1.55 ± 0.22
Pyruvate + oligomycin	0.55 ± 0.10	0.51 ± 0.16	0.43 ± 0.13	0.53 ± 0.41
Pyruvate + DNP	3.40 ± 0.22	1.53 ± 0.62	1.64 ± 0.27	1.64 ± 0.20
RCR	5.8	2.7	3.7	2.9
Succinate + ADP	4.25 ± 0.25	2.61 ± 0.18	2.82 ± 0.44	3.06 ± 0.61
Succinate + oligomycin	0.82 ± 0.17	0.97 ± 0.38	0.91 ± 0.15	1.20 ± 0.80
Succinate + DNP	5.93 ± 0.30	2.89 ± 0.36	3.24 ± 0.59	3.50 ± 0.50
RCR	5.2	2.7	3.1	2.6

Kidney cortex was used for all analyses and at least three kidneys were used in each case studied. RCR = respiratory control ratio which is the ratio of the rate of respiration with ADP to the rate of respiration with oligomycin; DNP = dinitrophenol; TAN = total adenine nucleotides; peroxide value = nmol malondialdehyde/mg wet tissue wt. Results are mean values with the SEM

* Respiration rates determined in homogenates = μmol O_2/min/g dry tissue wt

kidney cortex tissue. Perfusion with N_2 or cold storage prevents the accumulation of lipid peroxides. The maximal rate of pyruvate-linked respiration (in the presence of ADP) is reduced by about 50%. This results in a respiratory control ratio of about 50% less than in control homogenates. There was some degree of uncoupling of oxidative phosphorylation and the loss of maximal pyruvate-stimulated respiration may be related to a loss of cofactors necessary for pyruvate-linked reactions.

DISCUSSION

The reasons for developing this new perfusate were 3-fold. First, we wanted a perfusate that was isosmolar and would suppress cell swelling during hypothermic preservation. We have previously shown[9] that replacing Cl^- with less permeant anions (such as gluconate) prevented hypothermia-induced cell swelling. Second, although CPP provides adequate preservation for 3 days, it is difficult to modify without altering its composition away from normal physiological values. Third, perfusion under N_2 for 3 days with a perfusate containing primarily Cl^- as the anion produced a large decline in the pH of the perfusate (7.5–6.7) due to lactic acid accumulation. This pH drop prevented successful preservation unless the perfusate was replaced with fresh perfusate to raise the pH. The perfusate containing gluconate showed no such pH drop during 3 days of anaerobic perfusion.

To our surprise the results of the biochemical studies as well as post-operative renal function were similar in both groups except for the fact that peroxidation levels were lower in the kidneys preserved under anaerobic conditions. Three explanations can be given for these findings. First, Po_2 levels in the perfusion media could not be lowered below 10 mmHg, and even this low Po_2 might have been sufficient to sustain aerobic metabolism. Second, during the nitrogen perfusion studies anaerobic metabolism substituted for aerobic metabolism. However, the absence of a build-up of lactic acid makes this explanation unlikely. Third, and most likely, is that continuous perfusion is not especially important for continuous aerobic metabolism, but its main beneficial effect may relate to other aspects of organ homeostasis. One possibility is that perfusion allows maintenance of the intracellular pH by removing acidic end products of metabolism and H^+. In simple cold storage continuous anaerobic metabolism may lead to low intracellular pH levels, which are detrimental to kidney viability[13]. Perfusion at a pH of 6.5 or less produces severe renal damage even after a storage period as short as 24 h. Some enzyme systems, especially lysosomal enzymes, are more active at acid pH. The increase in lactate in cold stored kidneys is maximal within 24 h[14]. Why the kidney can tolerate this low pH well for 24–30 h but not for 72 h is difficult to explain. One possibility is that the release of lysosomal enzymes is time-dependent and requires 48–72 h for maximal activation. This activation may occur more rapidly in cold-stored kidneys, due to the low intracellular pH.

Another explanation is that perfusion removes toxic metabolites from the kidney, such as free fatty acids, formed by the action of phospholipases on phospholipids[15]. Albumin in the perfusate may enhance the removal of free fatty acids from the perfused kidney. Fatty acids are potent modulators of mitochondrial structure and function[16,17] and may also cause alterations in the properties of other membranous systems. The mechanism for loss of mitochondrial activity during preservation, in fact, appears related to the accumulation of free fatty acids (see Chapter 16).

Using this simple gluconate-based perfusate we have been able to obtain good 3-day preservation. This isosmolar solution can also be used for cold storage of dog kidneys for 24 h. However, we have been unable to obtain 5 days of preservation by perfusion under N_2 or air. It appears that improvements in perfusion preservation and simple hypothermic storage of kidneys both require a more complete understanding of the mechanisms that prevent cell viability, and the design of perfusates to suppress these destructive cellular reactions.

Acknowledgement

This work was supported by NIH Grant AM 16248.

References

1. Belzer, F. O., Ashby, B. S. and Dumphy, J. E. (1967). 24 hour and 72 hour preservation of canine kidneys. *Lancet*, **2**, 536
2. Collins, G. M., Bravo-Shugarman, M. B. and Terasaki, P. I. (1969). Kidney preservation for transportation. Initial perfusion and 30 hours ice storage. *Lancet*, **2**, 1219
3. Belzer, F. O. and Southard, J. H. (1980). The future of kidney preservation. *Transplantation*, **30**, 161
4. Marshall, V. C. (1980). Renal preservation prior to transplantation. *Transplantation*, **30**, 165
5. Collins, G. M. and Halasz, N. A. (1977). Current aspects of renal preservation. *Urology*, **10** (suppl. 1), 22
6. Southard, J. H., Senzig, K. A., Hoffmann, R. M. and Belzer, F. O. (1980). Toxicity of oxygen to mitochondrial respiratory activity in hypothermically perfused canine kidneys. *Transplantation*, **29**, 459
7. Tappel, L. and Falkin, H. (1959). Lipid peroxidation in isolated mitochondria. *Arch. Biochem. Biophys.*, **80**, 326
8. Bidlack, W. R. and Tappel, A. L. (1973). Damage to microsomal membrane by lipid peroxidation. *Lipids*, **8**, 177
9. Southard, J. H. and Belzer, F. O. (1980). Control of canine kidney cortex slice volume and ion distribution at hypothermia by impermeable anions. *Cryobiology*, **17**, 540
10. Southard, J. H., Senzig, K. A., Hoffmann, R. M. and Belzer, F. O. (1977). Energy metabolism in kidneys stored by simple hypothermia. *Transplant. Proc.*, **9**, 1535
11. Williams, J. A. and Woodburg, D. M. (1971). Determination of extracellular space and intracellular electrolytes in rat liver *in vivo*. *J. Physiol.*, **212**, 85
12. Ohkawa, H., Ohishi, N. and Yagi, K. (1978). Assay for lipid peroxides in animal tissues by thiobarbituric acid reaction. *Analyt. Biochem.*, **95**, 351
13. Bore, P. J., Sehr, P. A., Chan, L., Thulborn, K. R., Ross, B. D. and Radda, G. K. (1981). The importance of pH in renal preservation. *Transplant. Proc.*, **13**, 707
14. Cunarro, J. A., Johnson, W. A., Uehling, D. T., Updike, S. J. and Weiner, M. W. (1976). Metabolic consequences of low temperature kidney preservation. *J. Lab. Clin. Med.*, **88**, 873

15. Huang, J.S., Downes, G.L. and Belzer, F.O. (1971). Utilization of fatty acids in perfused dog kidney. *J. Lipid Res.,* **12,** 622
16. Hunter, D.R., Haworth, R.A. and Southard, J.H. (1976). Relationship between configuration, function, and permeability in calcium-treated mitochondria. *J. Biol. Chem.,* **251,** 5069
17. Zborowski, J. and Wojtzcak, L. (1963). Induction of swelling of liver mitochondria by fatty acids of various chain lengths. *Biochem. Biophys. Acta,* **70,** 596

36
The use of oncotic support agents in perfusion preservation

R. M. HOFFMANN, J. H. SOUTHARD and F. O. BELZER

Continuous perfusion of the kidney produces an increase in the extra-cellular space[1,2] usually accompanied by cell shrinkage leading to what has been termed the 'exploded view'[2]. This increase in extracellular space leads to tissue oedema which may have a detrimental effect on the distribution of intrarenal flow. The influence of fluid shifts in the tissue on perfusion para-meters is evident during the later stages of perfusion as indicated by an increase in perfusion pressure and decreased flow[3]. At present all perfusates used in experimental and clinical renal preservation contain serum albumin for oncotic support. Unfortunately, serum albumin (MW 66 000) escapes from the intravascular to the extravascular space during perfusion and thus with time intravascular oncotic pressure is diminished[1]. In addition, perfusion-induced denaturation of albumin can occur and produce endo-thelial damage[4]. Theoretically, intracellular fluid distribution in the perfused kidney could be controlled by the addition of compounds to the perfusate which provide oncotic support and remain intravascular.

During the past 2 years an extensive study was undertaken in our laboratory to evaluate the role of oncotic support substances in preservation in the hope of finding a compound that would be stable, provide sufficient oncotic support, remain intravascular and produce no direct endothelial cell damage. The object of this report is to present results using different polymers including hydroxyethyl starch, dextran, gum arabic, polyethylene glycol, cross-link albumin and cross-link haemoglobin as oncotic agents in continuous perfusion of canine kidneys.

METHODS

All studies were performed on female dogs weighing between 18 and 25 kg. The dogs were anaesthetized with halothane. Each dog was pretreated with 500 ml of normal saline containing mannitol (5 g). After dissection, the kidneys were allowed a 15 min *in-situ* recovery period and were removed in the diuresing state. The renal arteries were cannulated and the kidneys flushed with cold (4 °C) saline (0.9%) followed by preservation for 24 h and in some cases 72 h by pulsatile perfusion on the Belzer machine[5]. The kidneys were autotransplanted through the groin. Contralateral nephrectomy was performed following transplantation. In all experiments, post-transplant serum creatinine levels were determined daily and followed until the levels reached normal or the dogs died. Autopsies were carried out, and tissue sections of the kidneys were examined histologically with haematoxylin and eosin stain. The contralateral kidneys were preserved by similar methods and cortex tissue was analysed for total tissue water by oven drying.

The perfusate composition was similar to that described by Halasz and Collins[6] and used previously by our group[4]. Various combinations of polymers were added to this perfusate at varying concentrations. In some experiments human serum albumin (HSA) was also added to the perfusate. Final concentrations were Na^+ (130–140 mmol/l), K^+ (4–6 mmol/l) and osmolality (300–320 mosmol/kg). Bovine serum albumin (BSA) was cross-linked by glutaraldehyde. BSA (5 g%) was dissolved in H_2O and glutaraldehyde (10 mmol/l) was added slowly. The reaction was allowed to proceed for 1 h at which time lysine, equal to 5 times the concentration of glutaraldehyde, was added to complex any unreacted glutaraldehyde. This mixture was dialysed for 4 h against distilled water using the Dow-Cordis Dak Dialysis coil. The cross-linked albumin was lyophilized and re-dissolved in the perfusate at the level to be studied. The size of the cross-linked albumin was determined by column chromatography. Over 90% of the total protein eluted as one peak (OD 280 nm) with a molecular weight range of 200 000–300 000. Haemoglobin was prepared from dog red blood cells by the procedure of Rabiner et al.[7]. Haemoglobin was cross-linked by the procedure used for BSA and resulted in a protein of similar molecular weight. Hydroxyethyl starch (HES) (200 000 MW) was obtained as a gift from McGaw Laboratories. Dextran (2×10^6 MW), gum arabic (250 000 MW), polyethylene glycol (PEG) (4000 MW) and bovine serum albumin were obtained from Sigma Chemical Co.

RESULTS

The experimental results were compared to control experiments (Table 36.1) where 6 of 6 dogs survived with kidneys preserved for 24 h with our basic HSA perfusate. All the polymers tested resulted in post-transplant serum creatinine levels greater than controls after only 24 h of preservation. HES provided the best preservation for 24 h (4/4 survival). Dextran and PEG were somewhat less effective (3/12 and 6/9 survivals, respectively). Gum arabic was toxic to all kidneys studied (0/10) and caused severe endothelial cell damage. Only two kidneys were functional following 72 h of preservation with HES. All the other polymers caused endothelial cell damage after 72 h as indicated by the formation of black kidneys upon the release of the vascular clamps.

Pegg et al.[8] have shown that addition of albumin to dextran-containing

Table 36.1 Effects of perfusion preservation with polymers and albumin on post-transplant kidney function

	No. dogs	Perf. time (h)	Total tissue H_2O	Kidney colour	Survival	Highest serum creatinine (mg/dl)	Normal serum creatinine <2 (days)
HSA (control)	6	24	4.20	normal	6/6	1.8	—
HES 1–3%	4	24	3.67	normal	4/4	2.7	5
HES 2–6%	7	72	4.20	> 6% conc. black	2/7	6.5	10
PEG 2.5–5%	9	24	3.83	normal	6/9	4.3	6
Dextran 1–10%	12	24	3.85	dusky to black	3/12	4.6	7
Gum arabic 2–10%	10	24	3.35	black	0/10	—	—
Cross-link albumin 3–7%	7	24	3.50	black	0/7	—	—
Cross-link haemoglobin 3–7%	7	24	3.60	black	0/7	—	—

Experimental procedures are described in the text

perfusates improved preservation. However, we found that the combination of albumin and polymers did not improve significantly survival of kidneys after 24 h of preservation. Both cross-linked proteins were not effective even after only 24 h of preservation and produced severe endothelial cell damage.

The total tissue water was reduced by the addition of polymers to the perfusate. With the basic perfusate containing HSA, the total tissue water averaged 4.2 ± 0.2 kg/kg dry weight. Following 24 h of perfusion the total tissue water was consistently reduced to 3.0–4.0 kg/kg dry weight by the inclusion of the various polymers.

DISCUSSION

Although serum albumin can be used for successful 3-day preservation of dog kidneys, there is evidence to suggest that this colloid osmotic support agent may be a factor in limiting the quality or duration of preservation. A number of reports have indicated that successful preservation often depended upon the particular batch or supplier of albumin. We have shown that simple mechanical manipulation of albumin can lead to poor preservation and often direct toxicity to endothelial cells[4]. Furthermore, the primary role suggested for albumin, oncotic support, is lost with time due to the extravascularization of the albumin. These problems, inherent in albumin-containing perfusates, suggested to us that one reason successful long-term preservation (> 5 days) is not reproducibly attainable is the presence of albumin. We therefore attempted to find more suitable materials capable of providing oncotic support, which would remain in the vascular network, and produce no endothelial cell damage.

Although most of the polymers produced good intravascular oncotic support as evidenced by the lower level of total tissue water compared to albumin-perfused kidneys, all but the HES and PEG 4000 produced severe endothelial damage as demonstrated by the darkening of the kidneys shortly after implantation. Microscopic findings supported the presence of endothelial cell damage as indicated by extravascular haemorrhage. HES and PEG 4000, especially in combination with albumin, allowed 24 h preservation, but produced endothelial damage if preservation was extended to 72 h.

The precise mechanism of vascular damage induced by these polymers cannot yet be described. The damage does appear to be vascular-related since metabolic parameters determined on kidneys preserved by these methods (tissue oedema, electrolyte composition, levels of adenine nucleotides and mitochondrial function) appear to be similar to kidneys that are viable (unpublished observation). At this time serum albumin appears to be the only safe substance to provide oncotic support during kidney preservation.

The results we have presented, although essentially negative, will hopefully stimulate further consideration of important questions related to optimizing preservation of kidneys. For instance, is oncotic support a necessary characteristic of a perfusate or does albumin serve other roles in maintaining kidney viability? Do perfusates need formed elements such as platelets to aid in preserving the viability of the vasculature? Is endothelial cell damage related to mechanical or biochemical-induced cell damage? Will synthetic polymers provide non-toxic oncotic support if combined with an ideal perfusate?

Acknowledgement

This work was supported by NIH Grant AM18264.

References

1. Belzer, F.O., Hoffmann, R.M., Senzig, K.A. and Southard, J.H. (1979). Perfusion preservation of canine kidneys. In Pegg, D.E. and Jacobsen, I.A. (eds.) *Organ Preservation II*, pp. 207–219. (Edinburgh: Churchill Livingstone)
2. Pegg, D.E. and Farrant, J. (1969). Vascular resistance and edema in the isolated rabbit kidney perfused with a cell-free solution. *Cryobiology*, **6**, 200
3. Belzer, F.O., Hoffmann, R.M. and Southard, J.H. (1978). Kidney preservation. *Surg. Clin. N. Am.*, **58**, 261
4. Southard, J.H., Senzig, K.A., Hoffmann, R.M. and Belzer, F.O. (1981). Denaturation of albumin: a critical factor in long-term kidney preservation. *J. Surg. Res.*, **30**, 80
5. Belzer, F.O., Ashby, B.S. and Dunphy, J.E. (1967). 24 hour and 72 hour preservation of canine kidneys. *Lancet*, **2**, 536
6. Halasz, N.A. and Collins, G.M. (1974). Simplification of perfusion preservation methods. *Transplantation*, **17**, 534
7. Rabiner, S.F., Helbert, J.R., Lopas, H. and Friedman, L.H. (1967). Evaluation of stroma-free hemoglobin solution for use as a plasma expander. *J. Exp. Med.*, **126**, 1127
8. Pegg, D.E., Jacobsen, I.A. and Walter, C.A. (1977). Hypothermic perfusion of rabbit kidneys with solutions containing gelatin polypeptides. *Transplantation*, **24**, 29

37
Intermediate *ex-vivo* and *in-vitro* perfusion to prolong hypothermic kidney preservation up to 6 days

B. G. RIJKMANS, G. KOOTSTRA, J. VAN DER WIJK and A. NIZET

In experimental studies successful 3-day kidney preservation with hypothermic continuous perfusion has been reported by several authors[1-4]. The results of preservation for more than 3 days are less consistent[5,6]. We have shown that a few hours of normothermic *ex-vivo* perfusion halfway through a period of 6 days hypothermic perfusion has a beneficial effect on the preserved kidney[7,8]. Since this model is not applicable in the clinical situation we investigated whether this beneficial effect could also be achieved with perfusion in a heart–lung machine (*in vitro* perfusion).

METHODS

An autotransplantation model with immediate contralateral nephrectomy was employed. Mongrel dogs (21–24 kg) were anaesthetized and hydrated with 1 litre of 2.5% glucose and 0.45% saline solution. The right renal vessels were dissected free; 5 min before clamping, 20 g mannitol was given intravenously. After removal, the kidney was flushed with 500 ml Euro-Collins solution at 4 °C.

Group I

In group I (6 dogs) the kidney was preserved for 144 h on a preservation machine (Gambro®). The flow of the perfusate (an extracellular albumin (Kabi®) solution) was adjusted to 75/ml/min/100 g. The perfusate was kept between 5 and 7 °C. Oxygen (200 ml/min) was blown over the perfusate. Daily pH measurements were made at 37 °C. After 6 days the kidney was reimplanted in the neck with a ureterocutaneostomy and the contralateral kidney was removed.

Groups II and III

In group II (6 dogs) and in group III (8 dogs) the procedure was the same as in group I except that after 72 h the perfusion was interrupted by a normothermic perfusion for 3 h. In group II the donor dog was used for this perfusion[7,8]. In group III the normothermic perfusion was performed for 3 h in a heart–lung machine using whole heparinized allogeneic blood as perfusate. A detailed description of the perfusion machine, including a cylinder film oxygenator and a Dale Schuster-type pump, has been given previously[9,10]. The arterial blood pressure was kept between 110 and 120 mmHg.

After the normothermic perfusion the kidneys were flushed with Euro-Collins solution, and placed on the Gambro machine for another 72 h. The implantation technique was the same as in group I.

During the normothermic perfusion a saline solution with 0.020 mCi [^{125}I]iothalamate and 0.020 mCi [^{131}I]hippuran was infused. Hourly urine and blood samples were taken and counted on a dual channel scintillation detector. Kidney function was determined by calculating the clearance of [^{125}I]iothalamate (GFR) and [^{131}I]hippuran (ERPF) using the standard formula (UV/P)[11]. By dividing the GFR by the ERPF the FF was calculated.

RESULTS

In all groups a constant systolic pressure of 25 mmHg was recorded. The pH of the perfusate increased from 7.0 to 7.2. In the *ex vivo*-perfused

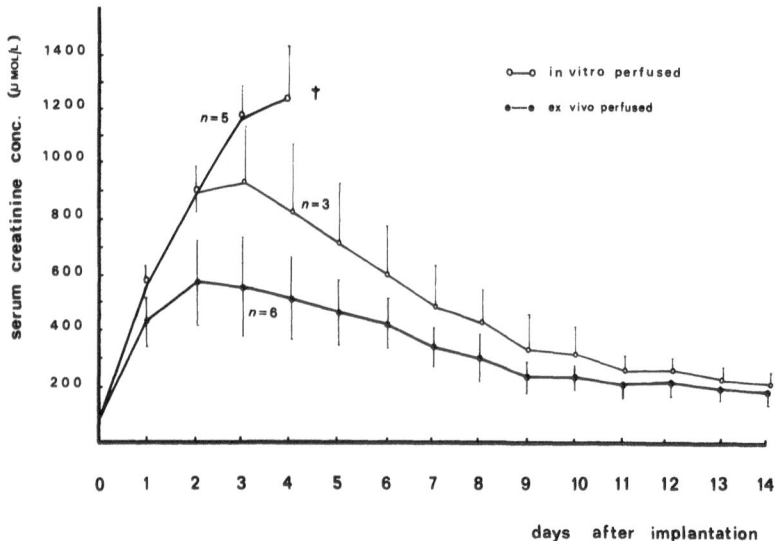

Figure 37.1 Mean values (± SD) of serum creatinine concentration after implantation for groups II (*n* = 6) and III (*n* = 8). The results of group III have been divided into two lines. Upper line: five dogs died; bottom line: three dogs survived

Table 37.1 GFR, ERPF and FF values during *ex vivo* perfusion (group II)

Dog	GFR (ml/min/100 g)			ERPF (ml/min/100 g)			FF		
	1st hour	2nd hour	3rd hour	1st hour	2nd hour	3rd hour	1st hour	2nd hour	3rd hour
7	n.d.*	n.d.	n.d.	n.d.	n.d.	n.d.	n.d.	n.d.	n.d.
8	0.57	0.55	1.58	4.3	3.7	13.6	0.13	0.15	0.12
9	0.03	0.58	1.14	0.13	5.0	8.3	0.23	0.12	0.14
10	0.06	0.20	0.39	0.29	4.1	6.2	0.20	0.05	0.06
11	0.21	0.94	1.61	0.8	6.6	10.7	0.26	0.14	0.15
12	4.39	5.46	4.39	22.0	22.7	15.8	0.20	0.24	0.28

* Not done: the urine collection failed during this perfusion

Table 37.2 GFR, ERPF and FF values during *in vitro* perfusion (group III)

Dog	GFR (ml/min/100 g)			ERPF (ml/min/100 g)			FF		
	1st hour	2nd hour	3rd hour	1st hour	2nd hour	3rd hour	1st hour	2nd hour	3rd hour
13*	2.9	4.2	3.1	13.7	23.8	19.1	0.21	0.18	0.16
14*	0.2	0.4	0.2	1.2	1.8	0.8	0.17	0.22	0.25
15	2.3	3.1	2.1	4.9	15.9	9.4	0.47	0.19	0.22
16	1.2	2.9	2.1	9.1	23.7	14.8	0.13	0.12	0.14
17*	4.2	3.1	2.4	19.6	24.7	18.8	0.21	0.13	0.13
18	3.0	3.4	3.0	24.6	30.9	23.5	0.12	0.11	0.13
19	2.7	2.8	2.6	17.6	16.4	12.9	0.15	0.17	0.20
20	8.1	10.1	7.1	32.7	39.8	28.4	0.25	0.25	0.25

* These dogs had life-sustaining kidney function after implantation

group (II) all animals had life-sustaining kidney function after implantation. In the *in vitro*-perfused group (III) three out of eight dogs survived, whereas in the control group (I) only one out of six had life-sustaining kidney function. The mean serum creatinine concentration reached a maximum value in the *ex vivo*-perfused group on day 2: 580 μmol/l ($n = 6$), in the *in vitro*-perfused group on day 3: 890 μmol/l ($n = 3$) (Figure 37.1) and in the survivor of the control group (I) on day 5: 1080 μmol/l ($n = 1$). During the 3 h of *ex vivo* perfusion the mean arterial pressure delivered by the donor dog varied slightly (range 90–110 mmHg). In the heart–lung machine the arterial pressure was kept between 110 and 120 mmHg. The renal blood flow in the *ex vivo*-perfused kidneys was constant at 110 ± 17 ml/min/100 g. In all *in vitro*-perfused kidneys the renal blood flow increased steadily from 165 ± 21 ml in the first hour to 260 ± 49 ml/min/100 g in the third hour.

The GFR and ERPF measurements during the *ex vivo* and *in vitro* perfusion showed different results. In four out of five measurements in the *ex vivo* group, GFR and ERPF increased to a multiple of the first hour values. (In this study the value of the ERPF should not be considered as an approximation of the true renal plasma flow but rather as a measure of the proximal tubular function) (Table 37.1). Since ERPF increased relatively more than GFR a decrease in FF was seen. In one case GFR and ERPF values were relatively high, and the ERPF decreased, whereas little change in GFR was observed.

In most experiments of group III, higher values for GFR and ERPF were measured in the first hour of the *in vitro* perfusion (Table 37.2); however after a slight increase in the second hour all values dropped to the same level or even lower levels than those in the first hour. No correlation could be demonstrated between the values of the GFR and ERPF and life-sustaining function after implantation. (In this study the value of the ERPF should not be considered as an approximation of the true renal plasma flow but rather as a measure of the proximal tubular function.)

DISCUSSION

Normothermic perfusion of organs as applied in group II was used in the 1960s for preservation and viability testing[12,13]. *Ex vivo* perfusion was used in combination with hypothermic perfusion by Pausescu *et al.*[14] in heart preservation experiments, and we have used it for the first time in kidney preservation. Although the perfusion characteristics were good during the *in vitro* perfusion (group III), this did not have the same beneficial effect as *ex vivo* perfusion. This may be due to detrimental mechanical effects on the blood, but the heart–lung machine has been applied successfully for physiological studies[10]. Other explanations for the poor results of the *in vitro* perfusion could be lack of nutrients or the accumulation of toxic metabolites supplied or removed respectively by the donor dog in the *ex vivo* perfusion. Since in group II the renal blood flow was constant during the *ex vivo* perfusion, the GFR and ERPF values indicate an improving extraction of [^{131}I]hippuran by recovering proximal tubules. This phenomenon has also been described in human renal allotransplantation during the first 24 h[15]. In the *in vitro*-perfused group the GFR and ERPF values dropped during the third hour of perfusion, and the extraction of [^{131}I]hippuran was impaired even more. A similar decrease in tubular function after several hours of normothermic isolated perfusion has been reported by others[16-18].

In nearly all perfusions in group II and III a subnormal filtration fraction (FF) was observed, probably due to low glomerular filtration pressures, as also reported in human allotransplantation[19-21].

From this study we conclude that it is possible to restore an 'ischaemically damaged' kidney by 3 h of normothermic *ex vivo* perfusion, but not *in vitro*. Further study is needed to determine whether the benefit is an intrinsic effect of the *ex vivo* situation, or whether an ideal heart–lung machine would be equally effective.

Acknowledgements

This work was supported by a grant from the Dutch Kidney Foundation (C 163). We are grateful to Mr K. Bel, Mr D. Meijer, Mr. H. Thoumsin and Mrs J. Thoumsin-Moons for technical assistance. We thank Miss M. van den Berg for her secretarial assistance.

References

1. Abouna, G. M., Lim, F., Cook, J. S., Grubb, W., Craig, S. S., Seibel, H. R. and Hume, D. M. (1972). Three day canine kidney preservation. *Surgery*, **71**, 436
2. Belzer, F. O., Ashby, B. S. and Dunphy, J. E. (1967). 24-Hour and 72-hour preservation of canine kidneys. *Lancet*, **2**, 536
3. Claes, G. and Blohme, I. (1973). Experimental and clinical results of continuous albumin perfusion of kidneys. In Pegg, D. E. (ed.), *Organ Preservation*, p. 51. (London: Churchill Livingstone)
4. Liu, W. P., Humphries, A. L. Jr, Russell, R., Stoddard, L. D., Garcia, L. A. and Serkes, K. D. (1973). Three- and seven-day perfusion of dog kidneys with human plasma protein fraction IV-4. *Surg. Forum*, **24**, 316
5. Woods, J. E. (1971). Successful three- to seven-day preservation of canine kidneys. *Arch. Surg.*, **102**, 614
6. Johnson, R. W. G., Cohen, G. L. and Ballardie, F. D. (1979). The limitations of continuous perfusion with plasma protein fraction. In Pegg, D. E. and Jacobsen, I. A. (eds.) *Organ Preservation II*, p. 18. (Edinburgh: Churchill Livingstone)
7. Kootstra, G., Van der Wijk, J. and Rijkmans, B. G. (1980). A new device towards intermediate term kidney preservation. An experimental study. *Scand. J. Urol. Nephrol.*, **54** (suppl.), 86
8. Van der Wijk, J., Slooff, M. J. H., Rijkmans, B. G. and Kootstra, G. (1980). Successful 96- and 144-hour experimental kidney preservation: a combination of standard machine preservation and newly developed normothermic ex vivo perfusion. *Cryobiology*, **17**, 473
9. Cuypers, Y., Nizet, A. and Baerten, A. (1964). Technique pour la perfusion de reins isolés de chien avec du sang hépariné. *Arch. Int. Physiol. Biochem.*, **72**, 245
10. Nizet, A. (1975). The isolated perfused kidney: possibilities, limitations and results. *Kidney Int.* (ed. review) **7**, 1

11. Smith, H. W. (1951). *The Kidney. Structure and Function in Health and Disease,* p. 43. (New York: Oxford University Press)
12. Baitz, T., Hallenbeck, G. A., Shorter, R. G., Scott, G. W., Owen, Ch. A. and Hunt, J. C. (1965). Preservation of kidneys for transplantation. *Arch. Surg.,* **91,** 276
13. Lavender, A. R., Forland, M., Rams, J. J., Thompson, J. S., Russe, H. P. and Spargo, B. H. (1968). Extracorporeal renal transplantation in man. *J. Am. Med. Assoc.,* **203,** 265
14. Pausescu, E., Mendler, N., Gebhardt, K. and Sebening, F. (1978). Exceptional performance in heart preservation with an amino acid-containing perfusion fluid. *World J. Surg.,* **2,** 109
15. Henderson, L. W., Nolph, K. D., Puschett, J. B. and Goldberg, M. (1968). Proximal tubular malfunction as a mechanism for diuresis after renal homotransplantation. *N. Engl. J. Med.,* **278,** 467
16. Rosenfeld, S., Sellers, A. and Katz, J. (1959). Development of an isolated perfused mammalian kidney. *Am. J. Physiol.,* **196,** 1155
17. Waugh, W. H. and Kubo, T. (1969). Development of an isolated perfused dog kidney with improved function. *Am. J. Physiol.,* **217,** 277
18. Schepper, J. de and Stock, J. van der. (1971). Een perfusie methode van de geïsoleerde hondennier. *Vlaams Diergeneeskd. Tijdschr.,* **40,** 373
19. Herdman, R. C., Vernier, R. L., Michael, A. F., Kelly, W. D. and Good, R. A. (1966). Renal function and phosphorus excretion after human renal homotransplantation. *Lancet,* **1,** 121
20. Herdman, R. C., Michael, A. F., Vernier, R. L., Kelly, W. D. and Good, R. A. (1967). Changes in phosphorus excretion and renal function after human renal homotransplantation. *Nephron,* **5,** 170
21. Kountz, S. L., Truex, G., Earley, L. E. and Belzer, F. O. (1970). Serial hemodynamics after renal allotransplantation in man. *Circulation,* **41,** 217

38
Is normothermic preservation an alternative to hypothermic preservation?

R. N. DUNN, F. K. MERKEL, D. ROSEMAN, M. HAKLIN and K. ENGLISH

Currently, clinical preservation is at a standstill, the approximate maximum safe cold periods for kidneys, livers and hearts being 72, $10\frac{1}{2}$ and $3\frac{1}{2}$ h, respectively; a tiny fraction of their *in vivo* lifespan[1-3]. Neither the exact nature of the limiting factors nor a method for circumventing them is at hand. It seems likely that inactivation of the sodium pump, depletion of respiratory chain nucleotides, cellular swelling and/or membrane injury result in deterioration of the organ over time[1].

Normothermia, on the other hand, would eliminate these difficulties and substitute a different set of problems, possibly more easily solved. A major obstacle has been finding a suitable method to support cellular respiration. Erythrocytes have not been satisfactory because of their fragility, rendering them incompatible with mechanical perfusion circuits[4]. However, other substances, such as fluorocarbon emulsions, can mediate oxygen transport[5].

This paper describes preliminary experiments designed to evaluate the efficacy of a fluorocarbon (FC-43)-Pluronic F-68 emulsion (Fluosol-43, Green Cross Corp., Osaka, Japan) in maintaining normothermically perfused canine kidneys. Our thesis has been to re-create a homeostatic milieu by relying on the FC-43 emulsion to enhance the oxygen-carrying capacity of a perfusate containing calf serum and specific metabolic substrates to fuel and regulate the organ's metabolic processes. In effect we are treating the kidney as a poly-layer tissue culture.

METHODS

Nine canine kidneys weighing 60–85 g were randomly assigned to two groups, whose perfusates differed only by the absence or presence of per-fluorotributylamine (FC-43). The final composition of the two perfusates consisted of: Pluronic F-68, 1.76 g%; hydroxyethyl starch, 2.06 g%; calf serum, 19.24 vol%; intralipid, 1.0 vol%; glutamine, 34.4 mg%; protamine, 17.2 mg%; insulin 2.4 U/l; cortisone, 1.37 mg%; ephedrine, 0.28 mg%; thyroxide, 6.87 mEq%; cephamandol, 0.39 mg%: electrolytes + albumin, 1455 ml; with FC-43 added to group A.

Perfusions were carried out in a circuit consisting of a Plexiglas chamber, bubble oxygenator/reservoir (Wm Harvey cardiotomy reservoir), heat exchanger, bubble trap with aneroid pressure manometer, and temperature probe. A VERSA-Therm Model 2158 temperature regulator (Cole-Palmer Co.) was used to maintain 37 °C throughout each perfusion. Flow was maintained at 5 ml/g/min by use of non-pulsatile roller pumps. The perfusate was gassed with a humidified 95% oxygen, 5% CO_2 mixture at 1.5 litres/min.

After preoperative treatment with sephamandol, 25 mg/kg, nephrectomy was performed on volume-expanded, diuresing, heparinized mongrel dogs through a midline incision under intravenous sodium pentobarbital anaesthesia. Prior to nephrectomy, a needle biopsy was taken. The kidneys were weighed, and placed on the perfusion circuit within 3 min after clamping the renal vessels. The first 150 ml of perfusate was used to wash out the kidney and was discarded; the remaining perfusate was re-circulated. To replace evaporative losses, sterile water was added to the reservoir at a rate of 4.5 ml/h. Neither the renal vein nor the ureter were cannulated; urine formed during the perfusion was recycled into the perfusate to prevent depletion of Pluronic F-68, which is rapidly excreted by the kidney[6].

The perfusion pressure was monitored continuously. Arterial and venous perfusate samples, as well as needle biopsies, were obtained at the 1, 3, 6, 12, 18 and 24 h intervals. Arterial and venous pH, PCO_2, HCO_3, total CO_2, and base excess were determined using an ABL-2 Blood Gas Analyzer. The O_2 consumption was calculated. The perfusate was also analysed for sodium, potassium, chloride, CO_2, BUN, creatinine, glucose, calcium, magnesium, phosphorus and albumin, using a Technicon SMA-11 Auto-analyzer and lactic dehydrogenase was determined using a DuPont Auto-matic Clinical Analyser. Osmolarity and oncotic pressure were measured by the Advanced Digimatic Osmometer Model 3D11 and a Weil Oncometer System 186.

RESULTS

Perfusate electrolytes were similar in both groups and the concentrations of sodium, potassium, chloride, CO_2, BUN, creatinine, glucose, calcium, magnesium, phosphorus, and albumin did not change in any perfusion.

All non-FC-perfused kidneys experienced a greater liberation of LDH than FC-perfused kidneys. This difference became statistically significant at the 3 h interval ($p < 0.01$; randomization tests) (Figure 38.1).

The osmolarity of the FC group ($n = 5$) was 300.6 ± 2.87 mosmol/l and that of the non-FC group ($n = 4$) was 295.5 ± 0.9 mosmol/l. The oncotic

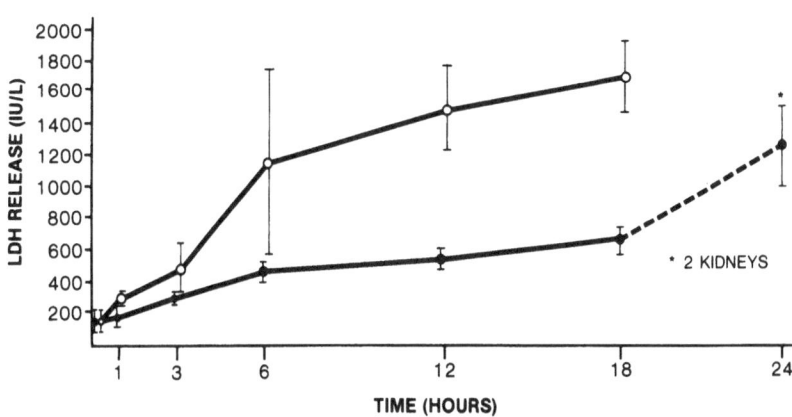

Figure 38.1 LDH release by FC and non-FC-perfused kidneys

pressure of the FC group ($n = 5$) was 23.4 ± 0.81 mmHg and the non-FC group ($n = 4$) was 22.75 ± 1.25 mmHg.

All kidneys were perfused for 18 h with the exception of two FC kidneys that reached the 24 h interval. All kidneys exhibited swelling in the final 3–5 h of their respective perfusions. The onset of visible swelling correlated to the onset of a rise in perfusion pressure for each kidney and mean weight gains of $56 \pm 5.3\%$ for the FC group and $51.9 \pm 4.1\%$ for the non-FC group.

The mean perfusion pressures for the two groups were similar. A perfusion run was terminated when the perfusion pressure reached 220 mmHg or when extravasation of perfusate from the cortical biopsy sites reduced the renal vein effluent sufficiently to preclude adequate sampling.

The oxygen-carrying capacity of each group was calculated from the ambient partial pressure of oxygen, the oxygen solubility coefficients of plasma and FC-43, and the respective volumes of the fluorocarbon and plasma phases (the fluorocrit = Fct).

[O_2]Group A at 37 °C and Po_2 500 mmHg

$$[O_2] = (0.06 \times Po_2 \times \text{Fct})_{FC} + 0.003 \times Po_2 \times (1 - \text{Fct}) \text{ plasma}$$
$$= 2.19 \text{ vol\%}_{FC} + 1.39 \text{ vol\%}_{Plasma}$$
$$= 3.58 \text{ vol\%}.$$

[O_2] Group B at 37 °C and Po_2 500 mmHg

$$[O_2] = (0.003 \times Po_2)$$
$$= 1.5 \text{ vol\%}.$$

Therefore, under identical conditions, the O_2 content of group A (FC) is 2.19 times as great as group B (non-FC).

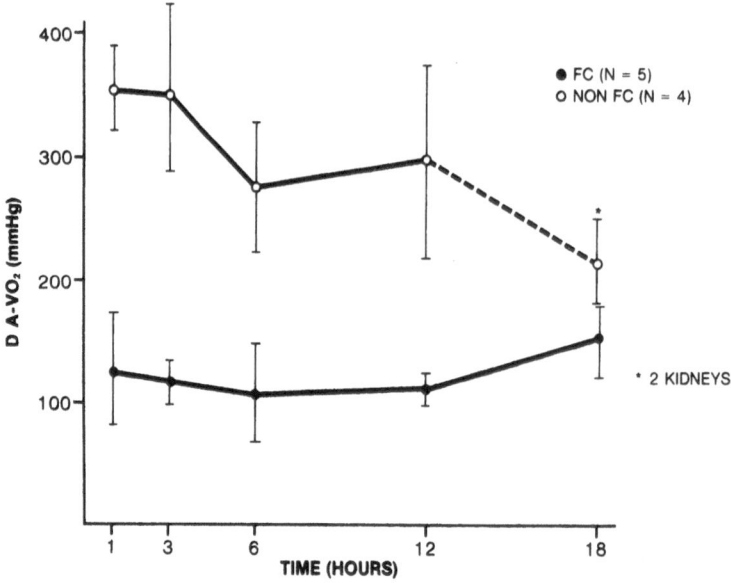

Figure 38.2 Arteriovenous Po_2 difference between FC and non-FC-perfused kidneys

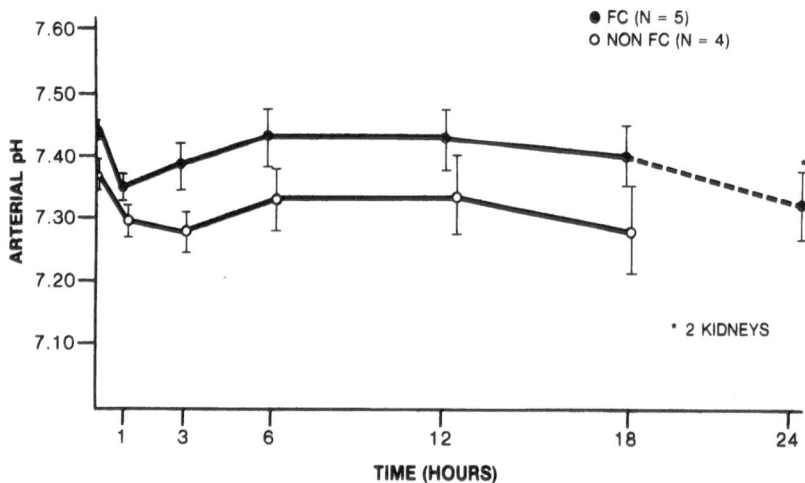

Figure 38.3 Perfusate pH measurements from FC and non-FC-perfused kidneys

The A–V O_2 differences were greater for the non-FC-perfused kidneys at each time interval (Figure 38.2). The differences are statistically significant ($p < 0.01$; randomization test), except at 18 h, when venous sampling was not possible in two of the non-FC kidneys.

When O_2 consumption is calculated from the perfusate flow rate, A–V O_2 difference, and respective O_2 contents, no difference between the groups was found. Values of 3.5–5.23 vol%/100 g/min approximate *in-vivo* values.

In both groups the pH fell after perfusion began. This drop in pH was more sustained in the non-FC group (Figure 38.3).

CONCLUSIONS

The FC-43 group was superior to the control kidneys in terms of LDH release, and maintenance of normal pH. No differences were found between the two groups with regard to weight increase, oxygen consumption, or perfusion pressure.

The more marked deterioration of the controls may be related to a relative tissue hypoxia, while deterioration of the FC-43 group seems more related to perfusate toxicity, lack of homeostasis, pathological flow dynamics, or oxygen toxicity. Further work is necessary to elucidate the reasons for failure.

Acknowledgements

This work was supported in part by funds from the Department of Surgery and Section of Transplantation, Rush-Presbyterian–St. Luke's Medical Center, Chicago, Illinois; Department of Surgery, Michael Reese Hospital, Chicago, Illinois; Alpha Therapeutics Corporation, Los Angeles, California; and The Green Cross Corporation, Osaka, Japan.

The authors wish to thank Betsy Trampe for her assistance in the preparation of the manuscript.

References

1. Belzer, F.O., Hoffmann, R.M. and Southard, J.H. (1978). Kidney preservation. *Surg. Clin. N. Am.*, **58**, 261
2. Calne, R.Y. (1978). Hepatic transplantation – 1978. *Surg. Clin. N. Am.*, **58**, 321
3. Thomas, F.T. (1978). Heart transplantation – 1978. *Surg. Clin. N. Am.*, **58**, 335
4. Waugh, W.H. and Kubo, T. (1969). Development of an isolated perfused dog kidney with improved function. *Am. J. Physiol.*, **217**, 277
5. Geyer, R.P. (1973). Fluorocarbon–polyol artificial blood substitutes. *N. Engl. J. Med.*, **289**, 1077
6. Grover, F.L., Amundsen, D. and Warden, J.L. (1974). The effect of Pluronic F-68 on circulatory dynamics and renal and carotid artery flow during hemorrhagic shock. *J. Surg. Res.*, **17**, 30

39
Measurement of tissue P_{O_2} during kidney perfusion with Fluosol®-43

O. RULAND, U. SPIEGEL, J. HAUSS, K. SCHÖNLEBEN and
H. THEMANN

Fluosol®-43 was used to maintain the oxygen supply to the tissue. It is a perfluorotributylamine (FC-43) emulsion with an average particle diameter of 0.085 μm. To furnish the emulsion with physiological osmolarity, oncotic pressure and buffer capacity, the addition of hypertonic modified Ringer's solution and human serum albumin is necessary.

Measurement of local oxygen pressure in different organs is possible by means of the platinum multiwire surface electrode (according to Kessler and Lübbers, 1966)[1]. In order to estimate the oxygen supply to the tissue no less than 100 individual measurements were used to construct a P_{O_2} histogram indicating the statistical distribution of local oxygen pressures. Compared to normal kidney P_{O_2} histograms, the recorded values during perfusion at 22 °C with Fluosol®-43 in an open system exceeded physiologically possible conditions (Figure 39.1).

The continuous registration of local tissue P_{O_2} provided the opportunity to detect changes in the microcirculatory bed immediately. The monitoring reflects the correspondence between tissue P_{O_2}, perfusion pressure and the extent of equilibration. In Figure 39.2, points A and B mark the increase or decrease of perfusion pressure. At point C, the gas flow was lowered provoking tissue hypoxia. Return to standard supply is signalled by A_1, B_1, C_1. Tissue P_{O_2} was not restored to initial levels, showing a marked damage due to hypoxia. The tissue damage is documented by a wider range of P_{O_2} values and a lower mean value, as compared to the initial level.

Arteriovenous P_{O_2} differences were in agreement with the other data which document a reliable correlation between P_{O_2} measurements and renal tissue status. Kidneys perfused with Fluosol®-43 at 22°C maintained an unchanged high level and physiological configuration of the P_{O_2} histogram, even beyond a 12 h period.

In light and electron microscopic examinations of kidneys after 12 h of Fluosol®-43 perfusion no hypoxic damage was found. The mitochondrial

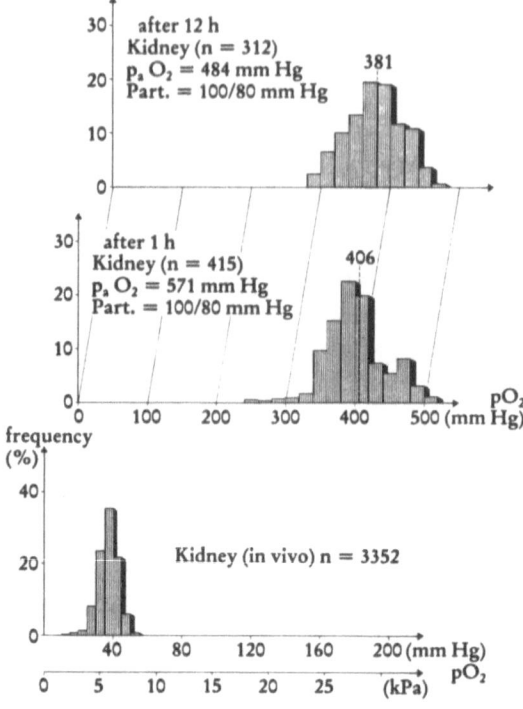

Figure 39.1 Kidney Po_2 histograms

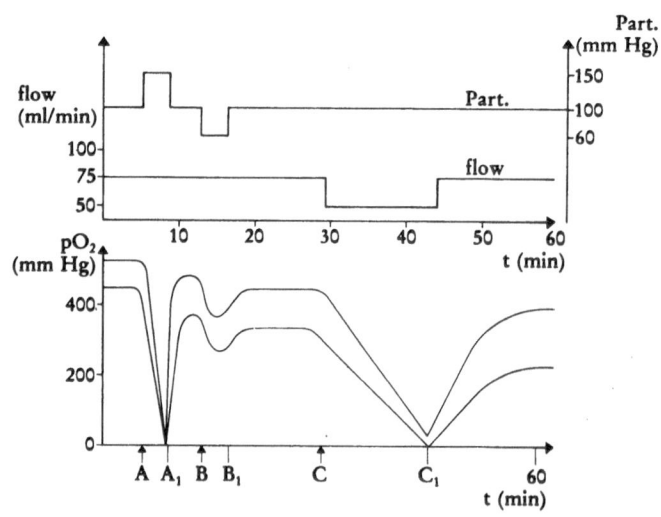

Figure 39.2 Continuous Po_2 measurement

structures were inconspicuous. No cell swelling was noted. In electrolyte and enzyme assessments from perfusate and urine no evidence of tissue damage was found.

Reference

1. Kessler, M. and Lübbers, D. W. (1966). Aufbau und Anwendungsmöglichkeiten verschiedener PO_2-Elektroden. *Pflügers Arch.*, **291**, 82

40
Liver preservation in the rat

N. KAMADA, R. Y. CALNE, D. G. D. WIGHT and B. J. ROSER

Small animals have been of limited use as models for liver preservation and subsequent transplantation because the surgery has been technically difficult. A cuff technique for the portal vein anastomosis was specially developed[1], which simplified vascular anastomosis after the isolated liver had been subjected to continuous perfusion. As a perfusate, fluorocarbon (FC) emulsion (Fluosol-43; Green Cross Co., Japan) was added to the basic perfusate[2], containing plasma protein fraction, which has produced the best results experimentally and clinically in our laboratory.

METHODS

Wistar rats of either sex between 250 and 350 g were used as donors and recipients in the experimental group and control group I, PVG rats between 200 and 280 g in control group II. The techniques of liver removal, perfusion and orthotopic transplantation have been published in detail[1,3] but certain modifications have been made.

Donor livers of the experimental group were perfused at 10-11 °C with added 8% (v/v) FC emulsion, control group I at 10-11 °C without FC emulsion and control group II at 20-25 °C with added 8% (v/v) FC emulsion.

RESULTS

In the experimental group, nine livers were perfused and the six recipient animals which survived more than 3 days are summarized in Table 40.1

Control group I consisted of six livers. Two recipients survived 4 and 5 days respectively. Control group II consisted of three animals all of which died during the first postoperative day.

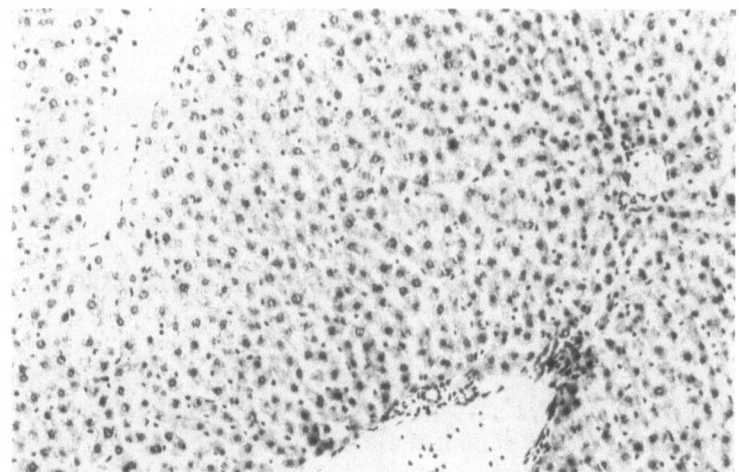

Figure 40.1 Experimental group (rat no. 1). Biopsy taken after revascularization. The liver is well preserved. H&E × 120

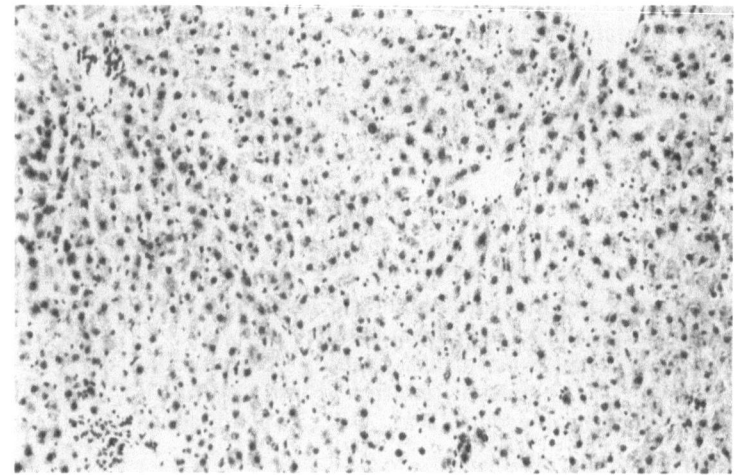

Figure 40.2 Control group I. There is widespread karyolysis and pyknosis of liver cell nuclei, especially in the mid zones. H&E × 120

DISCUSSION

As shown in Figure 40.1 (rat no. 1), livers perfused with added FC emulsion were well preserved and maintained recipient animals in good health. On the other hand, livers preserved for 20–22 h without FC emulsion showed extensive karyolysis and pyknosis of nuclei maximal in the centrilobular area (Figure 40.2), and could not maintain recipient animals for more than 5 days. In control group II, only three livers were perfused for 20–22 h at

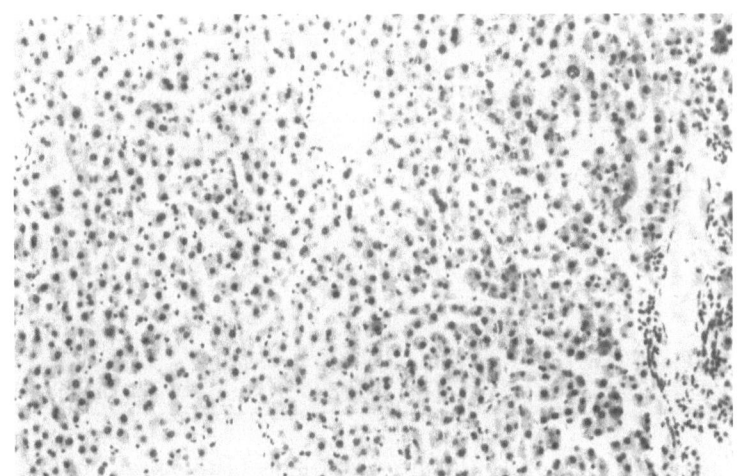

Figure 40.3   Control group II. There is some pyknosis of liver cell nuclei as well as separation of individual cells within liver cell plates. H&E × 120

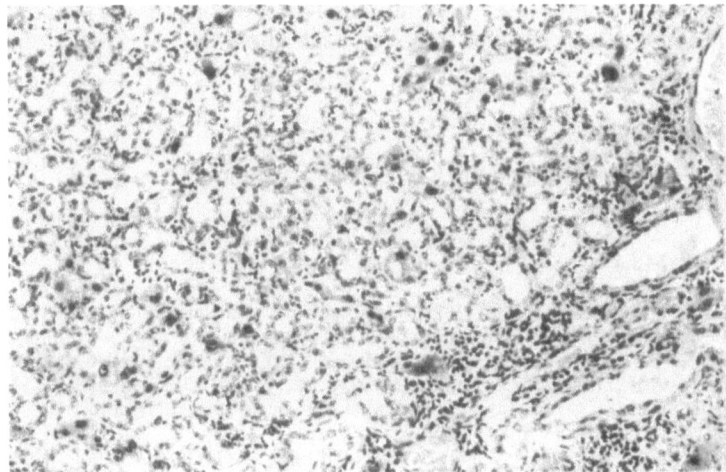

Figure 40.4   Experimental group (rat no. 2) (autopsy). Proliferating bile ductules have completely obliterated the normal liver architecture. This is the consequence of biliary obstruction. H&E × 120

20–25 °C with added FC emulsion and all of the animals grafted with these livers died within 24 h even though histologically (Figure 40.3) the degree of preservation seemed comparable to those of control group I. The cause of death could not be specifically determined in this group. It may be that the change from outbred Wistar to the more delicate inbred PVG strain was responsible for the failure to survive. This strain is known for example to be vitamin K-deficient and subject to postoperative bleeding.

In rat no. 2, autopsy showed almost complete replacement of the liver

Table 40.1 Results of transplantation of rat livers preserved with FC emulsion

Rat no.	Preservation time (h)	Bile production	Survival (days)	Cause of death
1	21	+ + +	420	Sacrifice
2	22	+ +	88	Biliary obstruction
3	22	+ +	3	Pneumonia
4	20	+ +	380	Sacrifice
5	21	+ +	395	Sacrifice
6	20	+ + +	268	Intestinal obstruction

with proliferating bile ducts (Figure 40.4). This histological finding has been produced by biliary obstruction.

We believe that the rat isograft model is particularly suited to studies of this type, and also that our current techniques of continuous perfusion might be usefully applied to immunological studies of the interaction between alloreactive cells and the liver as an allograft.

Acknowledgements

We thank Miss Anne Jones for secretarial assistance.

References

1. Kamada, N. and Calne, R. Y. (1979). Orthotopic liver transplantation in the rat. Technique using cuff for portal vein anastomosis and biliary drainage. *Transplantation*, **28**, 47
2. Calne, R. Y., Dunn, D. C., Herbertson, B. M., Gordon, E. M., Bitter-Suermann, H., Robson, A. J., MacDonald, A. S., Davis, D. R., Smith, D. P., Reitter, F. H. and Webster, L. M. (1972). Liver preservation by single-passage hypothermic 'squirt' perfusion. *Br. Med. J.*, **4**, 142
3. Kamada, N., Calne, R. Y., Wight, D. G. D. and Lines, J. G. (1980). Orthotopic rat liver transplantation after long-term preservation by continuous perfusion with fluorcarbon emulsion. *Transplantation*, **30**, 43

41
The effect of donor pretreatment on tubular function of the preserved canine allograft

A. SWISTEL, D. LORIEO and R. McCABE

Donor pretreatment (PT) with cytolytic drugs has been shown to have an additive effect with low-dose immunosuppression (LDI) in allograft prolongation[1] but may lead to serious tubular damage in the 24 h preserved kidney. Thirty-one nephrectomized male mongrel dogs received renal transplants and were divided into five groups. *Group 1* received an autograft preserved 24 h by perfusion with pooled autologous plasma. *Groups 2, 3 and 4* received renal allografts pretreated with cyclophosphamide (CY) 50 mg/kg and methylprednisolone (MP) 50 mg/kg 14 h before. *Group 2* kidneys were transplanted directly into LDI recipients that received azathioprine 2 mg/kg and MP 2 mg/kg daily. *Group 3* kidneys were cold stored in Collins' solution whereas *Group 4* were perfused for 24 h before allotransplantation to LDI hosts. *Group 6* kidneys were pretreated by perfusion with autologous plasma containing 1.0 g MP/800 ml for 24 h before implanting into LDI dogs. Animals were followed with daily serum creatinine and were considered to have rejected when the creatinine rose above 3 mg/dl. The results are tabulated in Table 41.1.

Table here

In these experiments PT caused a reversible tubular damage in the preserved kidney that was not observed in the directly transplanted kidney. The injury was more severe and prolonged in the cold-stored kidney and can be effectively eliminated by machine pretreatment with lymphocytolytic doses of MP. With larger doses of CY, up to 70 mg/kg, and the more prolonged preservation necessary to share PT kidneys, this injury may lead to oliguria and an increased risk of graft failure[2] that may negate the immunological advantages of pretreatment.

Table 41.1 Effect of donor pretreatment on serum creatinine in canine renal allografts

Group	Number of animals	Serum creatinine (mg/dl) post-transplant (± SEM)		Day of rejection (± SEM)
		Day 3	Day 7	
I Perfused autograft	6	2.9 ± 1.2	1.9 ± 0.4	NA
II Direct allograft	8	2.3 ± 0.3	2.4 ± 0.6	15.0 ± 2.9
III Cold-stored allograft	6	6.1 ± 0.8	3.9 ± 1.2	12.8 ± 2.2
IV Perfused allograft	6	6.2 ± 0.9	3.3 ± 0.5	18.4 ± 3.8
V Machine pretreated	5	2.7 ± 1.1	1.7 ± 1.0	16.8 ± 2.0

References

1. McCabe, R., Swistel, A., Lorieo, D. and Fitzpatrick, H. (1980). Prolongation of canine renal allografts in the immunosuppressed host by donor pretreatment with cytolytic agents. *Transplant. Proc.,* **12,** 355
2. McCabe, R. E., Lattes, C. G., Lorieo, D. R., Hashim, G. A. and Fitzpatrick, H. F. (1980). The protective effect of methyl prednisolone on the machine-preserved kidney. *Am. Surg.,* **46,** 335

42
Xenobanking

E. KEMP, G. KEMP, S. LARSEN, H. STARKLINT and C. J. GREEN

A possible although difficult method for organ preservation is xeno-banking, a term coined by Dupree in 1969[1]. As has been shown previously[2] and as will be shown in this chapter, preservation of an organ in an inter-mediate host is in fact possible for weeks. Indeed organ preservation by xenobanking allows longer periods of storage than any other method so far tried, but the obvious immunological problems have so far rendered it impractical. For this reason few workers have considered the possibility of storing organs in other species than the donor and most studies to date have been indistinguishable from investigations into xenografting[3-5]. Not until

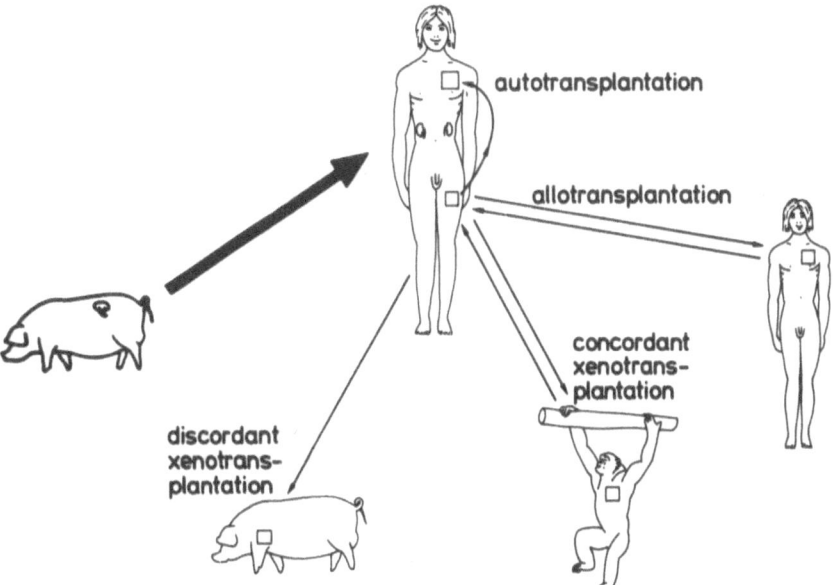

Figure 42.1 Different forms of transplantation: autotransplantation, allotransplantation, concordant xenotransplantation and discordant xenotransplantation

291

the early 1960s were more serious experiments carried out with clinical application in mind[2].

In the 1970s even less effort was committed to xenobanking or xeno-grafting, perhaps due to the attention focused on allografting and the relative success achieved in that situation with conventional immuno-suppressive treatment. Attempts at preventing the xenograft reaction with similar therapy proved discouraging[6].

However, the introduction of cyclosporin A[7] and the evidence that it is a highly potent suppressive agent suggested to us that it might prevent rejection of tissue transplanted between different but relatively close species (concordant xenograft–transplantation) even if it would be unlikely to affect rejection between discordant species (Figure 42.1). Since we already know that cyclosporin A (CS-A) prevents rejection of renal allo-grafts in rabbits[8], we decided to assess its value in protecting renal xeno-grafts donated by European hares (*Lepus europaeus*).

METHODS

A total of 21 renal xenotransplants were performed. Donor kidneys from European hares were transplanted into bilaterally nephrectomized French Lop-eared rabbits by previously described techniques[9,10].

Experimental groups

Group 1 (five experiments): control group, without CS-A or any other drug. *Group 2* (three experiments): 10 mg/kg body weight i.m. daily of CS-A from day 1 as long as the animals lived. *Group 3* (seven experiments): 15 mg/kg body weight i.m. daily of CS-A from day 1 for 30 days. Six experiments failed due to surgical or anaesthetic complications (e.g. ureteral blockage or renal artery thrombosis). These six cases have been classified separately into a 'failure group' after careful consideration between surgeon, nephrologist and two pathologists. Cyclosporin A was supplied dissolved in Miglyol 812 at 100 mg/ml and was administered by deep i.m. injection daily.

Light microscopy

The tissue was fixed in 4% formaldehyde buffered to pH 7.0, embedded in Paraplast®, cut into 4, 3 and 2 μm sections and stained with haematoxylin and eosin (H&E), PAS + H, silver methamine + H&E, Martius yellow scarlet blue and picro-Mallory V for fibrin. Weigert's resorcin fuchsin for elastic tissue and Giemsa stain for evaluation of the cell types in infiltrates were used.

Immunofluorescence microscopy

The methods, controls and equipment used have been described previously[11]. All kidney sections were examined by a direct IF staining technique using FITC-conjugated antisera obtained from Nordic Immunological Laboratories and used in dilutions 1 : 4–1 : 20. The following specific antisera were used: Rabbit anti-cat Ig, goat anti-rabbit Ig, swine anti-rabbit Ig, rabbit anti-duck Ig, goat anti-rabbit IgG, goat anti-rabbit C_3, and rabbit anti-duck IgG.

Electron microscopy

The tissue was immediately chopped and fixed in 2.5% glutaraldehyde in Tyrode's buffer modified to contain half of the sodium chloride given in the formula. Osmolarity varied in the range of 320–340 mosmol/l. The pH was 7.2. Tissue was post-fixed in osmium tetroxide, 1% in Tyrode, and Epon was used as the embedding medium. Ultrathin sections were stained with 1% uranyl acetate and 0.4% lead citrate.

Definitions

Hyperacute rejection was diagnosed when there were widespread, mainly glomerular, microthromboses. Acute cellular rejection was diagnosed when a mononuclear infiltrate (lymphocytes, lymphoplasmatoid cells, and immunoblasts) was found in the interstitial tissue, often gathered around the greater intrarenal vessels (Figures 42.6–42.8). All light and immunofluorescence microscopy was done without prior knowledge of the clinical or experimental data.

RESULTS

Renal function

Group 1 (recipients having no CS-A or other treatment). Renal function deteriorated rapidly and at day 4 to 6 the animals were severely uraemic and either died or were sacrificed. The serum creatinine levels of these animals are depicted in Figure 42.2. *Group 2* (recipients were given CS-A at 10 mg/kg i.m. daily from day 1 until they failed). Only three technically successful xenografts have so far been performed in this group so, although there is a tendency to prolonged survival (Figure 42.3), it is not statistically significant. *Group 3* (recipients given CS-A at 15 mg/kg i.m. daily from day 1 for 30 days). At this dosage the immunosuppressive effect of CS-A was striking. Several of the animals survived for weeks as shown in Figures 42.4 and 42.5, even though they received treatment for only 30 days.

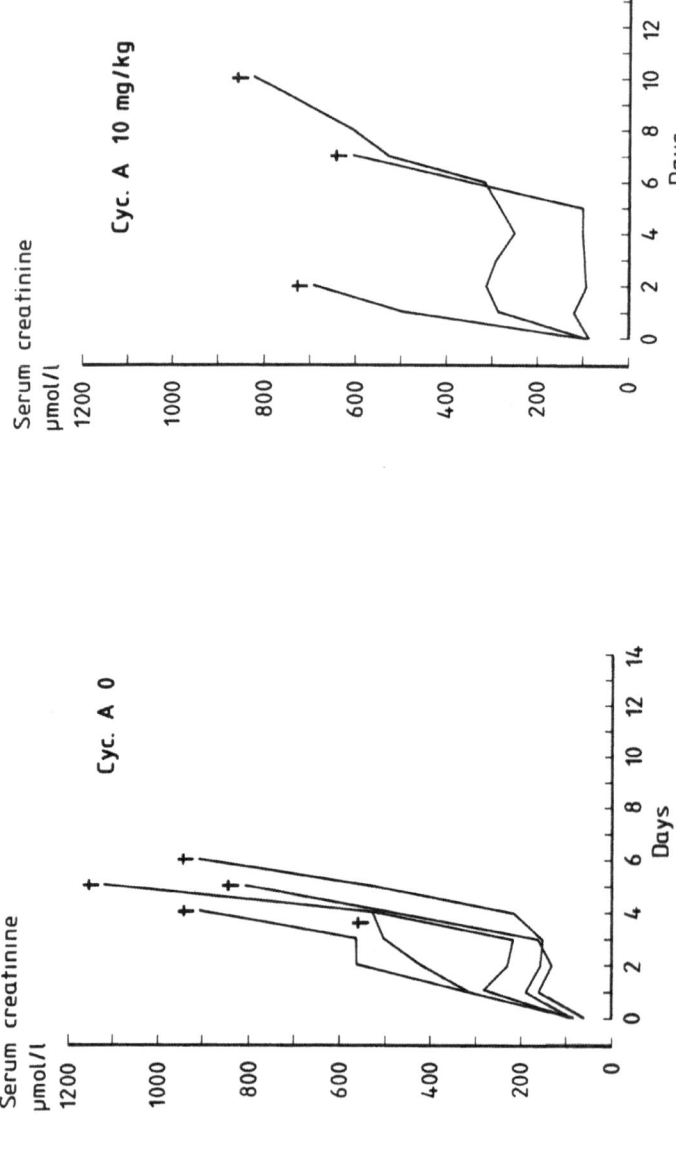

Figure 42.2 Renal function of five rabbits after bilateral nephrectomy and subsequent transplantation of hare kidneys

Figure 42.3 The serum creatinine levels of three rabbits treated with cyclosporin A 10 mg/kg body weight i.m. daily from day 1 as long as the animals lived. The animals were bilaterally nephrectomized and xenotransplanted with hare kidneys

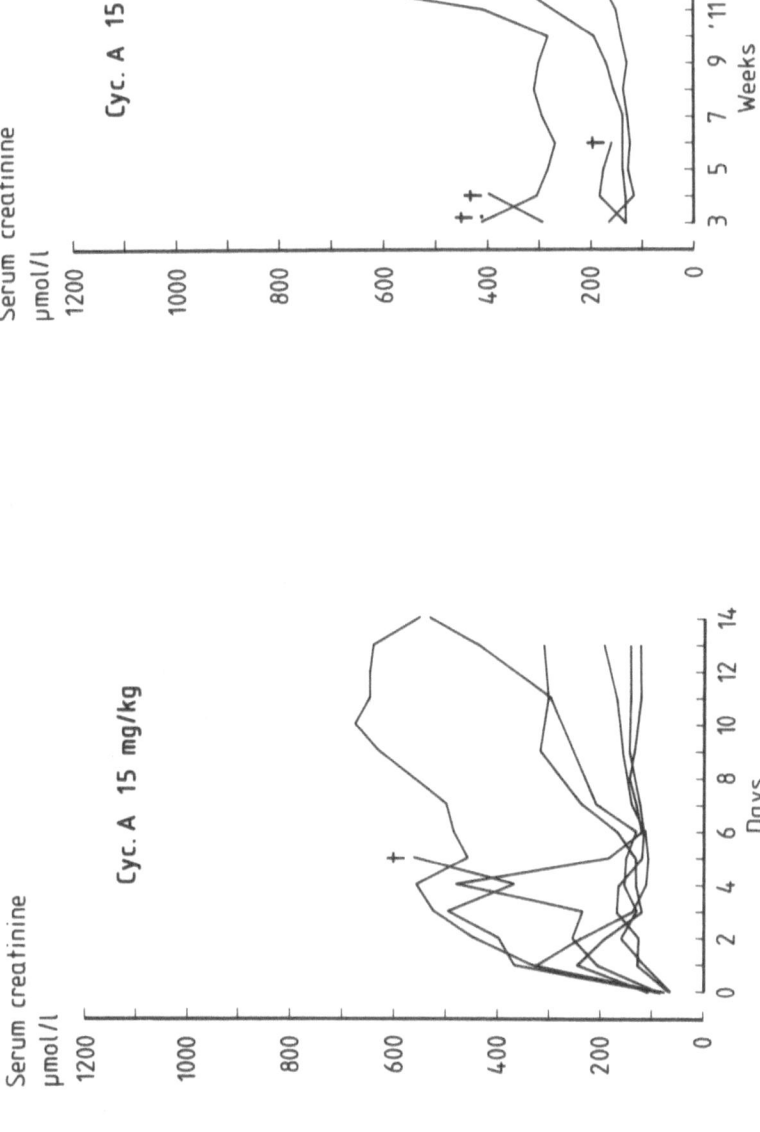

Figure 42.4 The serum creatinine levels of seven rabbits treated with cyclosporin A 15 mg/kg body weight i.m. for 30 days. The animals were bilaterally nephrectomized and xenotransplanted with hare kidneys

Figure 42.5 Serum creatinine in the same experiment as shown in Figure 42.4. Note the difference in abscissa (weeks) in comparison with the other figures (days)

Histology

Group 1. Two of the grafted kidneys showed hyperacute rejection. The greater intrarenal vessels showed fibrinoid necrosis with loss of elastic tissue. A sparse granulocytic infiltration was found in perivascular spaces. One showed signs of acute cellular rejection too, but microthromboses dominated. Three grafts showed only acute cellular rejection. There were no thromboses or necrosis of the vascular walls. Acute tubular necrosis was found in cortical tubules of one graft, and rather extensive calcification was seen in necrotic tubules. Four grafts were investigated by immunofluorescence. One of them showed a weak, diffuse, segmental, granular reaction along the glomerular basement membrane. Focally the tubular basement membrane was positive. Electron microscopy was done in one case with hyperacute rejection. The result was confirmatory. There was no accumulation of thrombocytes. Four of the corresponding not-transplanted right kidneys were normal. The fifth showed weak mesangial thickening. Immunofluorescence microscopy showed a weak, diffuse, global granular positivity for C_3 along the glomerular basement membrane. The corresponding left kidney was negative. Electron microscopy showed basement membrane material in mesangial area but no deposits.

Group 2. The grafted kidneys showed in two cases the aforementioned picture of hyperacute rejection. Their survival was slightly longer than the first group's. The third showed total infarction, probably as the result of an arterial occlusion after 2 days. All the grafts were investigated by immunofluorescence microscopy. One of them showed a weak focal, global positivity of granular type along the glomerular basement membrane. Focally the tubular basement membrane was positive. Electron microscopy of one case showed the same picture as in group 1. The corresponding right kidneys were normal on light microscopy. One case showed weak focal segmental fluorescence for C_3 along the glomerular basement membrane. The left kidney from this animal was negative.

Group 3. Acute cellular rejection was found in six animals. In three cases it was accompanied by acute tubular necrosis, predominantly of cortical tubules. Two of these, and one without acute necrosis, showed rather extensive calcification of tubules. The survival of the kidneys with acute tubular necrosis did not differ from those without it. The kidney with tubular calcification but no necrosis was the longest survivor. One kidney with acute cellular rejection showed glomerular alterations too. The glomeruli were infiltrated by polymorphs, mostly neutrophils but also some eosinophils. A slight proliferation of mesangial and endothelial cells was found. Scattered fibrin was found along the walls of glomerular vessels but no thrombosis or necrosis. The basement membrane showed duplication (Figure 42.9). Immunofluorescence microscopy showed diffuse global granular positivity for Ig from goat and swine against rabbit and for IgG and C_3 from goat against rabbit. The picture was very much like the post-transplant disease described in human beings[12]. In one case there was no sign of rejection, and only slight proliferation of mesangial cells. Immunofluorescence for C_3 was present. It was diffuse, global and granular in

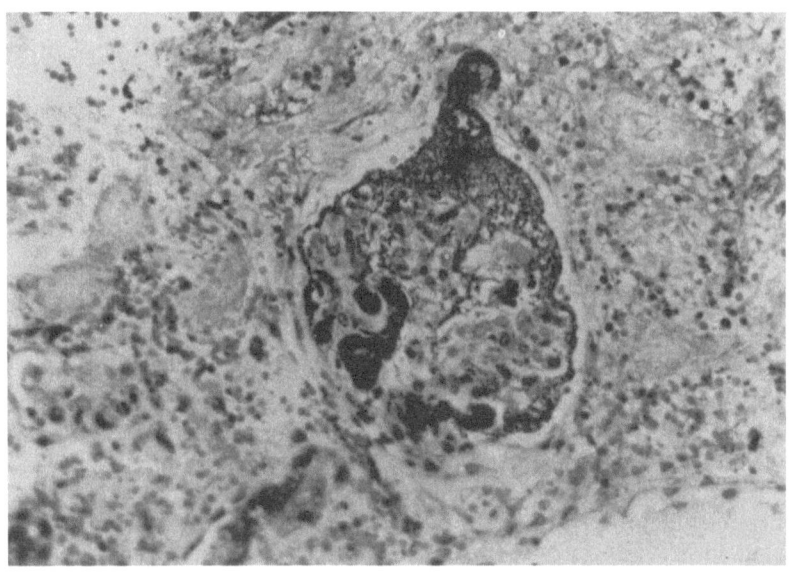

Figure 42.7 Acute cellular rejection. Interstitial perivascular infiltrates. (Giemsa stain; magnification × 53)

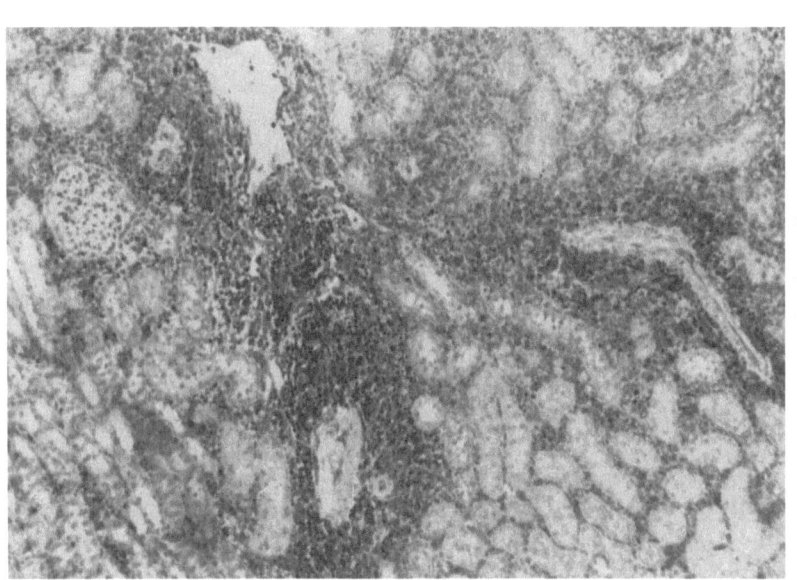

Figure 42.6 Hyperacute rejection. Glomerular microthrombosis and fibrinoid necrosis of artery. (Picro-Mallory V; magnification × 210)

glomeruli and accompanied by focal tubular positivity. The rest of the group showed no glomerular positivity by immunofluorescence, only focal tubular deposits of C_3. The right kidneys were all negative. Electron-microscopy in three cases with acute cellular rejection showed a mild non-specific widening of mesangial areas. Fibrin or thrombocytes were not found in the capillaries.

DISCUSSION

Comparing these findings with the results from the rather limited literature concerning xenobanking, the use of CS-A seems promising. Storage of kidneys for weeks to months was possible in the experiments presented here, whereas renal preservation with flushing or with continuous perfusion allows storage for a few days only.

Several aspects militate against the success of xenobanking in other than experimental situations. First of all we do not know whether the genetic differences between hare and rabbit are comparable with those between man and non-human primates such as baboons. Such a comparison can only be an educated guess at present. Further evidence of these genetic differences can be gleaned from the fact that attempts to cross-breed hares and rabbits have always proved unsuccessful. In terms of taxonomy rabbits and hares are considered as belonging to the same family but to a different genus, whereas man is considered to be one of four Old World monkey families and hence would be expected to present rather more genetic differences from, say, baboons which are classed in another family.

Another difficulty with xenobanking is the surgical problem likely to be encountered during retransplantation – a problem not faced after conventional preservation. Xenobanking on a bigger scale would also present economic problems. However, the additional expense would perhaps be outweighed in the long term by better survival after more care-ful histocompatibility matching and patient selection if it is possible for the organ to 'wait' for its recipient.

However fanciful the future of xenobanking might be[13] our studies have certainly shown that CS-A is capable of suppressing rejection across the major incompatibility barriers of concordant xenografts. This is not possible with conventional azathioprine–prednisolone therapy in the hare-to-rabbit model (Green, C. J., unpublished observations). Even the ability to prolong survival long after stopping CS-A administration was demonstrated. Although this was not so obvious as in earlier rabbit renal allograft experiments[8] it is nevertheless an extraordinary phenomenon.

Histologically, all forms of rejection were found ranging from that described in the allograft situation when using CS-A[14] to the morphology previously reported in xenografts[15,16]. In these rabbits we do not know if these alterations are reversible or not, or even if such cellular infiltrates are important. For instance, in one of our cases, a hare kidney kept a rabbit alive for more than 80 days with a serum creatinine below 200 μmol/l, even though the kidney showed every sign of cellular rejection. We would guess

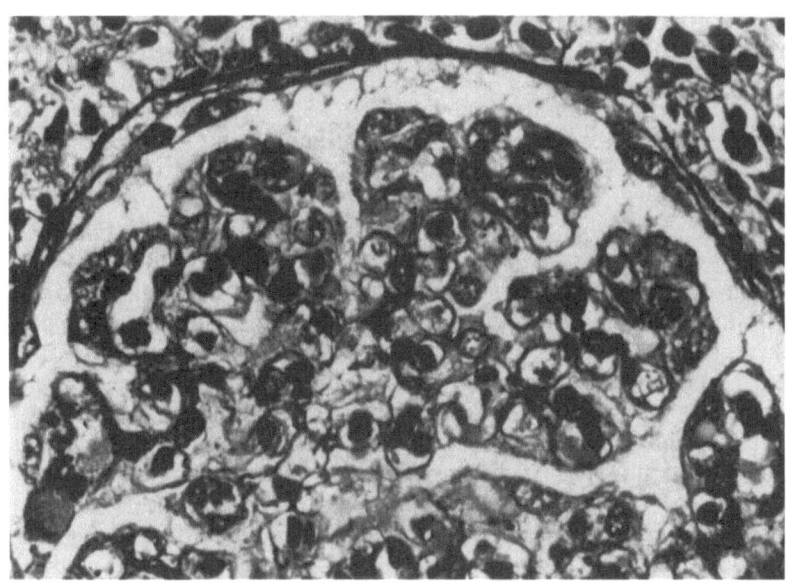

Figure 42.9 Chronic rejection, glomerular type (post-transplant disease). Reduplication of glomerular basement membrane and slight proliferation. (Methamine + H&E; magnification × 530)

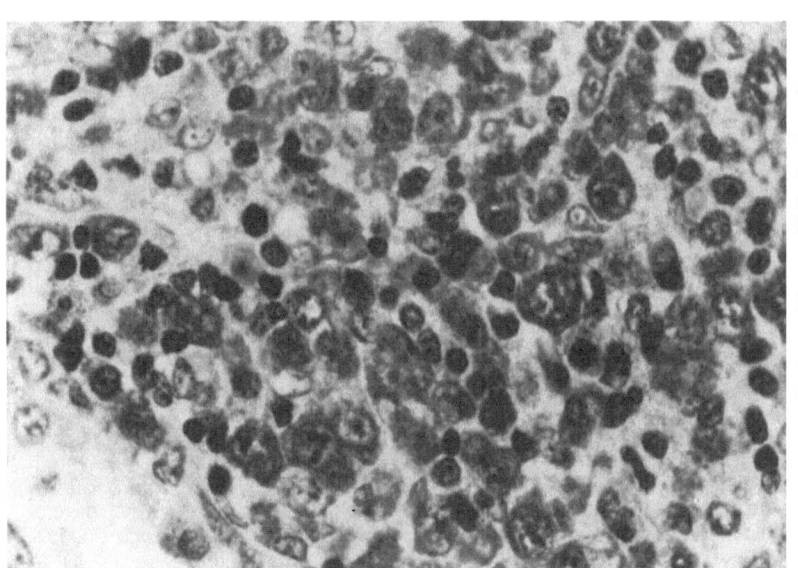

Figure 42.8 Detail from Figure 42.7 showing immuno-blasts, plasma cells and lymphocytes. (Giemsa stain; magnification × 530)

that these signs would disappear after retransplantation but at the present time the question is open. Although the number of experiments is small, a pattern in the pathological findings has emerged. In sum, hyperacute rejection was found in the untreated group and cellular rejection in the CS-A treated group. While hyperacute rejection was followed by rapid cessation of renal function, cellular rejection was compatible with life-sustaining although impaired renal function. The latter was probably associated with small areas of tubular necrosis. Immunofluorescence of the rejected kidney was neither pronounced nor consistent. Conversely, immunodeposits were found in some control hare kidneys which had not been transplanted, similar to those sometimes seen in untransplanted human kidneys[17].

While concordant xenografting thus seems possible, discordant xeno-grafting is still a much more difficult procedure[18-20]. Efficient depletion of complement still seems the only likely means of prolonging survival of discordant renal xenografts for days. In the laboratory in Odense, it has proved possible by a combination of therapy with cobra venom factor, the novel platelet anti-aggregation agent ticlopidine and CS-A to keep a rabbit kidney in good condition after transplantation into a bilaterally neph-rectomized cat for 4 days. During that time the serum creatinine of the cat rose only to $276\,\mu$mol/l. Histological examination revealed that glomeruli and most of the tubules were intact with necrosis in only about 10% of the proximal tubules. Even so the general condition of that animal and of all our animals in discordant xenograft experiments deteriorated within a few days so we must admit that xenobanking between discordant species is still far from a clinical possibility. However, since we found it possible to store hare kidneys in rabbits with reasonably good function and preserved morphology we are sufficiently encouraged to attempt further experimental xenobanking between concordant species.

Acknowledgements

This work was supported by the Danish Medical Research Council. We are grateful to Sandoz Limited, and ICI Limited for the gifts of cyclosporin A and ticlopidine respectively.

References

1. Dupree, E. L., Jr, Mills, M., Clark, R. and Sell, K. W. (1969). Xenogeneic storage of primate hearts. *Transplant. Proc.*, **1**, 840
2. Starzl, T. E., Machioro, T. L., Peters, G. N., Kirkpatrick, C. H., Porter, K. A., Rifkind, D., Ogden, D. A., Hitchock, C. R. and Wadell, W. R. (1964). Renal hetero-transplantation from baboon to man: experience with 6 cases. *Transplantation*, **2**, 752
3. Calne, R. (1963). *Renal Transplantation*. (London: Edward Arnold)
4. Reemtsma, K. (1969). Renal heterotransplantation from nonhuman primates to man. *Ann. N. Y. Acad. Sci.*, **162**, 412
5. Kemp, E. (1978). *Xenografting. The Future of Organ Transplantation*, p. 116. (Odense: Odense University Press)

6. Prange, C.H. (1980). Die Beeinflussung der Primärabstossung xenogener Nieren-transplantate im Speciessystem Fuchs – Hund durch Immunsuppressiva, Antiseren und Antigenaufbereitungen. *Wien. Klin. Wochenschr.,* **92** (suppl.), 110

7. Borel, J.F., Feurer, C., Gubler, H.U. and Stähelin, H. (1976). Biological effects of cyclosporin A: a new antilymphocyte agent. *Agents Actions,* **6,** 469

8. Green, C.J. and Allison, A.C. (1978). Extensive prolongation of rabbit-kidney allograft survival after short-term cyclosporin-A treatment. *Lancet,* **1,** 1182

9. Kemp, E., Kemp, G., Svendsen, P., Nielsen, E., Buhl, M.R., Jacobsen, I.A. and Lundborg, C.J. (1976). Prolongation of xenograft survival by infusion of heterologous antibodies against recipient serum. *Acta Pathol. Microbiol. Scand., C,* **84,** 342

10. Jacobsen, I.A. (1978). Renal transplantation in the rabbit: a model for preservation studies. *Lab. Anim.,* **12,** 63

11. Larsen, S. (1978). Immunofluorescent microscopy findings in minimal or no change-disease and slight generalised mesangioproliferative glomerulonephritis. *Acta Pathol. Microbiol. Scand., A,* **86,** 531

12. Olsen, T.S. (1979). Pathology of renal allograft rejection. In Churg, J. (ed.), *Kidney Disease – Present Status,* pp. 342–347. (Baltimore: Williams & Wilkins)

13. Homan, W., Williams, K., Fabre, J., Millard, P. and Morris, P. (1981). Prolongation of cardiac xenograft survival in rats receiving cyclosporin A. *Transplantation,* **31,** 164

14. Calne, R.Y. *et al.* (1979). Cyclosporin A initially as the only immunosuppressant in 34 recipients of cadaveric organs: 32 kidneys, 2 pancreases, and 2 livers. *Lancet,* **2,** 1033

15. Porter, K.A. (1964). Renal heterotransplants. Pathological changes in transplanted kidneys. In Starzl, T. (ed.), *Experience in Renal Transplantation,* pp. 345–357. (Philadelphia: W.B. Saunders)

16. Dubernard, J.M., Bonneau, M. and Latour, M. (1974). *Heterografts in Primates,* p. 189. (Frankrig: Fondation Merieux)

17. Larsen, S. (1981). *Immune Deposits in Human Glomerulopathy,* pp. 1–78. (Published by the author)

18. Kemp, E., Kemp, G. and Larsen, S. (1980). Survival of discordant renal xenografts up to 3 days. Assessment of function, light and immunofluorescent microscopy. *Scand. J. Urol. Nephrol.* (suppl. 54), 150

19. Green, C.J., Kemp, E. and Kemp, G. (1980). The effects of cyclosporin A, ticlopidine hydrochloride and cobra venom factor on the hyperacute rejection of discordant renal xenografts. *Invest. Cell. Pathol.,* **3,** 415

20. Green, C.J., Kemp, E., Kemp, G. and Larsen, S. (1982). The role of ticlopidine in delaying the development of a microcoagulopathy during hyperacute rejection of kidney xenografts: Experimental studies. *Proc. R. Soc. Med.* (In press)

PART VI
PRESERVATION OF CADAVER KIDNEYS

43
Factors influencing primary function in kidney transplants from brain-dead donors

H. BONDEVIK, A. JAKOBSEN and A. FLATMARK

The removal of kidneys from heart-beating cadaveric donors is legalized in Norway. Twenty hospitals are licensed for establishing the diagnosis of brain death, and performing donor nephrectomy, the technique and policy being established by the transplant team at Rikshospitalet (the National Hospital), Oslo. After donor nephrectomy, all kidneys are perfused and cooled (Perfudex), before transportation to Rikshospitalet for inspection and placement in a perfusion machine of the Gambro type. During a 2-year period, 1978–80, 175 Norwegian kidneys were harvested and used for transplantation: 66 were used locally at Rikshospitalet and 109 shipped to ten other centres within Scandiatransplant. Information has been gathered on all these, as to cold ischaemia time and primary function, the latter being defined as onset of diuresis within 24 h, assessed by the attending surgeon.

The locally used kidneys had an average cold ischaemia time of 22.8 h, none exceeding 30 h. Primary diuresis was seen in 85% of these kidneys. The ten other centres of Scandiatransplant received 28, 16, 13, 11, 9, 8, 7, 7, 7 and 3 kidneys respectively. Mean cold ischaemia time on these kidneys ranged from 17.7 to 35.2 h for each of the different centres. The percentage of primary diuresis ranged from 43 to 86, being 60 for the whole group of exported kidneys. There was no clear relation between length of cold ischaemia time and rate of primary diuresis for these machine-perfused kidneys.

During the same period of time we received 35 kidneys from abroad, 18 of these in perfusion machines (Gambro), and 17 in Collins' or Sacks' solution. The incidence of primary diuresis was the same, disregarding preservation technique, 83% and 88% respectively for the machine-perfused and the simply-cooled group. This is again the same as for the kidneys harvested in Norway and used at Rikshospitalet. Only in one case did the cold ischaemia time exceed 30 h. Thus, within our time limits, the mode of preservation does not seem to affect onset of function.

Of the 175 Norwegian kidneys 15 were single, the others constituting 80 pairs. In 43 of these pairs both kidneys had primary diuresis, in 11 none. In the remaining 26 pairs one of the kidneys had primary diuresis, the other not. Difference in cold ischaemia time was not correlated to the difference in onset of function, within these kidney pairs. Neither did the reported warm ischaemia time give any indication as to which kidneys would have a delayed start. Since all these kidneys were removed with a beating heart, the warm ischaemia time should always be short. We feel, however, that the reported warm ischaemia time may not give an accurate measure of the circulation and oxygenation of the kidney before flushing and cooling. The great variation in incidence of primary function between different centres may also indicate differences in handling of the kidney at the time of implantation.

Indications from this study are that cold ischaemia times of less than 40 h do not influence primary function in machine-perfused kidneys. Machine-perfusion and simple-cooling with Collins' or Sacks' solution functions equally well within 30 h. We have no data for longer ischaemia times. Handling of the kidneys at the time of nephrectomy and implantation, as well as the 'real' warm ischaemia at both these stages, is judged to be highly important.

44
Can immediate function of a cadaver renal transplant be predicted?

A. T. RAFTERY, L. HUNT, S. B. LUCAS and R. W. G. JOHNSON

Immediate function of a transplanted kidney proves the viability of the organ, makes the diagnosis of rejection less difficult and eases pressure on dialysis facilities. Further, there is evidence to suggest that delayed function may have an adverse effect on long-term graft survival[1,2].

Donor and storage details of cadaver renal transplants carried out over a 5-year period have been analysed to assess factors affecting immediate function. The following factors were studied: age of donor, period of ventilation, period of hypotension, urine output, type of premedication, warm ischaemic time, cold ischaemic time, type of storage, i.e. ice or hypothermic pulsatile perfusion, and anastomosis time. Univariate analysis showed that a young donor ($p = 0.014$), a short warm ischaemic time ($p = 0.011$) and premedication with phenoxybenzamine ($p = 0.040$) significantly increased the chances of immediate function. Univariate analysis, however, fails to take into account the variables in relation to one another. Multivariate analysis was therefore undertaken on data relating to 155 cadaver renal transplants using a linear logistic model[3]. This was used to estimate the coefficients (α) of the prognostic index (Z), $Z = \alpha_0 + \alpha_1 x_1 + \alpha_2 x_2 + \ldots + \alpha_p x_p$ where x represents the variables. This prognostic index is directly related to the probability that the kidney in question will function immediately. The probability that the kidney will function immediately for any one kidney is

$$P = \frac{e^Z}{(1 + e^Z)}$$

If $Z > 0$, there is a more than 50% chance that the kidney will function immediately, and if $Z < 0$ there is a less than 50% chance that the kidney will function immediately. Using this method factors which favour immediate function (increase Z) are good urine output, administration of a diuretic, ice storage and administration of an α-adrenergic blocking agent. Factors which are unfavourable (decrease Z) are increased ventilation time, older donor, long anastomosis time, long warm ischaemic time, administration of dopamine, long cold ischaemic time and a long period of hypotension.

Substituting values for the variables in individual cases into the equation it was found that, of the 95 kidneys that actually functioned immediately, prediction was correct in 77 (81%) whereas of the 60 which failed to function immediately only 24 (40%) were accurately predicted.

It is concluded that immediate function of a transplanted kidney cannot be accurately predicted. This may be due to (a) the large number of variables involved, (b) availability and accuracy of donor records and (c) possible factors in the recipient.

References

1. Anderson, C. B., Sicard, G. A. and Etheredge, E. E. (1979). Delayed primary renal function and cadaver renal allograft results. *Surg. Gynecol. Obstet.*, **149**, 697
2. Davidson, J. M., Uldall, P. R. and Taylor, R. M. R. (1977) Relation of immediate post-transplant renal function to long term function in cadaver kidney recipients. *Transplantation*, **23**, 3
3. Anderson, J. A., Whaley, K., Williamson, J. and Buchanan, W. W. (1972) A statistical aid to the diagnosis of keratoconjunctivitis sicca. *Q. J. Med.*, **41**, 175

45
Factors of consequence for graft survival: a statistical analysis

H. E. JØRGENSEN, S. KREINER, M. LARSEN, L. R. POULSEN and
S. WALTER

The background for the statistical analysis was 149 consecutive cadaver transplantations performed on 126 patients in the period September 1970 to March 1977 with a minimum period of observation of $3\frac{1}{2}$ years. The time of admittance into the material was onset of function of the graft, i.e. the verified urine production. Thus 19 never-functioning grafts were excluded. The exit of the material was rejection with cessation of function. Death of a patient with preserved graft function was not considered as cessation of function. The material is analysed with regard to risk factors for the first 3 months and for the following period separately. The Kaplan–Meyer estimation[1] of survival distribution is used for comparison of the time to rejection for the subgroups. A stepwise analysis based on the regression model proposed by Cox[2] is used to determine the influence on prognosis from more than one variable. The independent variables included in the analysis are shown in Table 45.1.

Table 45.1 Risk of rejection within and later than 90 days after onset of function

Variable	p-Value of correlation with risk	
	Within 90 days	Later than 90 days
Transplantation no. (1st or 2nd transplant)	0.747	0.800
Age at transplantation	0.967	0.264
Pregnancy/sex	0.102	0.476
Number of transfusions	0.002*	0.220
Duration of dialysis	0.795	0.452
Warm ischaemia	0.582	0.054
Cold ischaemia	0.838	0.006*
Time to onset of function	0.002*	0.325

* Statistically significant

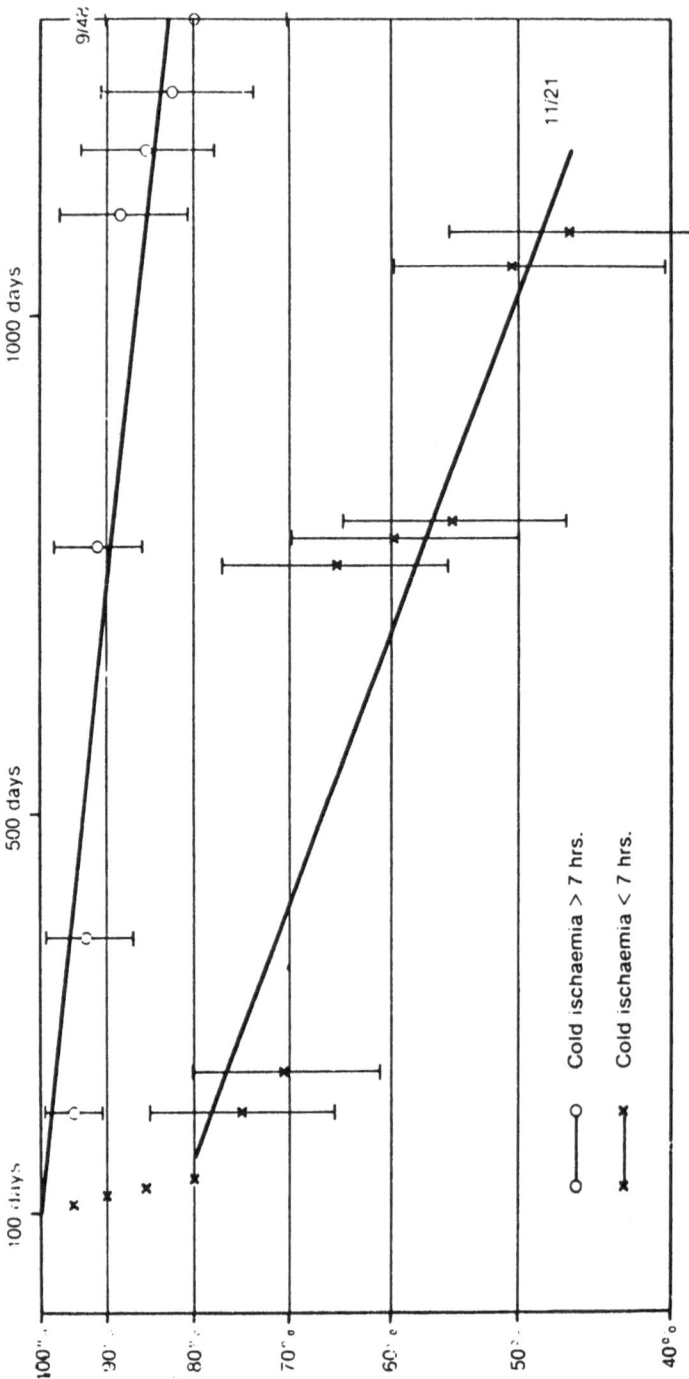

Figure 45.1 Graft survival later than 90 days after onset of function

The risk of rejection within the first 90 days after onset of function depends on the analysis of two factors: (1) time from transplantation to onset of function, (2) number of blood transfusions (Table 45.1). The risk of rejection within a given period of time, calculated for the two factors mentioned, is shown in Table 45.2

Table 45.2 Risk of rejection related to number of blood transfusions and time after onset

Onset of function		< 24 h		>24 h
Number of blood transfusions	0	1–10	> 11	
Number of patients/rejections	21/14	35/13	18/4	44/5
Time after onset				
10 days	24%	9%	0%	2%
30 days	39%	15%	6%	2%
60 days	61%	24%	17%	7%
90 days	67%	33%	17%	7%
120 days	72%	39%	23%	12%

After 90 days the duration of cold ischaemia was the only variable of prognostic significance for graft survival (Figure 45.1). Evidently in this material grafts with a cold ischaemia of > 7 h had a significantly higher survival rate than grafts with a cold ischaemia of < 7 h.

It has previously been shown that blood transfusions prior to transplantations improve the survival rate of the grafts[3]. We have no explanation why a delayed onset of function apparently improved graft survival among our patients, but we are convinced that analyses using the same variables in other transplant materials would reveal similar conditions[4]. It is our suggestion that the statistics here implied should be used in other centres and, perhaps most important, that future evaluation of graft survival is done with due consideration of factors influencing the first 3 months after transplantation and the subsequent period.

Acknowledgements

This work was supported by Det Lægevidenskabelige Forskningsfond for Storkøbenhavn, Færøerne og Grønland.

References

1. Kaplan, E. L. and Meyer, P. (1958). Nonparametric estimation from incomplete observations. *J. Am. Stat. Assoc.*, **53**, 457
2. Cox, D. R. (1972). Regression models and life tables. *J. R. Stat. Soc.*, **334**, 187
3. Uldall, P. R., Dewar, P. J., Morley, A. R., Hall, R. R., Wilkinson, R., Murroy, S., Boxly, K. and Taylor, R. M. R. (1977). Factors affecting the outcome of cadaver renal transplantation in Newcastle upon Tyne. *Lancet*, **2**, 316
4. Opelz, G., Sasaki, N. and Teresaki, P. I. (1978). Prediction of long term kidney transplant survival rates by monitoring early graft function and clinical grades. *Transplantation*, **25**, 212

46
Early and long-term function of cadaveric kidneys preserved by ice storage after flushing with Collins' solution

I. R. HARDIE and G. A. BALDERSON

Factors influencing immediate and long-term (1, 3, 12, 60 months) graft function were analysed in 440 cadaveric kidneys removed after cardiac arrest and stored in ice after flushing with Collins' C3 solution. Isotonic C3 was used in Group 1 (1970–75: 125 kidneys) and hyperosmolar C3 in Group 2 (1975–80: 315 kidneys). All donors received ventilatory support, adequate hydration, mannitol and heparin. Warm ischaemia was 14.4 ± 5.6 (SD) min; cold ischaemia averaged 6.0 ± 4.2 h in group 1 and 13.1 ± 7.5 h in group 2 (range 1.8–29 h).

Immediate function occurred in 74% of group 1 and 57% of group 2 ($\chi^2 = 9.13$; $p = 0.003$), due partly to longer storage in group 2 (total ischaemia: 14.0 ± 7.6 h vs 6.9 ± 4.4 h: $p = 0.001$). However, recovery from acute tubular necrosis (ATN) was faster in group 2 (four dialyses in 10 days vs five in 15 days: dialyses $p = 0.028$; days $p = 0.002$). Kidneys with poor early function had longer warm and cold ischaemia times (warm: 16 ± 6 vs 13 ± 5 min – $p = 0.01$; cold: group $1 = 9 \pm 7$ vs 5 ± 3 h – $p = 0.001$; group $2 = 16 \pm 7$ vs 11 ± 8 h – $p = 0.001$). Left kidneys, which were usually removed first, had shorter warm but similar cold ischaemia times to right kidneys and functioned better (group 1, R:L – 82% : 67%; group 2, R:L – 68% : 48%).

Chlorpromazine pretreatment allowed longer cold ischaemia without significantly increasing the incidence of ATN. Donor age, hypothermia, steroid pretreatment and the use of vasoconstrictors (pitressin or dopamine) had no effect on early function. The presence of hypotension (< 80 mmHg systolic pressure) in the last 24 h, terminal oliguria or diabetes insipidus in the donor were associated with improved early function ($\sim 33\%$ ATN if present; 50% ATN if absent).

Long-term function was worse in kidneys with poor early function in group 1 (21% vs 49% at 5 years: $\chi^2 = 5.2$; $p = 0.02$), but not in group 2 (38% vs 35% at 5 years: $\chi^2 = 0.8$; $p = 0.37$ – log rank test).

These results confirm the superiority of hyperosmolar Collins' solution and the safety of 24–30 h ice storage of ischaemically damaged cadaveric kidneys after flushing with this solution. The dialysis rates are among the best reported for this technique and are comparable to those obtained with similarly stored non-ischaemic kidneys from heart-beating cadavers. Chlorpromazine was the only useful pretreatment while hypotension or terminal oliguria in the donor were not contraindications to using the kidneys.

47
The effect of dopamine administered to kidney graft recipients

R. GRUNDMANN

When kidneys are transplanted from donors with excellent renal function, early function depends on the periods of warm and cold ischaemia to which they are subjected. With minimal warm ischaemia, ice storage for 24–48 h is possible[1,2]. However, under these conditions rather high rates of acute tubular necrosis are found. We have transplanted more than 200 human cadaver kidneys which were harvested under optimal conditions and thereafter stored in Collins' solution. The kidneys were shipped by Eurotransplant and then transplanted after a mean preservation time of 20 h. Despite the relatively short preservation period and a warm ischaemia time prior to nephrectomy of not more than 15 min, 65% of the recipients had to be dialysed in the first week. This varying quality of function, despite equal preservation periods, indicates that additional factors (for example, inaccurately recorded hypotension in the donor) influence function after transplantation. In the experiments presented here, therefore, the effects of the warm ischaemia period and of the hypotension prior to nephrectomy were studied.

In addition we have examined whether treatment of kidney recipients can ameliorate the effects of hypotensive and warm ischaemic injury to donor kidneys. While several methods have been used to treat donors who have been hypovolaemic (e.g. phenoxybenzamine[3,4] or dopamine[4,5]) treatment of recipients has not been fully investigated. Therefore we examined the effect of dopamine on recipients of kidneys that were harvested either under normal conditions or were pre-damaged by hypotension or warm ischaemia.

DOG EXPERIMENTS

Methods

20–25 kg mongrel dogs were used. Under general anaesthesia both ureters were cannulated. *para*-Aminohippuric acid (PAH) and inulin were injected intravenously and PAH- and inulin-clearance values were obtained for each single kidney (= initial kidney function) before removing the kidneys (group 1, *n* = 6) or subjecting the kidneys to 1 h of haemorrhagic hypotension at 60 mmHg (group 2, *n* = 6) or to 15 min of warm ischaemia (group 3, *n* = 6).

Immediately after nephrectomy the kidneys were perfused with Collins' solution at 4°C and then stored in ice for 24 h. Thereafter the kidneys were transplanted into fresh mongrel recipients in whom bilateral nephrectomy had been performed. For each kidney three measurements of PAH- and inulin-clearance were made in the first 3 h after transplantation. Dopamine (5 μg/kg body weight) was then infused intravenously for the next 3 h and three further sets of clearance measurements were made.

Results

The results are summarized in Table 47.1 and Figure 47.1. The dopamine infusion did not improve the function of kidneys which had suffered a warm ischaemia period of 15 min. In contrast dopamine was able to improve the renal function of those kidneys subjected to sufficient hypotension (i.e. 60 mmHg MAP for 1 h) before nephrectomy to make them anuric during the hypotensive period.

Table 47.1 PAH- and inulin-clearances (ml/min/100 g kidney weight) before dopamine treatment

	Before storage	After 24 h hypothermic storage		
	Initial function (n = 27)	No hypotension (n = 6)	Hypotension 1 h/60 mmHg (n = 6)	15 min warm ischaemia (n = 6)
PAH	183.3 ± 34.2	28.71 ± 8.43	15.3 ± 8.05	4.38 ± 3.66
Inulin	39.3 ± 7.6	8.65 ± 2.76	6.3 ± 3.27	2.32 ± 1.96

At least a part of the action of dopamine depends on control of renal vasospasm. When that vasospasm did not occur the dopamine was of doubtful merit. Thus the dopamine infusion of recipients did not significantly improve the function of those kidneys which had *not* suffered a hypotensive episode in the donor prior to cold ischaemia for 24 h.

HUMAN CADAVER KIDNEY GRAFT RECIPIENTS

Methods

Fifty human cadaver kidney recipients were examined in a prospective randomized study, 25 of these patients receiving dopamine treatment (2 μg/kg bodyweight/min) for 4 days after transplantation. All kidneys were shipped by Eurotransplant and stored in Euro-Collins solution for not more than 30 h. Warm ischaemia did not exceed 10 min and the serum

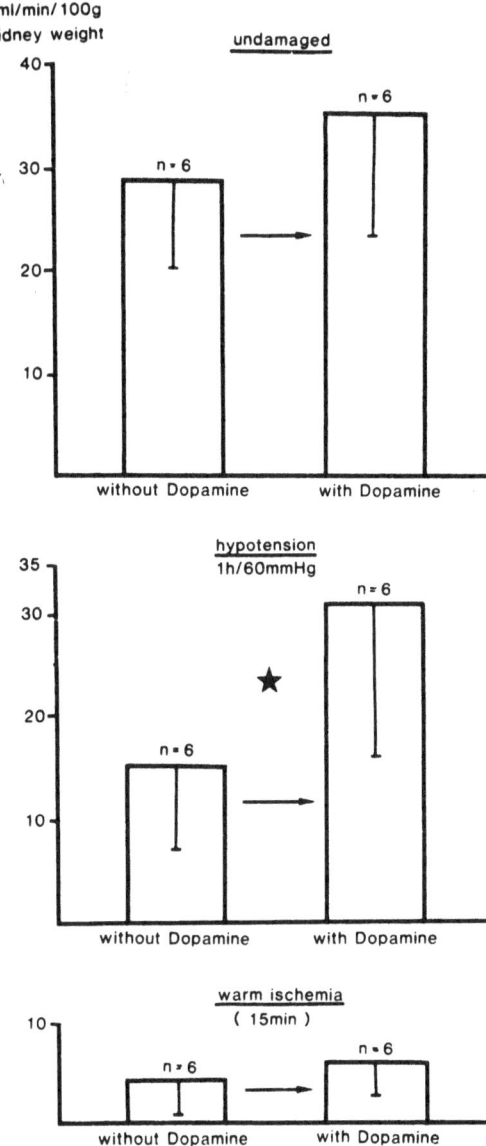

Figure 47.1 PAH clearance after 24 h hypothermic storage before and after dopamine treatment (dog experiments)

creatinine level in the donor was not more than 2.5 mg/dl. The blood pressure, pulse rate, urine production, creatinine clearance and dialysis frequency of the recipients was analysed postoperatively. The two groups (dopamine/no-dopamine) did not differ significantly regarding the condition of the donor or recipient. The preservation time averaged 21.3 ± 3 h in the dopamine group, and was also 21.3 h in the group with no

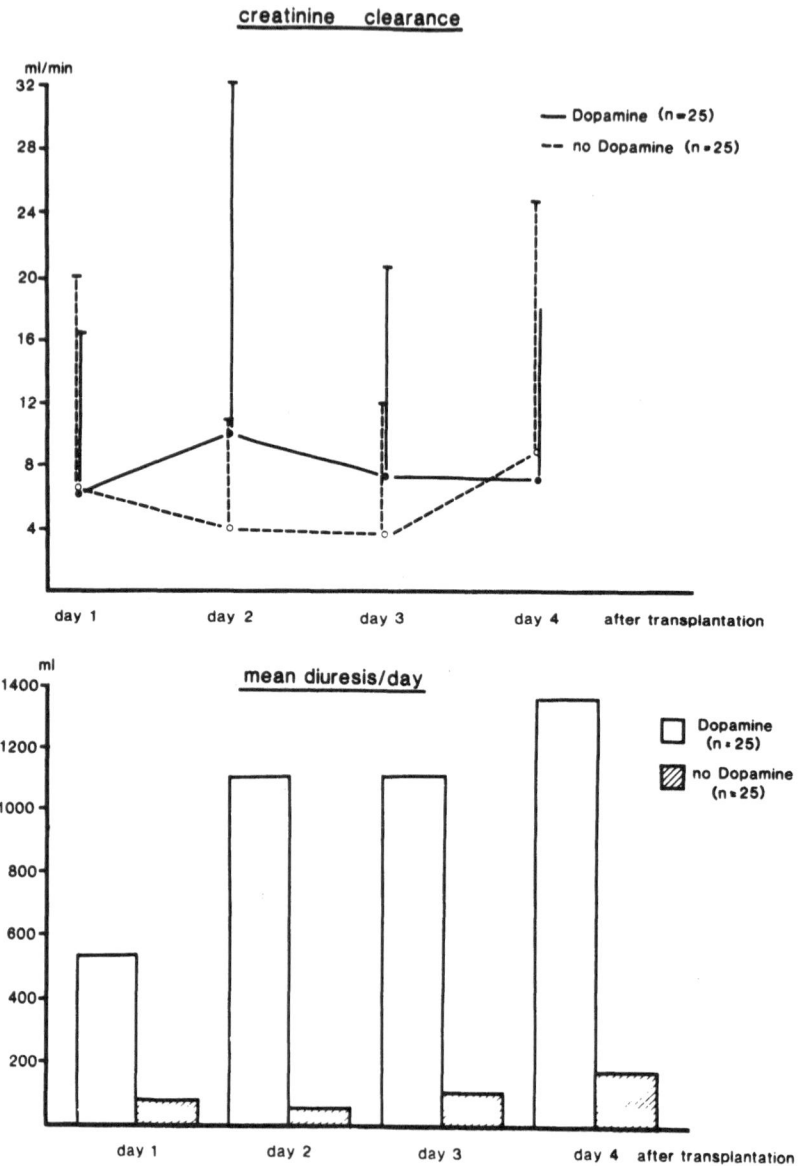

Figure 47.2 Creatinine clearance and mean diuresis/day in patients with and without dopamine treatment after transplantation

treatment. The warm ischaemia time prior to nephrectomy averaged 2 min in both groups.

Results

The dopamine infusion did not affect the dialysis frequency after transplantation; in each group 19 patients (76%) had to be dialysed during the first week after transplantation. This result corresponded to the clearance measurements, since the dopamine group had only slightly better clearances (Figure 47.2). However, urine production increased significantly when dopamine was given. In fact, in the dopamine group, 9 of 19 patients (47.4%) were dialysed although the diuresis rate was more than 11/day. In the group of patients that did not receive dopamine, only 3 of 19 patients (15.7%) were dialysed with such a diuresis rate.

Discussion

This analysis showed that the dialysis frequency in patients who received dopamine was identical with that of the control group. However, diuresis was increased after dopamine treatment. While dopamine was able to stimulate water excretion, the elimination of urinary constituents could not be increased, and renal ability to concentrate was not ameliorated. Since the kidneys were taken from heart-beating donors under optimal conditions, this result would be expected from the experimental data.

The experiments presented here show that dopamine treatment of the recipient would improve the function of kidneys only if they were subjected to hypotension before nephrectomy: the decrease of renal function due to cold ischaemia injury could not be influenced by the dopamine treatment of the recipient. The side-effects of dopamine were slight: thus we were able to use dopamine also in hypertensive patients and only in three patients was an increase of the pulse rate to 120–170/min observed, necessitating stopping the dopamine infusion.

References

1. Collins, G.M. and Halsaz, N.A. (1976). Forty-eight hour ice storage of kidneys: Importance of cation content. *Surgery*, **79**, 432
2. Grundmann, R., Strümper, R., Eichmann, J. and Pichlmaier, H. (1977). The immediate function of the kidney after 24–72h preservation. *Transplantation*, **23**, 437
3. Belzer, F.O., Reed, T.W., Pryor, J.P., Kountz, S.L. and Dunphy, J.E. (1970). Cause of renal injury in kidneys obtained from cadaver donors. *Surg. Gynecol. Obstet.*, **130**, 467
4. Dhabuwala, C.M., Bird, M. and Salaman, J.R. (1979). Relative importance of warm ischaemia, hypotension, and hypercarbia in producing renal vasospasm. *Transplantation*, **27**, 238
5. Raftery, A.T. and Johnson, R.W.G. (1979). Dopamine pretreatment in unstable kidney donors. *Br. Med. J.*, **87**, 522

PART VII
GENERAL DISCUSSION

48
Pretreatment

Marshall	In chapter 7 I described our ischaemia model in the rat. One of the first regimes we studied with it was chlorpromazine pretreatment, and we found that when untreated controls were compared with pretreatment with chlorpromazine, mannitol and saline, the chlorpromazine enabled the rats to survive (Jablonski, P., Howden, B., Marshall, V. *et. al.*, unpublished observations.)
Feinberg	I wonder if anybody has any thoughts about the persistence of chlorpromazine after pretreatment. We pretreated our animals 30 min before sacrifice, and perfused them for 30 min with a non-recirculating perfusion, so I wonder if there is any chlorpromazine left in those hearts; yet the effect is still there. An experiment with radioactive chlorpromazine would be very expensive because of the huge isotope dilution, but I really would like to know if there is still some chlorpromazine in those hearts.
Lambotte	Do you have any idea of the calcium uptake in those experiments?
Feinberg	No, we intend to study that.
Forsberg	Did you measure the water content of your hearts?
Feinberg	Yes, and there was no big difference.
	Mittnacht and Farber's data[1] are quite remarkable. They used 3 h of ischaemia, reperfused, and showed that the mitochondria looked terrible in both chlorpromazine-pretreated and control groups but chlorpromazine brought all indices of mitochondrial function back to normal.
Pegg	Could that be simply a vascular effect? Could it be that better perfusion enabled the mitochondria to repair? We have measured reperfusion in rabbit kidneys that had had 1 h of warm ischaemia, followed by preservation by Collins' solution. Without chlorpromazine pretreatment, there was only partial perfusion, and much retained blood remained, but if the animal was pretreated, the kidney was totally perfused[2].
Feinberg	I don't think that reflow would explain *our* results. Our coronary flows with constant reperfusion pressure were similar in the control and the chlorpromazine-treated groups.
Southard	Mittnacht and Farber[1] suggested that the mode of action of chlorpromazine was an inhibition of the breakdown of the phospholipids, and maintenance of membrane integrity in ischaemic organs. Concerning the vascular effects of ischaemia, they measured reflow by determining the distribution of a fluorescent stain in the liver, but only after 15 min reflow, and yet the total reperfusion time was 90 min. I wonder if good reflow was maintained during the 90 min. We tried a similar experiment with rabbit kidneys which were perfused for 30 min *in vitro* with or without chlorpromazine. Following perfusion the kidneys were left ischaemic for 120–180 min (37 °C) and we looked at the restoration of mitochondrial activities on reperfusion. We found

323

	that restoration of mitochondrial activity depended upon good post-ischaemic reflow, rather than upon chlorpromazine. If mannitol is included in the perfusate you get good mitochondrial activity and reflow after 2 h of ischaemia. Mannitol plus chlorpromazine, or chlorpromazine alone, gave the same results.
Collins	I would support that. Our experiments on the protection of the rabbit kidney from normothermic ischaemia[3] showed that vasodilator agents had no effect when superimposed upon a mannitol and sodium diuresis.
Belzer	Our studies also show that the major effect of chlorpromazine is its vasodilator action[4]. Dr Feinberg, you found a positive effect of chlorpromazine but if you used a really good reperfusion fluid, like albumin plus mannitol, the effect may not be there.
Feinberg	Well, I have used rabbit blood which is a pretty good fluid for perfusing rabbit hearts.
Belzer	Blood may not be the best. Using a poor perfusate, we had results similar to yours, but when our perfusate contained albumin and mannitol, we found no effect of the chlorpromazine[5].
Isselhard	There may be an energy-preserving effect in Dr Feinberg's protocol, because the ATP levels in the untreated controls were lower at the end of ischaemia than in the chlorpromazine group. Were the energy demands lower in the chlorpromazine-treated group?
Forsberg	I believe that chlorpromazine may inhibit sodium–potassium ATPase. Is that true?
Lambotte	We studied the effect of chlorpromazine on ATPase in the liver, and it had no effect on the ion gradient, or the membrane potential, so it seems to have no effect on the sodium pump at the concentration we used (50 mg/l)[6].
Jacobsen	The effectiveness of chlorpromazine in pretreatment raises the possibility of including it in the preservation solution. We studied 15 and 30 mg/l chlorpromazine with rabbit kidneys continuously perfused for 2 h, and then stored for 24 or 48 h. Both concentrations produced completely non-functioning kidneys.
Frödin	Does anyone know if phenoxybenzamine has the same action as chlorpromazine?
Collins	Only that in our model, phenoxybenzamine had no effect over and above that produced by a mannitol and sodium diuresis.

References

The discussion references are listed following chapter 51 on page 356.

49
Initial perfusion

REMOVAL OF BLOOD

Frödin   Karlberg in our laboratory has some work which is not yet published, measuring the regional red cell content of rat kidneys without ischaemia, after 45 min of warm ischaemia, and after recirculation. He found that 10–20 min after recirculation, 26% of the cells in the inner stripe of the outer zone of the medulla had remained from the period of clamping, 46% had accumulated 0–10 min after recirculation, and only 28% had entered this region 10–20 min after recirculation. In the cortex, 24% remained from the period of clamping, 32% had accumulated subsequently, and 44% remained circulating. It is suggested that red cell accumulation plays an important role in the medullary ischaemia found in acute ischaemic renal failure.

Johnson   We have looked at the effect of warm ischaemia on the time it took to cool dog kidneys down to 10 °C by perfusion of cold Collins' solution. With increasing warm ischaemia time it took progressively longer, and when we put the kidneys on the perfusion apparatus we found it was yet longer before the vascular resistance fell, and blood continued to be washed out for up to 10 h; it was often 4–5 h before the vascular resistance stabilized[7]. So even what we considered to be a 'successful' washout left considerable amounts of red cells trapped in the microcirculation. We also studied the effect of retained blood on the tolerance of kidneys to warm ischaemia. We used heparinized dogs, clamped the vessels *in situ*, and obtained immediate function, with low peak serum creatinine levels, after 1 h of warm ischaemia. However, if we washed out the kidneys before clamping, at 37 °C, with saline, or a number of other solutions, then we could get 2, 3, and occasionally even 4 h of warm ischaemia with immediate function[8]. It seems to me that we have ignored the problem of trapped red cells, and if we can only maintain the microcirculation, a lot of biochemical parameters may well be restored very quickly afterwards. So I think it is very important that we use the most effective perfusates for removing trapped blood.

Foreman   We found that the citrate solutions, both isotonic and hypertonic, gave the lowest residual haemoglobin levels in the kidney (see chapter 24).

Hoelscher   I think it is very important to note that in Foreman's experiments the haemoglobin level was still falling after 20 min, but we all use flush solutions for only 2, 3 or 5 min.

Feinberg   I would suggest that pretreating these kidneys with PGE$_1$ or prostacyclin would disaggregate or prevent the aggregation of platelets, and this would expedite washout.

Collins   When dealing with warm ischaemically injured kidneys one may need a more hyperosmolar flush solution than when dealing with fresh kidneys; there is some evidence that Sacks' solution may be better than Collins' solution when there has been significant warm ischaemia[9].

Pegg	I don't think the solution necessarily has to be hyperosmolar, but it must contain solutes that will retain fluid in the vascular system, so that there is more fluid to surround the red cells. I believe that dextran 40 is effective simply because it holds more fluid in the microcirculation[10].
Marshall	We find that you can increase the effectiveness of flushing a kidney either by increasing the osmolality of the solution, or by adding an oncotic agent. When we added albumin to the citrate solution it washed out even more rapidly and effectively and in fact was slightly more effective in preserving function. Another way of increasing the effectiveness of flushing is to do it normothermically. Again, we have used the citrate solution to do an initial washout: it is extremely rapid, but we have no evidence that it is better than hypothermic flushout.
Collins	One of the obstructions to flushing an ischaemically injured organ is the rigidizing effect of ischaemia on the red cell membrane, a point which Dr Pegg has raised[2]. Does anyone have any suggestions as to what might be added to flush solutions specifically to counteract this effect, excluding vasodilatory drugs?
Halasz	That might be an indication for using a normothermic flush.
Pegg	The rigidizing effect is due to calcium binding to the cell membranes[11]. Magnesium competitively inhibits this binding, and calcium chelators such as EDTA or citrate would also be effective. Both magnesium and citrate are important components of Ross and Marshall's solution, of course.
Feinberg	I would also suggest that dibutyryl cyclic AMP would be worth trying.
Merkel	It has been suggested that pulsatile perfusion of the kidney during flushing improves blood washout, but most of us just use a drip. Should we consider pulsatile flushing?
Cohen	We follow Belzer's suggestion, and use intermittent venous occlusion.

RATE OF COOLING

Green	I have done similar experiments to Dr Jacobsen (chapter 23) but not exactly mimicking his protocol. I flushed rabbit kidneys with 60 ml of hypertonic citrate solution at a constant pressure, which took around 3 min. I surrounded my whole perfusion apparatus in ice right up to the kidney in one group, and perfused the other group at 22 °C. I could not find any difference between the two groups. It may be significant that I did not pretreat my rabbits with chlorpromazine.
Belzer	Dr Green, you said you got no differerence? Did you get 100% survival in both groups?
Green	Yes, both were good.
Fahy	Fonteles and Karow[12] have shown more vasoconstriction in rabbit kidneys that were cooled rapidly, compared with ones that were cooled slowly, and it seems that one component of rapid-cooling injury is vasospasm. Perhaps this is why Dr Jacobsen found that, after rapid cooling, kidneys that were stored for 24 h had a higher survival rate (14/20) than kidneys stored for 45 min (6/20): the vasospasm may have declined. Of course, Dr Jacobsen used a different flush solution (hypertonic citrate) for his 24 h experiments, so these results may be due to the particular solution used. I certainly accept that the injury is not *all* due to vasospasm, since he has shown a direct injury to the tubular cells. Incidentally Fonteles did not chlorpromazine-pretreat his animals, but he found a cooling rate effect.
Jacobsen	Certainly there seem to be differences between hypertonic citrate and Collins' solution with the rabbit kidney; hypertonic citrate solution was much more successful in our hands.
	Fonteles looked at the response to catecholamines after rapid cooling

and slow cooling, but he did not show whether the low response to catecholamines in the rapidly cooled group was because of a genuine low response, or because of maximal vasospasm.

Fahy In 40% of his kidneys, the baseline resistance against which the catecholamine challenge was applied was actually up to about the level that he got when he applied the catecholamines to the slowly cooled kidney, suggesting that they could not vasoconstrict any more than they were. In the remaining 60% there was partial vasoconstriction and partial impairment of response not attributable to vasoconstriction.

Hoelscher I am worried about the pressures Dr Jacobsen used in his experiments on the effect of cooling rate (chapter 23) because the viscosity of the warm and cold fluids must have been different, and so if the flows were the same in both groups the actual renal resistances must have been different. Could it be that the more rapidly cooled kidneys developed more oedema because of the higher pressure, and therefore had less good function?

Jacobsen We allowed for the viscosity in the 2 °C environment being some 20% higher than at room temperature by increasing the height of the perfusate reservoir by about 20%. In fact the perfusion pressure and the vascular resistence were the same in the two groups.

Collins The resistance to flow in the tube leading to the kidney is only a small fraction of the renal vascular resistance. It is likely, therefore, that increasing the height of the perfusion to compensate for the temperature-dependence of viscosity would actually increase the pressure in the arterial system of the kidney.

Jacobsen The height was made different to compensate the pressure drop in the tubing, but the arterial pressure was the same.

Belzer I think Dr Jacobsen's results show that there is something like cold shock: in his first series, he found 30% survival versus 100% survival[13], and in his second series he still has a much better survival with slow cooling (chapter 23). It cannot be dismissed by saying the height is not enough and I think we had better remember it.

Isselhard I would like to support the idea that rapid cooling might be harmful. We have studied skeletal muscle in rats and dogs, and we found that rapid cooling to 0–2 °C in 4 min impaired both metabolism and survival, whereas cooling to the same temperature in 90 min had an excellent preserving effect. Our interpretation is that cooling depolarizes the cells, and the faster you depolarize the higher the energy demand is in relation to temperature[14].

Harness We have found that rat hearts perfused on a Langendorff column and maintained at room temperature (20 °C), take about 20 min to stabilize their vascular resistance. After that we can manipulate the temperature at about 1 °C/min without altering the vascular resistance.

Frödin The cooling rate in each part of a perfused kidney will depend on the flow rate in that particular part. If you use another perfusate you may get the same total flow, but you can still have different cooling rates in different parts of the kidney.

Jacobsen If what you say is true, Dr Frödin, there must have been a very major redistribution flow in the two groups, since the total vascular resistance was the same.

Fischer Another important factor, apart from the cooling rate of the whole organ, is the temperature of the perfusate entering the vessels. A cold solution may damage those parts of the tissue with which it comes in close contact, irrespective of the cooling rate of the whole organ. Does anybody here use initial warm perfusion with human kidneys, followed by a slow reduction of the perfusate temperature?

Marshall We have in experimental animals; it gives satisfactory function, but we haven't used it clinically.

Jacobsen   I think that most people really do perfuse with a warm solution, because they ignore the heat-exchanger effect of the tubing and the bottle itself.

SOLUTE EQUILIBRATION

Hoelscher   I am concerned we all flush kidneys for only 2, 3 or 5 min. We just don't equilibrate the extracellular space within this time. We have studied the equilibration of sodium using 'low-sodium' fluid and we found that equilibration within the vessels takes only 4–6 min, but equilibration of the tubular space with respect to the sodium concentration took 10–15 min. We now always use more than 10-fold the kidney weight of fluid to obtain equilibration of the extracellular and tubular space.

Fischer   I also think we should focus on the technique of flush perfusion, particularly with respect to equilibration of the whole kidney. In discussions with several participants at this meeting, I have heard about flush perfusion times from 5 to 15 min, in clinical practice, with perfusion via the renal artery or the iliac artery; there are enormous differences, which may be at least partly responsible for differing results – reports of life-supporting function after no more than 24 h preservation or up to 64 h. We should pay much more attention to the technique of flush perfusion.

References

The discussion references are listed following chapter 51 on page 356.

50
Hypothermic preservation

COMPOSITION AND VOLUME OF PERFUSATE

Fahy
I would like to say something about the selection of anions for preservation solutions: I don't think it necessarily matters whether you use a permeant anion or an impermeant anion, so long as *some* impermeant species is used. The cell has chloride and sodium outside and potassium, chloride and other substances I will call x inside. There is a membrane potential, which is negative inside and positive outside, because of the outward leakage of potassium. If you now shut off metabolism, sodium comes in and potassium continues to leak out, in equal concentration we'll say to a first approximation, so the exchange has no net effect on cell volume. Chloride also enters, and let's say that chloride distributes across the membrane so that there are equal concentrations on each side too. Now, if something is present on either side of the membrane in the same concentration the osmotic effect of that species is zero and it cannot have any further effect on cell volume. The fact that the membrane potential has been lost had no effect on cell volume. However, you still have x inside the cell, protein or whatever, that cannot exchange across the membrane to equilibrium. We can ignore the fact that chloride will be partially excluded because of the charge on intracellular anion: the important fact is that we have a certain number of milliosmoles of this material which is inside, and if there is nothing outside to correspond to it, water will come into the cell; this will then dilute the potassium, sodium and chloride, so these ions enter too, and the process will continue. If you add an impermeant substance outside, no matter what it is, until the number of milliosmoles of this substance outside is equal to the number of milliosmoles of x inside, the cell will not swell. You can then take into account the second-order effects – like charge effects – but these just change the magnitudes slightly, and the external impermeant solutes do not have to be charged. The membrane potential really doesn't have much to do with it.

Harness
If you have two solutions separated by a membrane, it is the chemical potentials you have to look at. The Second Law of Thermodynamics states that the Gibbs function must be a minimum, and when the concentration of one ion is changed, all the chemical potentials on that side of the membrane alter. Diffusion across the membrane then takes place in accordance with all the chemical potentials.

Fahy
I agree that there are slight differences between different compounds, but I don't think they are important in this case. It is the activity of water which determines where the water goes.

Harness
No, you must consider the activity of each ion, not just the activity of water.

Pegg
I am sure you are right. To understand the details of what happens.you

329

	must use a rigorous thermodynamic approach, but in the end, and here I agree with Dr Fahy, the fact that actually makes the cells swell is that they contain impermeant anion[2]. This raises an interesting question. Why does everybody use far more impermeant solute than there is inside? We should not need more solute than 25–30 mosmol/kg[15].
Fahy	Yes, I have asked myself the same question. I think it may be because the 'impermeant' solutes in question do cross the membrane, albeit slowly.
Fischer	I suggest it may be because you are not equilibrating the whole kidney with the flush solution. If you did it might be dangerous, but the short flush delivers only some of the glucose to the kidney. The extent to which you equilibrate the kidney may be very important, and this brings us back to the duration of the flush perfusion.
Pegg	That seems a likely explanation. We have done experiments with slices of rabbit heart, to determine the concentration of sucrose needed to prevent hypothermic swelling, and it is 30–40 mmol/l added to an isotonic salt solution.
Fahy	I want to make the point that you may raise the total osmolality by *adding* non-penetrating solute to an isotonic electrolyte solution to control cellular swelling, but *replacing* some of the ions with a non-penetrating solute achieves the same end. The osmolality itself is less relevant than what the solution is.
Lambotte	Professor Marshall, does your isosmolar solution contain mannitol? (chapter 31).
Marshall	Yes, but of course less mannitol than the hypertonic citrate solution.
Lambotte	The point is that impermeant molecules might be important.
Marshall	Yes, of course, it doesn't make any difference to the theory of impermeant solutes.
Fuller	I think we should stop talking about osmolality as Dr Fahy and Dr Lambotte have mentioned already; we should worry about what is slowly permeating and what is freely permeating. What was altered to change the osmolality in your solution, Professor Marshall? Was it citrate?
Marshall	It could be done in a lot of different ways, but the obvious one was to vary the amount of mannitol. We could not alter the concentration of citrate because citrate has a specific effect[16].
Fahy	Could I comment on the differences between RPS-2 solution and LIC solution (chapter 25). First, in LIC there is an increase in glucose content by 43 mmol/l. The more extracellular glucose, the more cell swelling will be retarded. However, RPS-2 and LIC are both solutions in which the inclusion of solutes that do not cross the membrane produces a 290 milliosmolal solution that retards cell swelling. We have also produced the same effect with albumin; a kidney slice placed in a 5% albumin solution that would otherwise permit swelling, will not swell. The other difference between RPS-2 and LIC is the replacement of chloride by phosphate. I should mention that sodium and potassium chloride are present in RPS-2 simply as osmotic fillers: when the kidney is transplanted it will be exposed to a 290 milliosmolal environment and it must have that concentration intracellularly if it is not to swell or shrink. A possible mode of action of phosphate concerns the prevention of cellular chloride loading, and the fact that energy is expended in returning to normal afterwards. I don't think phosphate acts as a non-penetrating solute; phosphate seems to penetrate more rapidly than glucose[17], but perhaps phosphate helps by preventing chloride loading in the loop of Henle where there is an active chloride pump, and reduces the work-load on that mechanism. The phosphate effect is not apparent in the kidney cortex.

Green	High phosphate would certainly give you a high buffering capacity, and surely that is important?
Fahy	Yes, that is true.
Belzer	Concerning phosphate, I think it does no harm in flushout solutions because it probably fails to reach the cells anyway, but in perfusion solutions I think it may be dangerous. If the membranes become permeable to phosphate, it causes a tremendous swelling of the mitochondria, and is a very potent uncoupler.
Collins	We have done quite a number of perfusions for periods up to 72 h, using quite high concentrations of phosphate anion with essentially the same results as with chloride anion[18].
Belzer	We could not repeat those experiments. Our high phosphate perfusions had an increasing perfusion pressure over the period of time and the kidneys did not function afterwards.
Cohen	We also studied phosphate buffered perfusates[19], and in fact the best of our 8-day stored kidneys were done with a phosphate buffer at a concentration of 15 mmol/l. We used air-gassing in these experiments: if we used CO_2 gassing the buffer was unable to hold the pH, which became alkaline.
Forsberg	Dr Collins, you mentioned that the glutathione in RPS-2 solution (chapter 25) might be important. Why?
Collins	The inclusion of glutathione came from Dr Fahy's experiments[20]. My only information is that removing it, together with other components, led to inferior results.
Fahy	The rationale behind glutathione is partly theoretical and partly experimental. Theoretically it may maintain the Redox potential and since it is an antioxidant it may prevent peroxidation. Another possibility is that glutathione can be used to generate ATP under anaerobic conditions, if it is broken down and then used through a pathway that diving mammals use[21]: in this pathway glutamate and aspartate are used to shuttle back and forth between mitochondria and cytoplasm in transamination reactions.
	On the experimental level, I find every time I add glutathione, the glutathione-treated tissue comes out with better function than the non-glutathione control, both in rabbit and in dog. Based on tissue slice experiments the optimum concentration is about 5 mmol/l. Much of my data has been from prolonged preservation, and I think that the effect of glutathione might be more pronounced after longer periods than 24 h.
Belzer	I think that glutathione is very good for aerobic perfusion because it does prevent peroxidation, but in simple cold storage you don't have any peroxidation. Also the dog does not possess the glutaminase enzyme, and thus cannot convert glutamine to ammonia[22]. Glutathione might have an effect in your slices, but not in cold storage.
Fahy	So the theory may not apply but empirically it works. I looked at it in the first place because 90 min perfusion of the rabbit kidney depleted almost all of the normally very high concentrations of glutathione[23]. I felt that it must be there for some reason, it is certainly important for amino acid transport in the kidney tubules[24], and washing out a lot of it can't be good. When I put it back again function was improved.
Southard	When I was studying enzymology, and had an unstable enzyme, the first thing I did was to add glutathione and that often stabilized the enzyme.
Pearson	Why glutathione; because it can't cross intact cell membranes? Unless the cell is damaged it shouldn't get in. Perhaps a highly permeant antioxidant would be better.
Fahy	Maybe things do cross membranes more than we think they do under hypothermic conditions. Glucose and mannitol certainly cross membranes; if you just wait long enough they will go in. You may say

331

the cells are damaged, but if the damage is reversible then is it significant?

Johnson
It has always interested me that simple cold storage and continuous perfusion are carried out at somewhere near the same temperature (we usually perfuse at about 6 °C, and cold storage is between 2 and 4 °C) and yet the two solutions that we use for each type of preservation are entirely different. If we try to perfuse at 6 °C with Collins' solution we have a total disaster, and if you try simple cold flush storage with PPF you will be very lucky to get 24 h. It seems to me that there are fundamental differences other than temperature involved.

Belzer
No, I disagree strongly. Our sodium gluconate solution (see chapter 35), which prevents cell swelling gives simple cold preservation as effectively as Collins' solution, but it is also very good for perfusion; we have good kidney preservation with this high-potassium solution for 24 or 48 h. It is true, you cannot use Collins' solution in perfusion, but you can make a solution that is suitable for both techniques, and you can make a solution that is high in mannitol or gluconate to prevent cells swelling, and get perfectly good cold storage[25]. I don't think there is a fundamental difference.

Marshall
I support Dr Belzer. The hypertonic citrate solution can also be used for continuous perfusion, providing you add an oncotic agent (Jablonski, P., Howden, B., Marshall, V. et al., unpublished observations). I must also query Dr Johnson's temperatures: in simple hypothermic storage the kidneys are put into a bag surrounded by ice and the temperature is 0 °C.

Johnson
I really do not believe that you are storing at 0 °C. If you were, you would have ice crystals in the kidney, and putting a temperature probe in I have never been able to measure 0 °C.

Pegg
Ice melting at atmospheric pressure is at 0 °C by definition and if the kidney is surrounded by melting ice it too will be at 0 °C. There are solutes in the kidney, so it must have a lower freezing point, and consequently there will not be any ice in it.

Collins
I do not believe that a solution which contains only an impermeant anion, but is otherwise a typical extracellular solution, will be as good as one with other modifications, such as increased potassium concentration; we could argue about magnesium perhaps, but we have shown that an increased potassium concentration is vital and I simply do not believe that the effectiveness of flushout solutions can be explained entirely by impermeant anions and non-electrolytes.

Marshall
I don't believe that either, but I do not know what the answer is.

Fahy
It seems eminently reasonable to me to try to apply some of these additives used in simple cold storage to perfusion preservation. Professor Marshall, do you know how long you can preserve rat kidneys using your new flush solution (chapter 31)?

Marshall
Not yet.

Southard
Could I raise a point made by Hans Krebs some time ago[26]: he said that for normothermic perfusion of rat kidneys, the smallest possible volume was the best, and for normothermic perfusion of rat livers, the incorporation of lysine in the perfusate gave better function. I think these observations both relate to washing out of important co-factors and other cell constituents, and with a small volume you may get less washout. I have noticed that if you try to make mitochondria from 5-day preserved kidneys, the homogenate is not as red or brown as homogenates from fresh kidneys, and I think this is due to the loss of cytochromes from the mitochondria. I think there's plenty of evidence that we wash things out of kidneys during perfusion, so maybe a small perfusate volume is important. Has anybody considered this?

Armitage
Some of the longest rat heart perfusions were performed by Linask *et*

	al.[27]; co-ordinated contractions were maintained for up to 9 days at 22 °C. They used a single-pass perfusion with, consequently, a very large volume of perfusate.
Lambotte	We have continued the work of Kestens[28] on isolated perfusion of the dog liver with whole blood, and we have found that one of the most significant factors for maintaining function is to use only a moderate volume of perfusate.
Pearson	In the analogous situation of cell-culture we always like to have a high cell density. We know that cells leak material which is retained near to them and helps them to grow: the use of conditioned media[29] in cell cultures is another way of using these released materials. Incidentally in quite a lot of cell culture media amino acids are the main energy source, and nearly all contain glutamine.
Forsberg	Dr Fischer, is there any difference in solubility of molecular oxygen in D_2O, as compared to H_2O?
Fischer	It is a little lower, but since we did not perfuse, there could not be enough oxygen for full oxygenation during storage in such an electrolyte solution anyway.
Harness	Could I ask the cost of D_2O?
Fischer	One litre of D_2O costs £200.
Ozaki	Do you think D_2O would be helpful if it were included in a perfusate for continuous perfusion?
Fischer	It should be, but we have not investigated it yet.
Lambotte	When you produce osmotic shock with D_2O does the water redistribute as quickly as H_2O?
Fischer	Our model is really not suitable to answer that question.

OPTIMUM TEMPERATURE

Belzer	We have done some studies to help decide what temperature is best for preservation. We cultured kidney tubule cells on cover slips for a brief period and then determined viability daily at temperatures of 37, 30, 25, 20, 15, 10, 6 and 2 °C. The best viability was at 6 °C. Interestingly enough, 2 °C was not as good as 6 °C. The advantages of using kidney cell cultures were that it avoided perfusion, the cells were all fully exposed to the medium, and the whole model was very well standardized.
Kemp	I find that a very effective method, but the problem is that other kinds of cell may behave differently, and it is really necessary to set up many different cell cultures.
Belzer	Yes, these were mostly proximal tubular cells as far as we could tell, but the studies could be repeated using endothelial cells. We have published a paper that looked at the ATPase system of endothelial cells[30]; it was quite different from the ATPase of kidney tubular cells, because it was completely inhibited at 10 °C, and ouabain had no effect at that temperature. I think it would be nice if some of these studies could be repeated on endothelial monolayers.
Collins	I think it is a matter of experimental fact that the acellular perfusion of kidneys for preservation does have a temperature optimum that is rather close to 6 °C as Dr Belzer mentioned. The classical perfusion solution doesn't seem to work very well at 4 °C for instance, or above 12 °C. Somewhere in the range of 6–10 °C seems to be optimal. I think we need to devote our attention to finding the explanation for this.
Lambotte	We have looked at the effect of temperature on conservation of ion gradients, and between 37 and around 10 °C, intracellular potassium is well maintained. We conclude that both active and passive ion movements are similarly affected by temperature down to 10 °C, but

below 6 °C we found that active transport is more affected than passive transport, and potassium is lost[31].

Fischer — I think there is a problem in deciding on one optimal temperature of preservation, because it may not only differ for endothelial cells and tubular cells in the kidney but also for the liver or the heart. They may all have different requirements.

Armitage — With cardioplegic arrest of the heart, which admittedly might not be really relevant, the temperature of the solutions being used has been going up in the last few years, and some workers are now proposing temperatures around 18-20 °C.

Isselhard — I would not agree with that. This idea comes from work on the rat heart[32,33], where the higher temperature was better, but for all the other hearts, including the dog heart, it is now clear that lower temperatures are better. Of course this is only protection for 2 or 3 h, not for 1 or 2 days.

Collins — It is interesting that the higher temperature seemed to be optimal for the rat heart; it may be another example of the cold shock that Dr Jacobsen mentioned. Presumably rat hearts cool very quickly if you put a cold cardioplegic solution through them, whereas dog hearts would cool more slowly.

Belzer — I make a prediction though, which I cannot really support, that continuous perfusion in the future will be at 18-20 °C. At the present time you cannot get good preservation at these temperatures because other harmful effects are greater than at 6 °C; for example, phospholipases are active, and fatty acids cause mitochondrial uncoupling. If we can get a handle on those things in the future, the whole situation may change. The one thing I don't think we will ever be able to change is lipid transformation, which occurs in the dog kidney at around 18 °C, so I think that the future of hypothermic preservation will be around 20 °C where the lipids are in their normal state.

Lambotte — I entirely agree with that. We have studied many functions of the liver and everything that occurs at 37 °C also occurs at 20 °C, but at a slower rate. I very much agree that this is going to be the way to preserve normal function.

pH

Collins — I was interested in Dr Bore's paper (chapter 13) because we have found that the surface pH of ischaemic kidneys changes quite rapidly at first and then stabilizes after about 15 min[34]. This is much more rapid than your overall model, and suggests that maybe the cortex and the medulla have a different time dependency of pH change.

Southard — Could I ask Dr Bore what proportion of the pH change he measures is in the blood and how much is in the cells?

Bore — The NMR measurements (chapters 13 and 14) are of intracellular pH, and we cannot usually say what happens to the extracellular pH. This system is dependent on resolution, and with very good resolution you can distinguish two separate P_i peaks, one representing intracellular pH and the other extracellular pH. You can sometimes do that under normoxic conditions, but as soon as the tissue becomes ischaemic, there is such an enormous amount of intracellular P_i produced that you can no longer resolve the two components.

Frödin — Could I ask Dr Bore how he put the Bis-Tris-Propane buffer into the kidneys (chapter 13).

Bore — At the onset of ischaemia. We clamped the aorta, above and below the renal artery, injected the buffer into the clamped segment within

	seconds of the start of ischaemia and then clamped the pedicle to keep the buffer in the kidney during the ischaemic interval.
Collins	Dr Bore, do you have any controls that would take account of the fact that there might also be an effect of impermeant buffer anion in preventing cell swelling? The classical flush solutions such as the Sacks' or Collins' really work not so much by pH control as by controlling cell swelling.
Bore	No, we attempted to set up a control using a similar compound which lacked any buffering capacities, but we have not yet been able to do that.
Marshall	I wouldn't want to quarrel that pH is important, but your model can be criticized, Dr Bore. First of all you have a very high mortality for rats after 60 min of warm ischaemia, it is a complicated model, and you have only compared two solutions, one of which, saline, cannot be expected to be effective. Like Dr Collins I think you have got to show that your bis-tris-propane solution is better than a flush solution that we know to be better than saline.
Hoelscher	For 3 years we have been trying to develop a flush solution for *in situ* surgery, and have measured the extracellular pH in an *in vitro* model, at the level of the outer medulla. We think the pH changes within the kidney are different in the cortex, the outer medulla and the deep medulla, and since glycolysis is most active in the outer medulla we made the measurements there. We have compared the pH changes during pure ischaemia and after flushing with a solution which does not contain any sugar (the HTP solution of Bretschneider[35]) and with Euro-Collins' solution. Our data suggest that if the solution contains sugar, glycolysis is enhanced, acidotic products, mainly lactate, are released into the extracellular space and the pH falls. When we compared the pH data with function after 60, 120, 180 and 240 min of warm ischaemia, we did not see immediate function in any of the kidneys stored with a sugar solution, but we did find immediate function in the kidneys having a pH above 6.5.
Johnson	Dr Hoelscher, if you use the Bretschneider solution, which has a histidine–tryptophan buffer that keeps a very tight control of pH, you obtain immediate survival, but what happens if you use the Euro-Collins' solution with mannitol in place of glucose?
Hoelscher	We have not studied that. We have tried to raise the ATP levels by adding sugars to the HTP solution, and when we did so we obtained exactly the same results as we did with Euro-Collins' solution. Even a very small amount of sugar, 5–15 mmol/l, causes enhanced glycolysis at 37 °C, sufficient to prevent the kidneys from functioning.
Johnson	So you infer that sugar is bad, rather than that buffering must be good.
Hoelscher	Yes, sugar is bad, and you cannot put enough buffer into the kidney at 37 °C to hold the pH.
Bore	We did look at a couple of kidneys that had been flushed with Collins' solution and we would agree that the pH fall is more than in kidneys flushed without glucose.
Grundmann	We have done an experiment similar to the one proposed by Dr Johnson. We stored kidneys in Collins' solution containing glucose and in another solution containing mannitol for the same periods, and then immediately after storage we washed out the kidneys with 100 ml of Ringer's solution and measured the lactate concentration in the washout; we found significantly higher lactate concentrations in those kidneys stored in medium which contained glucose, but this did not correlate with function after transplantation[36].
Hoelscher	I don't want to disagree with Dr Grundmann, but we must differentiate between hypothermic storage and normothermic ischaemia. We all know that Euro-Collins' solution works very well for hypothermic

storage, and we find that kidneys preserved at 0 °C with a sugar solution have about the same extracellular pH after 10 h as kidneys preserved with a solution without sugar. At cold storage temperatures it does not matter whether you include sugar or not because glycolysis cannot be enhanced at this temperature. But if you have, for example, 10 min of warm ischaemia before the kidney is cooled, a sugar-containing solution will cause the pH to drop to ~5.0, where we find irreversible damage. We can show that the pH change at this time correlates very well with an increase of renal vascular resistance after reflow, there is an accumulation of cells in the vessels, and there is no immediate urine output. After 3–5 h, the urine output picks up again because the pH gradually returns to normal.

Halasz An interesting exception to that is the diving mammal, which has an enormous glycogen store which it breaks down while it is not perfusing its kidneys. The pH drops down to 5.8–5.9 at normothermia, yet the kidneys open up and function immediately[37]. Granted the vascular response in those animals is different, and in that setting there is a preplan for glycolysis and it works.

Could I also make the point that in hypothermic systems a pH drop of 0.2 or 0.4 units is considerably more important than in a normothermic system, because the dissociation constant of water changes as one cools and the neutral point rises, adding another four- or five-tenths of effective pH drop. In other words, a pH of 7.85 at 0 °C is equivalent to 7.40 at 37 °C.

Green What range of pH did you study in the rat model, Professor Marshall, and what was the optimum?

Marshall The range was 6.5–8.0 and the optimum was 7.0 (see chapter 31).

Fischer Was that measured at 37 °C?

Marshall No, at 0 °C. All the pH values were measured at the temperature of preservation.

Halasz Dr Fischer, is it possible to measure pH in D_2O solutions?

Fischer No you can't measure the pD directly with electrodes calibrated in H_2O buffer solutions, but you can calculate it if the D_2O/H_2O ratio of the solution is known[38].

Frödin We have considered the possibility that pH changes could be limiting during perfusion preservation. Has anybody any views on this?

Grundmann The pH was always stable under our hypothermic perfusion conditions. When the kidneys were perfused for longer than 96 h they did not function after transplantation, but the lactate concentration did not increase except when there had been significant ischaemia prior to perfusion[39], and there was no correlation with viability.

Johnson It is really remarkably easy to maintain pH control up to 3 days, but after this time the progressive release of bicarbonate pushes the pH gradually upwards whatever buffering we have used. You need warm ischaemia periods of 30 min or more to pull the pH down.

Southard Why do you need 30 min of warm ischaemia? The lactate concentration rises within 120 sec, and the pH is already down at that time[40].

Johnson Yes, but I am saying that a kidney subjected to a significant warm ischaemia interval causes a profound fall in pH *of the perfusate* as soon as it is put on the circuit. If the pH does not recover and there is a high lactate level, then the kidney does not function, whereas kidneys with warm ischaemia times up to 30 min that do correct the pH fall, and in which the lactate does not rise any further after 3 or 4 h, are perfectly viable.

Van der Wijk We did not adjust the pH of the perfusate in our experiments (chapter 37). The pH decreased slightly, but there was no correlation with life-sustaining renal function afterwards.

Ozaki In my experience in dog experiments, the pH decreases when the kidney on the machine is dying but when the kidney is viable the pH increases. We actually use a pH controller to add carbon dioxide to the perfusate to maintain a stable pH (see chapter 33).

Cohen In most of our kidney perfusions the pH increases continuously but there is no correlation between viability and that increase in pH.

Hoffmann I think the pH changes you see are also dependent on the perfusion system you use. With an oxygenator in the circuit the tendency is for the pH to increase, because of constant CO_2 leakage from the circuit. However in systems that simply rely on a buffer, the tendency is for the pH to fall, depending on the strength of the buffer.

Frödin If the perfusate does not reach all regions of the perfused organ, you could then have regions where the pH changed with time without you knowing it.

Belzer About 10 years ago we reported an experiment where we varied the pH of the perfusate in dog kidney preservation experiments, and above pH 8.0 or below pH 6.5 we had only non-viable kidneys after 24 h storage[41]. In chapter 35 I showed that anaerobic perfusion with a chloride medium caused severe acidosis because of continuing glycolysis: those kidneys did not survive, but when we did an identical experiment but maintained the pH, we had viable kidneys. So I think that, from the experiments, I would say that with marked pH changes, not 7.1 or 7.2 but 6.0 or 8.0, there is no question that the kidneys do not do as well. Now Dr Bore and Dr Hoelscher have shown that it is very difficult to buffer out a large pH drop; it needs at least 120 mmol of HEPES per litre to do this. I think we have to look at the detrimental effects of low pH, and try to block those effects, rather than the fall in pH. But a low pH does not seem to disturb the mitochondria that much: perhaps it activates lysosomal enzymes; this might be a very fruitful area for future research.

Southard One paper that has concerned me regarding the effect of low pH on preservation is one that came out of Wisconsin[42]. It showed that the lactate concentration in cold-stored kidneys reaches a maximum in about 4 h, and yet you can preserve those kidneys for up to 48 h. Those kidneys have been exposed to that low pH for 24–48 h and yet it apparently did not damage them, so what is so damaging about pH?

Hoelscher From our work on myocardial preservation, it seems that an extracellular pH below 6.0 is damaging in itself, in addition to the other breakdown products. We have data on the Q_{10} for the extracellular pH in anoxic kidneys and from 35 to 25 °C it is about 4.0, decreasing to 2.8 at lower temperatures. With a sugar-containing solution the Q_{10} is very different, but we do not have all the data right now. We are collecting it from 25 to 15 °C and from 15 to 5 °C also, and are studying how it compares with immediate function.

Bore I do not think it a valid assumption that constancy of lactate equals constancy of pH. There are many ways that protons can accumulate other than from glycolysis.

Johnson What we originally showed with regard to lactate and non-viability of kidneys that had been subjected to deliberate periods of warm ischaemia was this: kidneys that had their blood supply cut off, had blood trapped in them and were kept at 37 °C for up to 2 h, did show profound falls in pH, and there was a washout of lactate as the microcirculation opened up. Also there was no doubt that the depth to which the pH plummeted correlated with whether or not the kidney survived[7]. We then put these two things together, and found with human kidney transplants that the washout of lactate correlated with immediate function. That was all we were able to show.

Chan I think we should consider pH in relation to the other metabolic changes that occur in cells during ischaemia. The fall in pH alone may not be particularly toxic, but the drop in pH in the presence of a low energy supply, limitation of substrates, and the release of lysosomal enzymes, and other things may cause deterioration in the cell function; these may act together to limit the energy that is available in the cell.

Fischer I do not think that the basis of the early pH change is the lactate accumulation. In our experiments using hypothermic ischaemic storage with Collins' solution, the lactate concentration increased continuously during the first 24 h, but in the heart, free fatty acids accumulate during ischaemia and this may be the basis of the pH change[43].

Southard I would mention the results of a study[44] where heart mitochondria were suspended in a simulated 'ischaemia' environment. Lactate, pH, sodium and potassium in ischaemic cells were determined and mitochondria suspended in a similar medium. They found that the mitochondria swelled and lost respiratory control under these conditions. They therefore concluded that the intracellular environment in ischaemia could be sufficient to cause those mitochondrial changes, but whether or not this takes place in a whole cell exposed to ischaemia may be another question.

Feinberg To some extent a moderate increase in protons can be looked at as a conservation step, because protons can be used by functioning mitochondria to generate ATP, just like the protons that the mitochondria produces itself. So I think that to a certain extent a small fall in pH might be very useful, from an energetic viewpoint, but when you go beyond that you are probably looking at shifts in enzyme activity just as we would with temperature; for example, adenine translocase may become limiting at a different pH. There is certainly some indication that it does, and I think that it is the kind of thing that has to be looked at.

Pegg Maybe we should seriously question the widespread assumption that accumulation of lactate and hydrogen ions is harmful. Apart from gross pH changes, the evidence really is unclear: Dr Ross said that he had some experiments where exceedingly high lactate concentrations had no harmful effect, and Professor Feinberg points out that hydrogen ions can be energetically useful. Perhaps we should re-examine our ideas with some care.

Feinberg I would like to make a point about the smooth muscle that is around small vessels and how it is responding to Po_2 and Pco_2 and pH. This may in fact be determining much of the survival data you are looking at here, and not the metabolism of the kidney cell itself. I am thinking of some experiments that we are doing right now with platelets, where we are looking at the internal pH by radioactive methylamine distribution. We can measure pH differentials across the platelet membrane, and when we plunge them into very acid conditions they can hold on to their intracellular pH unless we raise the Pco_2; then it changes very rapidly. I haven't heard about anybody trying to alter renal intracellular pH by buffering it with a CO_2-bicarbonate buffer; people usually use HEPES or Tris, and that may make a big difference.

Fahy I do not know how relevant it is, but in the turtle the pH actually goes up to around 8 or so as the temperature falls, although in hibernators it does not. The question is, should we imitate the turtle or the squirrel?

Halasz Essentially turtles follow the $\Delta pH / \Delta t$ correction for the neutral point of water whereas hibernators vary a great deal; some follow the $\Delta pH / \Delta t$ quite closely, but others, the pocket mouse for instance, shift very little[45]. It is not a homogeneous distribution in the hibernating group.

Johnson Concerning the turtle, I think John Hunter a very long time ago showed that cold-blooded animals are not in fact privileged in the cold. Their temperature varies with the surroundings, but they are not protected when the ambient temperature falls.

Green   You are right: a snake will die at a low temperature if exposure is prolonged.

CONTINUOUS PERFUSION

Fischer   I think it is important to distinguish the two preservation methods: in continuous perfusion you try to hold a near-normal metabolic state and membrane function, but in simple hypothermic storage you want to block metabolism. The difference is very important; for example, you may welcome a pH fall in hypothermic ischaemic storage because it helps to block metabolism, but you cannot tolerate a pH drop in continuous hypothermic perfusion.

Grundmann   Yes, the two situations, hypothermic storage and hypothermic perfusion, are really not comparable. Another example is this: we have tried to improve on simple hypothermia by intermittent perfusion with Collins' or Sacks' solution, but even perfusing the kidneys every 12 h with only 100 ml Collins' solution, when storing at 0 °C, was always worse than single flush-storage in Collins' solution. Two flushings are *not* as good as one[36].

Fischer   That finding could also mean that prolonged flushing is not as good as brief flushing.

Collins   Dr Marshall, was the continuously perfused oxygenated citrate solution better than a single flush of non-oxygenated citrate solution in your rat kidney model (chapter 31)?

Marshall   Yes, when we added albumin and oxygenated the perfusate, continuous perfusion with recycling was better.

Halasz   What is your 5 ml/h in the rat kidney in terms of ml/g/min?

Marshall   That is quite a low perfusion rate, but we did improve our results by using a higher rate of perfusion which is analogous, in terms of organ weight, to the flows we use with the human kidney.

Jacobsen   I think the question of flow rate is important. In fact I think that Dr Frodin (chapter 30) used such low flows that he was really studying simple hypothermic storage. Temperature is also very important in relation to flow, and I am not surprised that he got worse results with higher flows because he perfused at a very low temperature.

Frödin   It is possible that this result was peculiar to the model, as I did say.

Cohen   Have you compared simple hypothermic storage and continuous perfusion at the same storage temperature?

Frödin   No, the simple hypothermic storage was at 2–4 °C and perfusion was at 4–6 °C.

Cohen   Has anyone done hypothermic storage at temperatures usually used for continuous perfusion, say 8 °C?

Pegg   I don't think so, but Dr Fuller and I compared continuous perfusion at 4 °C with a variety of flush solutions, also at 4 °C[46]. Using the normo-thermic perfusion assay and the rabbit kidney, we found simple hypo-thermia with a high osmolality solution was better than the usual isosmolar, extracellular perfusion.

Johnson   There are technical problems with very low flow rates used in small animals; for example, stagnation of the perfusate: we had to actually agitate the perfusate reservoir in order to keep it stable and well mixed.

Jacobsen   I really don't think that the problems are major. We can certainly obtain the same flow/g kidney weight/min in the rabbit kidney as you do in the dog kidney, and I would be surprised if it were different in the rat kidney. We see just the same sorts of damage in the smaller kidneys as in larger ones: if the 'jet effect' were a problem (see page 356) we would end up with lots of vascular thrombosis, but that does not happen.

Belzer   We have attempted to combine the good things of simple hypothermia, particularly the decreased vascular endothelial damage, with the good things of continuous perfusion. We have tried, for instance, to perfuse at 8 beats/min, which should be sufficient for oxygenation and removal of waste products, or to perfuse initially with pharmacological agents at an increased temperature and then drop the temperature and continue with cold storage, but so far we have had spectacularly poor results – not even 24 h storage. But we still think that this could be possible in the future.

CELL MEMBRANE PERMEABILITY

Belzer   One important factor that I think Dr Pegg did not discuss (chapter 6) is leakage of membranes. I think one of the problems in preservation is that the loss of ATP causes a rearrangement of the proteins and lipids of the cell membrane and they become very leaky. This may be a particular problem on reperfusion of the organ, because if the membrane pumps do not function properly, and there are membrane leaks, the cells just go awry. The same problem has been shown in shock. There has been a great deal of interest in the use of ATP complexed with magnesium in shock, but I am always amazed how a large charged molecule like that could get into the cells. It has been shown, however, that although it doesn't have any effect on normal cells it does have a definite effect on ischaemic, damaged cells[47].

Isselhard   Do you conclude that the ATP does get into the cells?

Belzer   Yes, ATP that is complexed with magnesium does get into the damaged cells and does improve their function[47].

Feinberg   I don't think we should be too dogmatic about the entry of ATP into cells, because there may be an advantage of giving ATP that is different from what you might think. That is, that as phosphorylated adenosine it may be protected against deaminases that would otherwise destroy it, and therefore it is able to persist and enter the cells as adenosine, not as ATP. If you gave it as adenosine it would be almost instantaneously deaminated. If you do find an advantage of giving ATP, you may be seeing that effect, although one cannot be sure that it does not also get in as ATP.

Lambotte   I agree with Dr Belzer about the importance of leaky membranes. At the Odense meeting[48] I showed that liver cells preserved with a sucrose-rich solution had a normal ion concentration at the end of an anoxic period, but if they were perfused, they gained sodium very rapidly because of the leaky nature of the cell membranes. I now have some more recent data which compare the effects of anoxia with those of ouabain, and we found very similar changes in sodium and potassium, but much more chloride was gained in anoxia than with ouabain. This seems to mean that something is lost from the cell in anoxia to maintain electrical equilibrium. The change in membrane potential is also greater in anoxia, which indicates an increase in permeability, and in fact the permeability for sodium is as high through the membrane as it is in free solution; there is no restriction at all to the movement of sodium. Cell swelling is also important in relation to membrane permeability. Recently I tried to use vanadate instead of ouabain to block the sodium pump but in the liver, vanadate does not enter the cells and it had no effect. But when we gave vanadate to osmotically swollen liver cells it inhibited the sodium pump, and we have shown with radioactive vanadate that it was able to enter the cells in those conditions. We conclude that anoxia, both by itself and as a consequence of the swelling it produces, increases cell membrane permeability[49].

340

Frödin	Can anybody tell me how a cell can swell when the membranes do not function and are leaking?
Pegg	Surely that depends on how leaky it is: if the internal impermeant anion is retained it will swell, unless that anion is balanced either by active pumps, or external impermeant solute.
Southard	I don't think we ever see swollen cells in our perfusion preservation experiments. We always see the 'exploded view', where the cells are collapsed and it is the interstitial space which is expanded. Even when we perfuse with perfusates of low oncotic pressure we still do not see swollen cells: the only time we have ever seen cell swelling was when we perfused with Ringer's lactate, and then we saw it within 4 h. One problem in perfusion preservation is the exploded view: we think it may be due to leaky cell membranes allowing material to leak out of the cells into the interstitial space, and we do not know how to prevent that yet.
Belzer	Yes, I agree that we don't see swollen cells during preservation, but we do see tremendously swollen cells right after implantation; that is when the cells start to swell.
Frödin	Has anyone seen cell shrinkage in preservation?
Pegg	Yes, I have seen it in kidneys preserved with Sacks' solution. One of the indications of increased membrane permeability that has been studied quite extensively is loss of intracellular enzymes into the perfusate. I have been concerned that these reports rarely, if ever, show the proportion of the particular enzyme that is lost[50], and I would like to ask Dr Cohen (chapter 34) just what proportion of the total NAG contained in the kidneys was released in his experiments? It is difficult to assess the magnitude of the loss unless such a 'latency' figure is provided[51].
Cohen	We don't know that. We have not allowed the kidney to break down totally and actually the lysosomes still appear intact.
Southard	We think that the role of lysosomes in kidney preservation is a neglected area, perhaps because it is difficult to study. We have been interested in looking at the fragility of lysosomes in homogenates of preserved kidneys. Kidneys were perfused for 3 days and homogenates incubated at 37 °C for 2 h. The homogenates were spun down at high speed and the release of lysosomal enzymes determined in the supernatant fraction. With β-glucuronidase, we measured 19% release in the control unpreserved kidney homogenates and 35% release in the homogenate from a perfused kidney, which suggested that upon perfusion the lysosomes were more fragile. There was also a loss in the total amount of lysosomal enzymes in the perfused group, which I think is indicative of leakage into the perfusate but we did not measure that. However, when we used cathepsin D as the marker enzyme, we found a 29% release in the controls, and only 12% release in the homogenates from perfused kidneys. So, depending upon which enzyme system we used, we found either an increase or a decrease in lysosomal fragility. This just emphasizes some of the difficulties of studying lysosomes, but I think it is something we should concentrate on, especially the role of lysosomal damage in long-term preservation.
Feinberg	I think we ought to determine the mechanism of enzyme leakage in the systems we are talking about: it can be surprising. For example, if you expose heart cells or a perfused heart to media containing no calcium for a very short time you will get enormous leakage; this is the calcium paradox, and it is not a function of a long storage time, it is a function of what you have exposed it to for just a very short time. Another point is that we have found that you can get enormous leakage of creatine phosphokinase from perfused hearts, but by the time you test them many hours later, as far as we can tell there is normal creatine phosphokinase activity within the cells. So there is a certain amount of leakage

341

that cells seem to be able to tolerate, but there must be other kinds of leakage which they cannot. My point is that we have to determine systematically, not just at random, whether we are dealing with a change in the composition of the perfusate that affects cell permeability, or with ischaemic changes or some other sort of change. There must be several different mechanisms for producing leakage and we should begin to discriminate.

Armitage
Holland and Olsen made the interesting point that hypothermia protects hearts against the calcium paradox[52]. So this is an example of a rapid and dramatic change in membrane permeability that happens at 37 °C, but not at 4 °C.

Johnson
Enzyme leakage certainly can be a very trivial injury. One thing that happens within minutes of starting continuous perfusion of canine kidneys is that the enzymes of the microvilli of the brush border are lost. It is completely recoverable and trivial, but nevertheless, it cannot be a favourable circumstance.

Lambotte
The rationale for Professor Fischer's D_2O study (chapter 27) was an attempt to stabilize membranes, but he looked only at water content and adenine nucleotide content. These things are important but may not be related to the permeability of the membrane. Has Professor Fischer measured the effect of D_2O on ion movements or the leakage of enzymes?

Fischer
No, we have not yet, but we know from the erythrocyte experiments that cell membranes are more stable in D_2O.

ONCOTIC AGENTS

Pegg
One effect of ischaemia and of hypothermic preservation is that the capillaries become leaky to protein. In the rabbit kidney preparation that we have studied, relatively brief periods of warm ischaemia produce a massive leakage of protein from the perfusate into the urine[53]. With kidneys undamaged by warm ischaemia there was greater protein leakage at 22 °C that at 37 °C, and this persisted, but did not worsen throughout 48 h hypothermic perfusion at 10 °C[54]. Do you find similar protein leakage in the rat model, Professor Marshall?

Marshall
Yes.

Cohen
In hypothermic perfusion of dog kidneys with PPF, we have shown that albumin progressively leaks through the perfusion; it increases linearly from 0 to 8 days, until the urine and perfusate albumin concentrations are equal.

Frödin
If you have more and more albumin outside the capillaries you must come to a point where there is no oncotic force at all. For how long is there any oncotic pressure in hypothermic renal perfusion?

Hoffmann
I agree with you Dr Frödin (see chapter 36). I would say we have oncotic support for up to 5 days only, and we think that this is one of the problems in prolonged perfusion, besides the metabolic problems.

Frödin
I think so, because in human kidneys we have found that after 24 h perfusion, the albumin concentration is the same in the perfusate, the tubular lumens, the lymph and the urine. But I would like to stress the dynamics of this process: there is very little leakage of albumin at the beginning of the perfusion, but it gradually increases during the first 24 h. And when there is no more oncotic force you ought to produce oedema.

Forsberg
But Dr van der Wijk (chapter 37) reported only minimal oedema in his study. Was histological judgement the only measure of oedema, Dr van der Wijk, or did you correlate histology with weight?

Van der Wijk
In some experiments we weighed the kidneys and there was no increase

	but the histologist could sometimes see tissue oedema when we could not detect it by weight.
Frödin	There is something peculiar about this, and I wonder if the fluid is passing out through the interstitium, into the lymphatics, and then out of the kidney.
Van der Wijk	I cannot say where the fluid goes.
Johnson	The albumin also moves through the glomeruli down the tubular lumen, out along the ureter, and back into the perfusate: it moves through the kidney, not just into a compartment to stay there.
Frödin	Yes, I agree.
Cohen	I think it is very interesting that we never see the 'exploded view' that Dr Belzer refers to. Apparently the basic difference between our perfusate and his is that he uses ten times as much mannitol.
Hoffmann	That's true. We have about 7 g/l of mannitol in our cryoprecipitated plasma (CPP) perfusate, and Dr Halasz's formula for human serum albumin perfusate that we used for this study required 20 g/l of mannitol[18].
Southard	But we see the 'exploded view' with almost every perfusate we use, including the gluconate solution (chapter 35), CPP, and human albumin solution, whether with or without mannitol.
Hoffmann	The only time we don't see the 'exploded view' is when we perfuse a kidney without oncotic support.
Pegg	Are your perfusion pressures the same as Dr Cohen's?
Cohen	We start at 60 mmHg using the same sort of machine.
Southard	We use the same.
Pegg	Dr Hoffmann, I wondered why, in your study of oncotic support agents (chapter 36) you did not include any of the gelatin plasma volume expanders. Haemaccel (Hoechst) is the one we have looked at, and it is the only plasma substitute that gave results with rabbit kidneys that were equivalent to the dextran–albumin mixture[55,56]. Have you looked at this material?
Hoffman	No, because you had problems with Haemaccel for prolonged preservation.
Armitage	With rabbit hearts we found that Haemaccel greatly improved normothermic perfusion[57], but at 10 °C it was better not to have this oncotic agent[58].
Grundmann	Why should a normal oncotic pressure be deleterious at 10 °C, providing you have low viscosity, I don't understand.
Halasz	I understood that cardiac perfusion really did not depend on an oncotically active substance, and that you can perfuse hearts with Collins' solution with no oncotic material at all. Is Haemaccel specifically toxic?
Armitage	The most important characteristic of a heart perfusate is its ionic composition, but you can improve perfusion at 37 °C by including Haemaccel. What is happening at 10 °C during perfusion with Haemaccel I wouldn't like to say.
Collins	It should be mentioned that Proctor published a paper reporting 72 h of preservation of kidneys and hearts without any oncotic agent at all[59].
Grundmann	Could Dr Collins repeat Proctor's experiments? We could not, and I don't know of anybody else who could.
Lambotte	There are clear indications that the oncotic pressure of albumin is of value, but it may have other valuable properties, such as the binding of fatty acids, which might prevent toxic effects. Maybe too, you do not need so much oncotic pressure at low temperature.
Fahy	You also find that the vascular resistance is less when the perfusate contains a colloid than when it does not, even when the colloid has leaked out of the vascular space, and I would suggest that may be because the colloid helps to control cell volume. Also, I wonder why nobody has

	studied PVP as a possible candidate. It is a perfectly good plasma expander as far as I know.
Pegg	I agree that colloids do reduce vascular resistance[60]. We have studied PVP but it produced glomerular damage in rabbit kidneys[60] and was worse than no colloid in rabbit hearts[61].

VASCULAR DAMAGE

Jacobsen	I was surprised to see that Dr van der Wijk (chapter 32) found a continuously decreasing vascular resistance during hypothermic renal perfusion. Is that the experience most people find, or does the vascular resistance increase slowly during long periods of perfusion?
Van der Wijk	We took our initial baseline flow measurement during the flush with Euro-Collins' solution, and when we put the organ into the Gambro perfusion machine, we got the lowest flow rate, but in the next hour it increased.
Cohen	We find that the vascular resistance of canine kidneys falls for about 48 h, and after that they are usually stable. Occasionally we do see a rise in resistance, even in viable kidneys.
Frödin	I would like to ask if there are any studies on regional perfusion at different periods during hypothermic perfusion.
Pegg	We certainly find a progressively developing corticomedullary vasodilation in rabbit kidneys perfused at 5–10 °C, but I don't know whether that is a general phenomenon in all species.
Fahy	Dr Cohen mentioned that endothelial cell swelling could be a problem, but it is very difficult to see in light micrographs (chapter 34). Have you done electron micrographs, Dr Cohen?
Cohen	We cannot say very much about electron micrographs: the endothelial cells do show swelling, but our pathologists are not too certain what is going on. One problem is that we can find areas that look completely normal, when other areas show swelling or damage: unfortunately one needs an awful lot of electron micrographs to get an accurate picture of what is going on. In the light micrographs we occasionally see fibrinoid necrosis in the larger vessels, and there was some fibrin in the glomeruli, presumably from endothelial damage.
Van der Wijk	Studies have been published that show perfusion nephropathy: light microscopy revealed fibrin deposits, which correlated very well with the endothelial disruption found in electron microscopic studies[62], but we did not find fibrin deposits, and we did not do an electron microscopic study.
Hoffmann	In our studies (chapter 36) a clear sign of endothelial dysfunction was blood extravasation throughout the kidney after reflow, causing the kidney to turn black.
Frödin	One thing that could be done is to use the micropuncture technique of Steinhansen; that is, direct puncture of the capillaries with injection of coloured substances to see what the flows really are after reimplantation.
Halasz	One thing that often strikes me about preserved kidneys is the patchiness of damage; one area can look beautiful and 2 cm away there is diffuse tubular necrosis and calcification.
Wheeldon	I want to ask a general question. In myocardial preservation it has become recognized that a so-called reperfusion phenomenon can occur after ischaemia: whatever parameter we look at, it becomes worse after reconnecting the blood supply than it was at the end of the ischaemic period. The question is, does the same thing happen in the kidney?
Bore	Yes, Sheehan and Davis[63] described what they called the no-reflow

Pegg
kidney; that is, after a period of ischaemia, blood did reflow briefly but then stopped and the kidney turned black.

Pegg
I don't think that this reperfusion phenomenon is the same thing as the no-flow phenomenon. No-reflow occurs after total ischaemia, when the vessels were full of blood during ischaemia, and it is immediate.

Bore
Yes, Sheehan and Davis did describe the no-flow phenomenon as an immediate event, but they also described a stage before that where the blood reflowed for a period of time and then failed.

Fischer
I would say that the reperfusion injury you see in the heart is a myocardial contracture, similar to the 'stone heart', but due to the calcium paradox[64]. All that can contract in the kidney is the muscle of the vessels.

Wheeldon
No, I'm not talking about anything as gross as no-reflow. The heart does in fact usually recover, but it is demonstrably worse histologically, biochemically, and functionally after reconnecting the circulation than at the end of a moderate ischaemic period, and it may remain so depending on the conditions of reperfusion. This has become known as reperfusion injury.

Collins
I would say that a damaged kidney tested in a blood circuit in our rabbit model or by transplantation, gets better with time, not worse.

Bore
Perhaps the analogous phenomenon in the kidney is when a transplant produces urine well at first, but then shuts down in 1, 2 or 3 days.

Frödin
A shutdown in 3 days is obviously due to medullary dysfunction, a failure to concentrate urine and so on.

BIOCHEMICAL FACTORS

Pegg
I was struck by Dr Zimmermann's results showing quite dissimilar effects on different systems collewd to the same degree (chapter 15). It has tended to be assumed that the effects on all systems are going to be roughly the same, and that cooling just produces a general retardation, but I think it is very clear now that that is not the case. Clearly, much more dats is needed to sort out this problem.

Zimmermann
In chapter 15 I showed that there was a break in the Arrhenius plot for glucose production in rat livers at $11\,°C$. We concluded that there must be something happening at this temperature and we therefore decided to see whether this might be an important temperature. In these experiments we perfused livers for 24 h at 11 or $4\,°C$. The rate of glucose production after 24 h at $11\,°C$ is about 80% of control ($100\,\mu mol/g/h$) but after $4\,°C$ perfusion production was only about 40%. From this experiment I could conclude that $11\,°C$ is going to be a better temperature for a liver preservation than $4\,°C$, but unfortunately the results were different when I used urea production as the criterion: with urea production the reduction was almost the same after perfusion at 4 and $11\,°C$.

Armitage
Could I just ask Dr Zimmermann whether he used a computer to fit the lines in his Arrhenius plots? If so, then presumably you included in the program, the number of lines that you wanted to fit to the data, thus assuming a particular number of break-points. My point is, is there really a true single break-point, or is the plot really a curve? And if so, does that have any relevance to possible phase transitions in lipids?

Zimmermann
We only see these breaks when we look at processes that are going on inside the mitochondria; with glycolysis for example we had a single straight line. That suggested that the breaks could be due to phase changes in the mitochondrial membrane, but I agree there may be other reasons.

Lambotte
The difference between the plots for glycolysis and glucose production

	may be connected with the availability of ATP, and the fact that glycolysis is ATP-producing. Reactions which consume ATP will be depressed if there is some anoxia at 37 °C due to the use of haemoglobin-free perfusate, and this will modify the Arrhenius plots, in addition to the effect of temperature.
Pearson	A simple question perhaps, but my understanding of Arrhenius plots is that theoretically a curved plot just can't happen. Can anybody clarify this point for me?
Armitage	I don't see why there can't be curved Arrhenius plots in highly complicated biological systems; this only indicates that the Arrhenius equation is inadequate to describe the effect of temperature on such complex systems.
Harness	In straightforward chemical reaction kinetics all Arrhenius plots give straight lines indicating a particular activation energy, and if you get a break it is because you are going from one reaction to another. Theoretically you must have a straight line.
Pegg	But there are examples of curved plots in biological systems[65].
Harness	Perhaps, but I am talking about straightforward chemical reactions where you know what is going on, and there you must get a straight line.
Isselhard	I want to point out that the Q_{10} of many processes, for example, lactate accumulation or ATP decay, is always above 2, but all the processes you measure by oxygen consumption have a Q_{10} below 2[66-69]. The overall slowing factor for an organ or even in a cell is therefore very difficult to predict.
Johnson	Mr Cohen, what happens to oxygen consumption during prolonged hypothermic kidney perfusion?
Cohen	Oxygen consumption seems to steadily decrease over the 5 days that we have measured it.
Johnson	Dr Pegg, you said in chapter 6 that at the temperatures used for continuous perfusion, that is 8 or 10 °C, that there is a possibility that active ion exchanges are still going on at the cell membrane. I am not sure that that is true, and even if it is, it may not be the maintenance of active transport in aerobically perfused kidneys that protects them during preservation.
Pegg	That was in my list of the assumptions I suggested were behind Dr Humphries' and Dr Belzer's original development of hypothermic perfusion. Indeed, they both used a low potassium concentration in their perfusates whereas you, of course, have increased the potassium concentration, assuming that potassium will be lost[2].
Collins	I think it is quite clear from the published literature[70] that active transport persists in separated renal tubules down to 0°C, so that I don't think there is any question that there must be some active transport which is oxygen-dependent at the usual perfusion temperatures.
Pegg	I think the question is whether or not it is sufficient to maintain the normal water and electrolyte balance or whether you have to assist it in some way.
Fuller	Certainly in the liver perfused at 10 °C, there is sufficient ion transport to partially maintain the sodium potassium ratio but it is not a normal ratio after 24 h at 10 °C[71].
Lambotte	In the isolated perfused liver we can demonstrate ouabain-sensitive transport of potassium down to 2 or 3 °C[72] but of course it is not adequate to maintain normal ion content.
Halasz	Some nerves will conduct down to 10 °C, although many cut out at 12-14 °C and that depends on an essentially normal metabolism.
Pegg	There can be no question that active metabolism does continue at around 10 °C, and not only membrane ion pump mechanisms. We, for instance, have shown that rabbit kidneys damaged by warm ischaemia

	can resynthesize adenine nucleotides under appropriate perfusion conditions at 10 °C[73].
Isselhard	We attempted to raise the ATP levels of normal cells beyond regular levels by the continuous infusion of high dosages of adenosine and all that we could get into the rat or the rabbit was, for instance, in the heart a 40% increase and in the dog only a 20% increase[74].
Feinberg	That is because there is a limiting mechanism in the normal cell where the ATP actually inhibits its own further synthesis. Even if you cut out the utilization of ATP altogether you would never go above 5 or 6μmol/g wet weight.
Southard	We attempted to increase the ATP levels in perfused kidneys, following the work in shock (see page 340), by adding Mg-ATP to the perfusate but we found it disappeared in about 4 h, and was all in the form of adenosine in the perfusate. I don't see how it could get into the cells because of the external ATPases.
Belzer	I enjoyed Dr Green's paper on hibernation (chapter 19), but the question is, can you show whether the hibernator really has different enzymes or other mechanisms, or is it a question of lipid unsaturation? I think that would be a major contribution which might help us in preservation.
Feinberg	Do hibernators cut off thermogenesis by shivering as well as from brown fat?
Green	They are capable of shivering, but they cut out both when they go down in temperature.
Collins	Dr Green, do you know whether it is possible to take a non-hibernating anaesthetized ground squirrel and simply cool it down to 4 °C, and have it survive at that temperature? If that were possible it would show that there is a mechanism already in place, that works as soon as there is a temperature change.
Halasz	It can be done with the sleep factor in a brain extract, without any adaptation.
Feinberg	It would be interesting to study the pentose shunt in these hibernators.
Bore	ATP levels are obviously a function of both ATP production and ATP utilization, and if one can postulate that the mechanisms of ATP utilization can be modified, then one can equally postulate that mechanisms of its production can be modified as well. If this is so, then high levels could simply result from reduced utilization.
Belzer	It might be interesting to look at the haemoglobin saturation at different temperatures and find if the haemoglobin is adapted in hibernators.
Green	It is interesting that if the body temperature of these thirteen-line squirrels starts to drop below 4 °C the brown fat comes into play, and they pick up in temperature and wake up.
Gooszen	Has anybody looked at reptiles, because they have very large diurnal whole-body temperature variations that can be accentuated even further by adaptation. Is that something that would be interesting?
Isselhard	I agree that we should be looking at poikilothermic animals, because snakes show temperature changes in 24 h between 10 °C and maybe 35 °C, and even more.
Green	I am assuming that the hibernator is not adapting, but that we have crept away from the poikilothermic state. I do not think that reptiles are too relevant: if you cool a snake down its whole metabolic rate falls and, for example, the amount of anaesthetic it needs is very low. It is totally different from these hibernating animals.
Pearson	Surely all the points that have been made show how different the hibernators are from us, and suggest that the poikilothermic creatures do something that is much more analogous to what you are trying to do when you preserve a kidney.

Feinberg	What intrigues me is what does the yoga do? These people can do something to their metabolism, perhaps through the autonomic nervous system or some sort of conditioning, so that they can then be put away in a block of ice and are able to tolerate these low temperatures.
Merkel	There was a case in Minnesota where a woman spent a night in a snow bank and was frozen, with rigid limbs, though she had a detectable heart beat at something like 20 a minute, and when she was rewarmed she woke up, and is fine[75].
Pegg	That was partial freezing, as the fact that she had a heart beat shows. Audrey Smith has reported extensive studies of partial freezing in whole animals that recovered, but if more than about a half of the body water was frozen, they did not survive[76].
Feinberg	I was not suggesting that yogas are completely frozen either.
Southard	This may not be relevant to our discussion, but has anybody tried to preserve a hibernator's kidney?
Green	That is exactly what I plan to do.
Belzer	We have been interested in another idea, and that is pharmacological freezing. This is an approach that Dr Halasz has talked about (chapter 20). I think that if we can get our biochemistry friends interested in this area and look at specific enzyme reactions, it might be possible to 'freeze' damaging processes by pharmacological manipulation.
Pegg	It seems to me that we still know so little about the effects of hypothermia on metabolism as a whole. There are a lot of data on temperature effects on purified enzyme systems, and masses of information about normothermic biochemistry, but really, we are still in the dark when we talk about what we would like to change, because we don't even know what is there before we change it. I would just hope that this discussion might have stimulated some of us to go away and do some experiments with our biochemical colleagues to obtain more basic data of the kind we need to think about and act upon.

LIMITING FACTORS

Collins	I would like to ask this question of the participants: do you think it is ever going to be possible to extend the period of hypothermic preservation beyond the time one could predict from the extent to which metabolism is depressed by cooling. I pointed out in chapter 22 that simple hypothermic storage seems to depress metabolism by a factor of 20–40 times, and also to extend the tolerance to ischaemia by 20–40 times. Should we then expect any technique of hypothermia to go beyond this 40-fold prolongation?
Southard	Certainly it is possible to preserve a kidney for longer than 3 days: Dr Cohen and Dr Johnson's data (chapter 34) show that some kidneys are viable for 7 or 8 days.
Collins	That is not the question. The assumption made in cold storage is that the prolongation of preservation depends upon a reduction of metabolism. That reduction of metabolism is about 40-fold which represents something like 48 h storage. Is there any technique which is dependent upon the depression of metabolism that will permit one to extend preservation beyond that maximum?
Marshall	I would say that the figures do support, more or less, a 40-fold increase; 2 h normothermic ischaemia is about the limit and 40 times that is 80 h, which is the limit we have now reached. That is indirect evidence, admittedly, but it does suggest that what we are doing is depressing metabolism to that extent.
Bore	Theoretically, you could attempt to stop metabolism pharmacologically, rather than hypothermically.

Pegg Equally, the correspondence could be fortuitous; years ago the prolongation factor was perhaps 20, subsequently it has progressively increased, so it was bound to coincide with your figure of 40 at some time. Actually I don't think there is any evidence for the assumption that survival is proportional to the reduction of metabolism. If that were so, you would get infinite preservation if you could arrest metabolism completely, and if the prolongation we do see was simply due to cooling, then the flush solution formulations would not make any difference. All you would have to do is cool the kidney, slow metabolism down, and then you would get your 40-fold prolongation. Until we can actually identify the mechanisms that limit preservation under these conditions, I really don't see how the question can be answered.

Collins I think that the most one can expect from flush cooling is protection equal to the extent to which metabolism is slowed by comparison with warm ischaemic conditions. The reasons why simple surface cooling does not achieve this expectation are (1) it does not cool very rapidly, so there is always some ischaemia especially with a large organ, and (2) hypothermia alone is damaging and the organ needs to be supported by an appropriate composition of solution in the extracellular space. If this reasoning is correct, then perhaps we have reached the best composition. No matter how hard we look or how much we manipulate the concentration of components in wash solutions, we have already reached the limit.

Fahy I think this is pretty much a matter of opinion.

Frödin I can only say that hitherto I have never done anything so well that I don't believe I can do it any better! If we now use the knowledge that we have learned here, about the pH, and metabolism, and so on, we will achieve better and better preservation results.

Johnson One of the fundamental things about cold storage is that it is damaging from the moment it starts, and the evidence for this is that whatever enzyme system you look at, it starts to be lost, from that very moment. Now many of these things don't correlate with the organ's ability to recover immediately, but the fact that they are released suggests a damaging process. So I think that the hypothesis that Dr Collins put forward is wrong. That is to say, the 40-fold reduction of metabolism certainly does not mean that there is going to be a 40-fold extension of tolerance to ischaemia, and if that is so, then there is no reason why the opposite should not be true, and there may be no fundamental barrier to extending preservation beyond 40 times the maximum warm ischaemic time.

Belzer I honestly do not believe that we have reached the limit of hypothermic preservation either. So far all we have done is to cool without damage, and I think most of the flush solutions do only this. The difference between Ringer's lactate and Collins' and hypertonic citrate is that Ringer's lactate produces direct damage while the others are non-damaging. The basis of these solutions is questionable: for instance, most of the things in a flushout solution never get to the cell; if you put radioactive inulin in the solution, flush out the kidney, and then measure where the inulin is, you find it is not even in one-third of the extracellular space (unpublished data). I think, however, that with a greater knowledge of which enzyme systems are involved and in what way, we should be able to get pharmacological inhibition of the damaging processes. Now this might require an initial period of perfusion for 1 or 1.5 h to get it to the cells, and I still think it may be possible to prolong hypothermic storage, if we understand the processes which are deteriorating under hypothermia.

Pegg Dr Collins' question is part of what I think is the most interesting question in hypothermic organ preservation today: what is responsible for limiting preservation time? If we consider preservation by continuous perfusion, one of the studies that may provide some clues as to what the mechanism is, is the work which Kootstra and his colleagues have done on intermittent warm perfusion (chapter 37), where it seems that something is happening, which enables the organ to repair damage that has occurred during hypothermic perfusion.

Kootstra We certainly hope that our *ex vivo* perfusion model can give us some insight into the mechanisms of damage, and actually the thing we are working on now is to see if we can do the same thing by hooking the kidney onto a heart-lung machine. If we are able to find the perfect machine and the perfect whole blood perfusate, but we still do not obtain the same good results as with the *ex vivo* perfusion, the question will be: do we need a whole animal? or just an intact liver or another organ?

Pegg That would be difficult to tackle experimentally. The obvious attraction of using a heart-lung machine is that if you can get an equivalent improvement to the *ex vivo* perfusion, then you can alter the composition of the fluid with which you're perfusing, to look at the role of the red cells, platelets, lymphocytes and different serum factors and dissect it all out. If you can't repair kidneys with the heart-lung machine, you first have to be sure that the problem is not simply technical, and if you can be quite sure about that, then I guess you have to consider designing very complex experiments with a liver or a lung or whatever in the circuit. Potentially, I think you have a very powerful, if difficult, tool.

Collins Returning to the initial question of why perfusion does not work for ever, I am sure that, as others have pointed out, damage begins at the moment when the organ goes on to the machine. Any parameter, the more sensitive it is the better, will indicate decreasing function with time, so I don't think we necessarily need long perfusion records to find what goes wrong with the organ; what we need is to study the metabolic processes which are deranged within perhaps just a few hours of perfusion.

References

The discussion references are listed following chapter 51 on page 356.

51
Experimental models

TYPES OF MODEL

Pegg
A constantly recurring question is the choice of a model. We have advocated, and used extensively, a normothermic bloodless perfusion assay for the rabbit[46,53,77,78,79], and Bishop and Ross[80], and now Marshall (chapter 31) have used a similar model in the rat. With these models you can get considerable amounts of work done rather inexpensively with nice quantitative data, although they certainly have limitations.

Collins
I think that is a valid point. All of us are looking for models that will be less expensive and will provide us with means of testing various hypotheses, with the ultimate plan of applying the best techniques to human kidney preservation. We have a difficult situation now, with a whole variety of techniques being applied in several species. The question arises as to which of these models is acceptable as a test for the application in man. This I suppose is the ultimate aim.

Marshall
Any, or all of them, may be applicable, but none of them is the proven optimal test. We are going to correlate our findings in the rat normothermic perfusion assay with transplantation in the rat in the first instance, and then later in other species before man. We visualize this only as a screening system to look at a lot of factors. Of our various findings so far, two have now also been looked at in transplantation models; first, we have completed a double-blind randomized trial of isosmolar citrate versus hyperosmolar citrate in the dog, and we found the same 24 h preservation results with both solutions; second, another group has studied continuous perfusion with the citrate albumin perfusate, also in the dog, and that solution works as well as conventional perfusion

Bore
Professor Marshall showed us (chapter 31) that measurements of creatinine clearance in his isolated perfused rat model would not distinguish between a kidney that had suffered 30 sec of warm ischaemia, and a kidney that had suffered 45 min of warm ischaemia.

Pegg
We found a very high sensitivity to warm ischaemia of several functions in the isolated perfused rabbit kidney[53] and in the same species we have done quite extensive comparisons between the normothermic perfusion assay and autologous transplantation after the same range of preservation methods, and the agreement was really excellent[46,81].

Jacobsen
I wondered whether Professor Marshall's findings regarding the osmolality of the flush solution could be to do with the testing system. I agree that this is a beautiful system, which gives you a lot of information, but one thing that it is not very sensitive to, is vascular integrity, and maybe the osmolality has its major significance with that part of the kidney.

Guttman	Neil Segal has set up a very similar system to that of Fuller and Pegg[77] and Marshall (chapter 31) and has attempted to assay rabbit kidneys on the normothermic perfusion apparatus and then test the same kidney in the *ex vivo* perfusion model that Dr Collins described in chapter 25. None of those kidneys functioned on *ex vivo* blood perfusion although they functioned pretty well on the *in vitro* perfusion apparatus for 3 h.
Pegg	And was the problem vascular?
Guttman	Yes, I assume so. We also found that dextrans were very damaging in our system, and 0.5% albumin was better than 1% albumin, so there is still a lot of variation, even in this *in vitro* system.
Pegg	I'm sure that all protagonists of the normothermic perfusion assay would agree that it does not reveal vascular injury. Moreover, the vascular injury you detected in the *ex vivo* blood perfusion may have been produced by the preceding bloodless perfusion. So I think the sequential comparison may not be valid.
Kootstra	I think these models might be useful for screening, but if you want to look at what the problems would be in long-term preservation, then you always have to use a transplant model, because after 3 days you get quite different problems with the endothelium and probably other things too. Could I also comment on Dr Collins' *ex vivo* rabbit kidney model (chapter 25)? In our *ex vivo* canine kidney perfusions we found different degrees of renal function in the first, second and third hours, so it would be interesting to see if measurements made throughout 3 h of perfusion would show any recovery of the kidney after cold storage.
Collins	Well, actually, it's not so easy to perform these perfusions for 3 h, for technical reasons. However, the general pattern of recovery with both of the preservation solutions we studied does not suggest that C2 is going to get progressively better and overtake LIC: they both improve in a parallel fashion.
Guttman	We set up Dr Collins' *ex vivo* rabbit kidney model 2 years ago, and at first we had inconsistent results, but when we made the connecting tubing extremely short, so that we could actually leave the kidney in the pelvis of the rabbit and close the abdomen during the perfusion, we had very good results up to 2 h, and even got some to 5 h, but that was inconsistent.
Fischer	Could it be a theoretical disadvantage of Dr Collins' model that you are working in an allogeneic system?
Collins	I don't think that is a problem unless there are natural preformed antibodies in the New Zealand rabbit. I suspect that most of the preservation transplant experiments have been allotransplants. Is that correct Dr Green?
Green	Most of them have been autografts, but we did do some allografts, and they functioned very similarly for the first 5 or 6 days before we got obvious rejection.
Bore	Are you sure, Dr Collins, that measuring creatinine clearance in your model is a sufficiently sensitive index to pick up the differences that you are seeking?
Collins	Yes it is very sensitive: we see very clear differences between kidneys that have had different periods of ischaemia. After all, this is really the equivalent of observing transplanted kidneys for the first 1–2 h post-transplant; these kidneys are being perfused with blood and the only difference is that they are not sewn in – they are plugged in, just for the sake of convenience.
Pegg:	What worries me about the model, Dr Collins, is that you reach different conclusions than we reached with the rabbit using actual transplantation. Of course, we did not look at the same solutions as you, but in studying variations in flush solution composition, we came to the conclusion that increasing the osmolality with glucose improved

352

function, decreasing ionic strength made virtually no difference and increasing the potassium concentration worsened function[81]. Those results were with standard transplantation and immediate opposite nephrectomy.

Collins   I would predict that if you test some of the LIC solution in the rabbit transplant model, it will do better than C2.

Halasz   What we all need is a cheap, consistent and predictable model, and the attempt to develop this *ex vivo* rabbit model was with the intention that it would be supersensitive over the first hour. We assume that if we show good early function then it is unlikely that there would be deterioration after that. We have had some problems in making it consistent; that probably has to do with the inherent problem of small animals, but in the United States dogs have become prohibitively expensive and one just has to do small animal work. I think it would be very valuable if this group could come up with a model which is consistent but not expensive.

Belzer   Dr Southard yesterday described the test model which we have been using (chapter 16), and that is the tissue homogenate. At least this gives you an opportunity to obtain twenty samples and test twenty different things on one kidney. The final test will always be transplantation, but we are using homogenates to screen out different compounds, and if a particular compound, for instance, produces a complete uncoupling of the mitochondria, I can tell you that the same compound will do very poorly during perfusion of the whole organ.

Collins   Do you consider that a transplant in the rabbit or the rat is an appropriate model from which to go straight to man, or do we have to go on to the dog, the pig or the horse? What do people think?

Johnson   I would like to make the point that the transplant model itself is not as good as it has been claimed to be. There are enormous variations in results with the same transplant model in different laboratories, with different surgeons and variations in protocol. One thing, for example, that Mr Cohen has shown, is that what we call a 'success' following a long term of preservation, may in fact be a seriously injured kidney, which only just makes it. Transplantation has a reputation beyond its true value, although I would agree that many of the other models are worse!

Marshall   I don't want to throw the dog transplant model out just yet; it has provided quite a lot of good data, not only on preservation but also on immunology.

Green   I would have thought that as a screening model, Dr Pegg's method, using a warm perfusion circuit to measure function after a period of cold storage, was one approach, but because that leaves out the problem of vascular integrity, it should be calibrated against Dr Collins' *ex vivo* perfusion model, in the rabbit, in the same laboratory, at the same time, using the same anaesthetics and pretreatment. That is what people never do! Then, within weeks, not a year, the experiments should be repeated in the autograft transplantation model with exactly the same pre-treatment and so on. Then you should go to the baboon, which is an expensive but not a difficult animal, and do just a few experiments in the baboon before you go to man, and get away from pigs and dogs.

Southard   It seems to me that it does not particularly matter which model system you study. You are after mechanisms, and the main thing is to have precise control so that you can see whether your changes improve anything, and if they do, you can say what mechanism is responsible for that change. In our studies, for instance, we are using rabbit kidneys to find out if the fatty acids go into the mitochondria, and what drugs inhibit it. We don't assume that the same thing will happen in the dog kidney, but we start with a small animal, work up to the dog kidney,

	and then maybe go on to the human kidney. It doesn't matter what model you use, as long as the appropriate controls are done.
Bore	You may also have to use different models to look at different aspects of the problem. As you progressively increase a period of ischaemia, for instance, you move through a series of magnitudes of damage, from kidneys that are almost normal to kidneys with impaired function, to kidneys which are temporarily non-functional, to kidneys which are permanently non-functional. It is unreasonable to assume that the mechanisms involved in the transition between normality and temporary loss of function are the same as those which are involved in the transition from temporary loss of function to permanent loss of function. You have to decide which model system is best to look at each particular part of the spectrum. I think that the quest for a single model system to examine everything is probably unreasonable.
Grundmann	I cannot agree at all that the models for temporary loss of function should be differentiated from models for permanent loss. If you are storing kidneys by simple hypothermia there is very good function after 12 h of preservation, perhaps 40–50% of normal, but the function decreases as preservation is prolonged in a logarithmic manner. In our model, after 48–72 h the PAH clearance falls to zero[82], but renal function can recover after 2 or 3 weeks if you don't do a contralateral nephrectomy, whereas after longer periods of preservation there may be no recovery at all. I think the important thing is to follow this logarithmic decay of function.
Thaw	An important point that has been missed, though, is that model systems should be standardized between laboratories, so that when you come to a meeting like this you can be sure that you are using similar baselines for comparison.
Southard	I disagree. I think you should use whatever model suits the needs of your experiments at the time. As Dr Bore just said, you may have to change models, depending on where your mechanisms lead you. I don't think there should be any standardized model.
Thaw	Well, in that case it will be very difficult for you to compare your results if you have to take into account all the similarities and differences between the many different systems you are using.

SPECIES DIFFERENCES

Collins	I think it is interesting and important to note that you will find differences depending on the species that you use for your model. I have already mentioned the species difference that we have detected between dogs and rabbits in comparing C2 and LIC flush solution (chapter 25). We also found that it is much more difficult to wash out dog kidneys than rabbit kidneys: a canine kidney that has been subjected to 1 h of warm ischaemia could not effectively be perfused with a solution containing 1% dextran, whereas a rabbit kidney could. If we raised the dextran content to 4% then the dog kidney could be perfused as readily as the rabbit. Another situation where there is a disparity is between man and the dog in relation to magnesium in flush solutions. When we used the C2 solution *without* magnesium in the dog, it was quite clear that this solution was not as satisfactory as C2 solution *with* magnesium, whereas in man, comparison of data from Euro-transplant with the American data would suggest that the magnesium content is quite unnecessary. I would suggest that the dog may indeed not be the ideal model to use for human kidney preservation and if there is any message here, it is that the final studies have to be done in man. I really don't know what we should use as a testing system in future studies.

Marshall	I want to respond to Dr Collins' comparison of the results in Eurotransplant and America. I don't think that's allowed any more. You can do prospective trials in clinical transplantation, and unless you can show a difference in a preservation system by such a trial, it is just anecdotal.
Hoffman	I would like to mention my experience of vasospasm in the kidneys of different laboratory animals. I find the rabbit kidney is like the pig kidney; when it is partially vasospastic, it stays vasospastic, while the dog kidney will open up during the washout procedure.
Belzer	I think this is absolutely true. When we did our original studies on vasospasm in the agonal period, we used dogs, but we could not get the vasospasm no matter what we did, and we had to go to the pig kidney to show the same response as the human kidney[83,84].
Fischer	I agree that there are species differences, not only in the vasculature but also in metabolism. For instance there is 100% difference in the maintenance of adenine nucleotides between different species[85].
Isselhard	In the heart it can be demonstrated that if you use the same procedure for inducing cardioplegia, the solution LK 352, which is the precursor of the present Bretschneider HPT solution, is much less effective in the rabbit than it is in the dog. We all know that the function of the heart is about the same in both species, they do the same amount of work per gram and so on, so I don't think the difference can be correlated with a different work load.
Collins	I think Professor Marshall's observations in his rat model (chapter 31) raise very difficult questions because he has found that an *isosmolar* citrate solution is the best solution for kidney preservation. In the dog, however, I believe he has reported that the *hyperosmolar* citrate solution is better.
Marshall	No, they were the same; there was no significant difference between the two solutions in the dog.
Collins	But if the rat model was the appropriate one, you would immediately apply the isosmolar solution to human kidney preservation.
Pegg	Which is what has been done in Cambridge (see chapter 24).
Marshall	That's right, and it seems to work.
Pegg	I think we should be cautious when suggesting that species differences can explain experimental results. For example, we have repeated some of the experiments on blood washout (chapter 24) in the dog kidney after the same period of warm ischaemia and they perfuse with our WF5PD perfusate or hypertonic citrate in the same way as rabbit kidneys. So we don't find a difference there. Also we have compared the fall in adenine nucleotides with increasing periods of warm ischaemia in the dog and the rabbit, and we find that the rabbit falls slightly more rapidly than the dog, but the difference is small and of doubtful significance. I have already mentioned that the results of our transplantation experiments in the rabbit do not square with your *ex vivo* perfusions in the same species. So I think there are many variables in these systems apart from variations between species.
Foreman	We have also studied the resynthesis of adenine nucleotides by the dog kidney during continuous hypothermic perfusion after 60 min of warm ischaemia, and when we added the same substrates that we used in the rabbit, we were unable to get back to baseline when we used a PPF perfusate, but if we used the same Haemaccel perfusate that we used in the rabbit, the results were much closer. So what at first appeared to be a species difference was actually due to another aspect of the experimental design that we thought was unimportant at first.
Marshall	I don't think the species difference is too great either.
Ozaki	Does anybody know if the optimal pH differs from species to species?
Grundmann	We studied the effect of pH in the hypothermic perfusion of canine

kidneys 9 years ago[86], and we found that the optimum was about 7.0, which is the same result as Professor Marshall found with the rat here (chapter 31).

Jacobsen I want to make a comment on the apparent species difference Dr Collins reported between dog transplants and *ex vivo* perfusion in rabbits (chapter 25), because he has added quite a considerable amount of plastic tubing to the very apparent differences between dogs and rabbits. Studies on extracorporeal circulation show that complement can be activated by plastics and there may be plasticizers in the tubing, so you have a lot of unknown factors in your rabbit model which you do not have in your dog model.

Collins Well, the tubing is Silastic, and I doubt if that contains any plasticizers at all. A freshly isolated rabbit kidney placed on the *ex vivo* circuit behaves exactly the same as the kidney left *in situ*, so the plasticizers, if there are any, do not appear to cause any loss of function during the period of our test.

Jacobsen But my point is that you don't know, and there may be an apparent species difference because you include plastic in the rabbit.

Collins Well, I think that is a red herring.

Belzer There can be technical problems with the rat and the rabbit; we found that if we used 8 kg dogs, we didn't get as good results as when we used 20 kg dogs, and one of the problems was that the cannulae were so small that we got a jet effect of the perfusate hitting the artery wall, which we don't see in the bigger model.

Marshall This point is important, but it can be overcome. We always calibrate our cannulae and make certain that they are equal and matched.

Merkel You see the jet effect in human kidneys also if you cannulate the renal artery; the endothelium becomes damaged over 24–48 h, and this is avoided by cannulating the aorta. I don't know whether the effect is more pronounced in small arteries, but I would assume that it may be so.

Johnson But nobody has ever succeeded in getting really long-term storage in small animal models. I think the longest I have ever seen for the rabbit is 48 h, so this does suggest that there is a difference between small and big animals.

Frödin I am very confused about the whole situation. I just want to say that if you compare two species after the same ischaemic periods and you find differences this could just be due to the dynamic changes in the systems; they could still be anatomically the same.

References

1. Mittnacht, S., Jr, Sherman, S.C. and Farber, J.L. (1979). Reversal of ischaemic mitochondrial dysfunction. *J. Biol. Chem.*, **254**, 9871
2. Pegg, D.E. (1978). An approach to hypothermic renal preservation. *Cryobiology*, **15**, 1
3. Green, R.D., Boyer, D., Halasz, N.A. and Collins, G.M. (1979). Pharmacological protection of rabbit kidneys from normothermic ischaemia. *Tranplantation*, **28**, 131
4. Southard, J.H., Lutz, M.S., Pavlock, G.S. and Belzer, F.O. (1981). Effect of chlorpromazine on mitochondria from rabbit kidneys exposed to ischaemia and reflow. *Biochem. Pharmacol.* (Submitted)
5. Pavlock, G.S., Southard, J.H., Lutz, M.S., Belzer, J.P. and Belzer, F.O. (1981). Effect of chlorpromazine and mannitol on rabbit kidneys following *in vivo* ischaemia and reflow. *Life Sciences*. (Submitted)
6. Lambotte, L. (1973). Use of hepatic cell membrane potential measurement to evaluate new method of liver preservation. *Surgery*, **74**, 509
7. Johnson, R.W.G. (1972). The effect of ischaemic injury on kidneys preserved for 24 hours before transplantation. *Br. J. Surg.*, **59**, 10

8. Hoffmann, R. M., Steiper, K. W., Johnson, R. W. G. and Belzer, F. O. (1974). Renal ischaemic tolerance. *Arch. Surg.*, **109**, 550
9. Halasz, N. A. and Collins, G. M. (1975). Forty-eight hour preservation. A comparison of flushing and ice storage with perfusion. *Arch. Surg.*, **111**, 175
10. Wusteman, M. C., Jacobsen, I. A. and Pegg, D. E. (1978). A new solution for initial perfusion of transplant kidneys. *Scand. J. Urol. Nephrol.*, **12**, 281
11. Weed, R. I., La Celle, P. I. and Merrill, E. W. (1969). Metabolic dependence of red cell deformability. *J. Clin. Invest.*, **48**, 795
12. Fonteles, M. C. and Karow, A. M., Jr (1977). Vascular alpha adrenotropic responses of the isolated rabbit kidney at 15 °C. *Arch. Int. Pharmacodyn.*, **227**, 195
13. Jacobsen, I. A., Kemp, E. and Buhl, M. R. (1979). An adverse effect of rapid cooling in kidney preservation. *Transplantation*, **27**, 135ᵗ
14. Isselhard, W., Eisenhardt, H. J. and Prangenberg, G. (1981). Preservation of skeletal musculature by hypothermia. (In preparation)
15. Robinson, J. R. (1971). Control of water content of non-metabolizing kidney slices by sodium chloride and polyethylene glycol (PEG 6000). *J. Physiol.*, **213**, 227
16. Jablonski, P., Howden, B., Marshall, V. and Scott, D. (1980). Evaluation of citrate flushing solution using the isolated perfused rat kidney. *Transplantation*, **30**, 239
17. Aquatella, H., Perez-Gonzales, M., Morales, J. M. and Whittembury, G. (1972). Ionic and histological changes in the kidney after perfusion and storage for transplantation. *Transplantation*, **14**, 480
18. Halasz, N. A. and Collins, G. M. (1974). Simplification of perfusion preservation methods: colloid and buffer studies. *Transplantation*, **17**, 534
19. Cohen, G. L. and Johnson, R. W. G. (1980). Perfusate buffering for 8-day canine kidney storage. In *Proceedings European Society for Artificial Organs*, **VII**, 235
20. Fahy, G. M., Hornblower, M. and Williams, H. (1979). An improved perfusate for hypothermic renal preservation. I. Initial *in vitro* optimization based on tissue electrolyte transport. *Cryobiology*, **16**, 618
21. Hochachka, P. W. and Storey, K. B. (1975). Metabolic consequences of diving in animals and man. *Science*, **187**, 613
22. Kamm, D. E. and Strope, G. L. (1973). Glutamine and glutamate metabolism in renal cortex from potassium-depleted rats. *Am. J. Physiol.*, **224**, 1241
23. Leibach, F. H., Fonteles, M. C., Pillion, D. and Karow, A. M., Jr (1974). Glutathione in the isolated perfused rabbit kidney. *J. Surg. Res.*, **17**, 228
24. Meister, A. (1973). On the enzymology of amino acid transport. *Science*, **180**, 33
25. Downes, G. L., Hoffmann, R., Juang, J. S. and Belzer, F. O. (1973). Mechanism of action of washout solutions for kidney preservation. *Transplantation*, **16**, 46
26. Krebs, H. A. (1974). Metabolic requirements of isolated organs. *Transplant. Proc.*, **6**, 237
27. Linask, J., Votta, J. and Willis, M. (1978). Perfusion preservation of hearts for 6–9 days at room temperature. *Science*, **199**, 299
28. Lambotte, L. and Kestens, P. J. (1971). Liver perfusion in the study of hormone effects on the ionic content and membrane potential of liver cells. In Diczfalusy, E. (ed.), *Karolinska symposia on research methods in reproductive endocrinology. Perfusion techniques*, p. 217. (Stockholm: Karolinskà Institutet)
29. Ham, R. G. and McKeehan, W. L. (1979). Media and growth requirements. In Jakoby, W. B. and Pastan, I. H. (eds.) *Methods in Enzymology. Cell Culture*, **58**, 44 (New York: Academic Press).
30. Belzer, F. O., Hoffmann, R., Huang, J. S. and Downes, G. L. (1972). Endothelial damage in perfused dog kidney and cold sensitivity of vascular Na-K-ATPase. *Cryobiology*, **9**, 457
31. Lambotte, L. (1973). Persistence of active and passive ionic transport during low-temperature liver preservation. *Surgery*, **73**, 8
32. Hearse, D. J., Steward, D. A. and Braimbridge, M. V. (1976). Cellular protection during myocardial ischaemia. *Circulation*, **54**, 193
33. Tyers, G. F. O., Williams, E. H., Hughes, H. C. and Todd, G. J. (1977). Effect of perfusate temperature on myocardial protection from ischaemia. *J. Thorac. Cardiovasc. Surg.*, **73**, 766

34. Hardie, I. R., Clunie, G. J. and Collins, G. M. (1973). Evaluation of simple methods for assessing renal ischaemic injury. *Surg. Gynec. Obstet.*, **136**, 43
35. Hoelscher, M., Kallerhoff, M., Klaes, G., Helmchen, U. and Bretschneider, H. J. (1980). Successful dog kidney preservation for 4 hours of warm ischaemia or 48 hours of cold ischaemia using the histidine-tryptophane–buffer solution of Bretschneider. ESAO Abstracts of the 7th Annual Meeting
36. Grundmann, R., Kürten, K., Bromberger, G. and Pichlmaier, H. (1979). Nierenkonservieurng durch intermittierende hypotherme. Perfusion mit einer Collins-bzw. Sacks-Lösung. *Res. Exp. Med.*, **176**, 37
37. Halasz, N. A., Elsner, R., Garvie, R. S. and Grotke, G. (1974). Renal recovery from ischaemia: a comparative study of harbor seal and dog kidneys. *Am. J. Physiol.*, **227**, 1331
38. Bates, R. G. (1973). *Determination of pH. Theory and Practice*, pp. 251 and 375. (New York: Wiley)
39. Grundmann, R., Eichmann, J., Keckstein, J., Raab, M. and Meusel, E. (1977). Relationship between the prolongation of warm ischaemia and the maximum available preservation period. *Surgery*, **81**, 542
40. Hems, P. A. and Brosnan, J. T. (1970). Effects of ischaemia on content of metabolites in rat liver and kidney *in vivo*. *Biochem. J.*, **120**, 105
41. Belzer, F. O., Ashby, B. S., May, R. E. and Dunphy, J. E. (1968). Isolated perfusion of whole organs. In: Norman, J. C. (ed.), *Organ Perfusion and Preservation*. (New York: Appleton-Century-Crofts)
42. Cunnaro, J. A., Johnson, W. A., Uehling, D. T., Updike, S. J. and Weiner, M. W. (1976). Metabolic consequences of low-temperature kidney preservation. *J. Lab. Clin. Med.*, **88**, 873
43. Gercken, G., Trotz, M. and Bischoff, H. (1979). Lipid metabolism in arrested ischaemic heart. *Pflüg. Arch. Physiol.*, **379** (suppl.), R5
44. Jurkowitz, M., Scott, K. M., Altschuld, R. A., Merola, A. J. and Brierley, G. P. (1974). Ion transport by heart mitochondria. Retention and loss of energy coupling in aged heart mitochondria. *Arch. Biochem. Biophys.*, **165**, 98
45. White, F. N. (1981). A comparative physiological approach to hypothermia. *J. Thorac. Cardiovasc. Surg.* (In press)
46. Fuller, B. J. and Pegg, D. E. (1976). Assessment of renal preservation by normothermic bloodless perfusion. *Cryobiology*, **13**, 177
47. Bhandry, L. H., Sayeed, M. M. and Bave, A. E. (1972). Evidence for the enhanced uptake of ATP by liver and kidney in hemorrhagic shock. *Am. J. Physiol.*, **233**, R83
48. Lambotte, L., Wojcik, S. and Pontegnie-Istace, S. (1979). Investigations on the mechanism of action of hyperosmolar intracellular solutions used in liver preservation. In Pegg, D. E. and Jacobsen, I. A. (eds.) *Organ Preservation II*, p. 292. (Edinburgh: Churchill Livingstone)
49. Lambotte, L. and Jamart, J. (1981). Vanadate inhibition of hepatocyte sodium pump. *Arch. Int. Physiol. Biochem.*, **89**, 21
50. Pegg, D. E. (1981). Viability assays of preserved cells, tissues and organs. In Aso, K. and Sumida, S. (eds.) *Low Temperature Medicine*. (Tokyo: Asakura Publishing Co.)
51. Lee, D. (1972). The effect of glycerol, ethanol and dimethylsulphoxide on rat liver lysosomes. *Biochim. Biophys. Acta*, **266**, 50
52. Holland, C. E., Jr and Olsen, R. E. (1975). Prevention by hypothermia of the paradoxical calcium necrosis in cardiac muscle. *J. Molec. Cell. Cardiol*, **3**, 917
53. Wusteman, M. C. (1977). The effect of warm ischaemia on the function of rabbit kidneys measured by isolated normothermic perfusion. *J. Surg. Res.*, **23**, 332
54. Foreman, J., Dvořák, R. and Pegg, D. E. (1981). Measurement of function during hypothermic renal perfusion. *J. Surg. Res.*, **31**, 246
55. Pegg, D. E., Jacobsen, I. A. and Walter, C. A. (1977). Hypothermic perfusion of rabbit kidneys with solutions containing gelatin polypeptides. *Transplantation*, **24**, 29
56. Pegg, D. E. and Green C. J. (1978). Renal preservation by hypothermic perfusion. IV. The use of gelatin polypeptides as the sole colloid. *Cryobiology*, **15**, 27
57. Armitage, W. J. and Pegg, D. E. (1977). An evaluation of colloidal solutions for

normothermic perfusion of rabbit hearts: an improved perfusate containing Haemaccel. *Cryobiology*, **14**, 428

58. Armitage. W. J. and Pegg, D. E. (1978). The influence of gelatin polypeptides, potassium, calcium and osmolality on the hypothermic perfusion of rabbit hearts. *Cryobiology*, **15**, 537

59. Joyce, M. and Proctor, E. (1974). Hypothermic perfusion-preservation of dog kidneys for 48-72 hours without plasma derivatives or membrane oxygenation. *Transplantation*, **18**, 548

60. Pegg, D. E. and Farrant, J. (1969). Vascular resistance and edema in the isolated rabbit kidney perfused with a cell-free solution. *Cryobiology*, **6**, 200

61. Armitage, W. J. (1979). *The Effects of Low Temperatures and Cryoprotective Agents on the Isolated Rabbit Heart*. Ph.D. thesis. London: CNAA

62. Hill, G. S. and Light, J. A. (1976). Perfusion-related injury in renal transplantation. *Surgery*, **79**, 440

63. Sheehan, H. L. and Davis J. C. (1959). Renal ischaemia with failed reflow. *J. Pathol. Bacteriol.*, **78**, 105

64. Jynge, P. (1980). Protection of the ischaemic myocardium: calcium-free infusates and the additive effects of coronary infusion and ischaemia in the induction of the calcium paradox. *Thorac. Cardiovasc. Surg.*, **28**, 303

65. Russell, J. C. and Peach, D. M. (1974). The temperature dependance of (Na$^+$-+K$^+$)-ATPase. *Physiol. Chem. Physics*, **6**, 225

66. Kübler, W., Hähn, N., Reidemeister, C. J. and Spieckermann, P. G. (1964). Ruhigstellung des ischämischen Myokards durch extrazellulären Natriumentzug und Novocaingabe als Methode zur Verlängerung der überlebens – und Wiederbelebungszeit des Herzens. *Pflüg. Arch. Ges. Physiol.*, **281**, 53

67. Bonhoeffer, K. (1967). Sauerstoffverbrauch des normo-und hypothermen Hundeherzens vor und während verschiedener Formen des induzierten Herzstillstandes. *Biblio. Cardioplegica Fasc.* **18**. (Basel: Karger)

68. Isselhard, W., Berghoff, W., Schüler, H. W. and Apostolopoulos, C., (1968). Temperaturabhängigkeit der Änderungen im Stoffwechselstatus des küstlich stillgestellten anaeroben Herzens. *Z. Exp. Med.*, **145**, 30

69. Kübler, W. (1969). Tierexperimentelle Untersuchungen zum Myokardstoffwechsel im Angina-pectoris-Anfallund und beim Herzinfarkt. *Bibl. Cardio.*, **22**. (Basel: Karger)

70. Burg, M. B. and Orloff, J. (1964). Active cation transport by kidney tubules at 0 °C. *Am. J. Physiol.*, **207**, 983

71. Fuller, B. J. and Attenburrow, V. D. (1979). Effects of temperature and method of storage on hepatic function. Presented at the *British Transplantation Society*. 4 April, London (UK)

72. Lambotte, L. (1973). Persistence of active and passive ionic transport during low-temperature liver preservation. *Surgery*, **73**, 8

73. Pegg, D. E., Wusteman, M. C. and Foreman, J. (1981). The metabolism of normal and ischaemically injured rabbit kidneys during perfusion for 48 hours at 10 °C. *Transplantation*, **32**, 437

74. Isselhard, W., Eitenmüller, J., Mäurer, W., DeVreese, A., Reineke, H., Czerniak, A., Sturz, J. and Herb, H. G. (1980). Increase in myocardial adenine nucleotides induced by adenosine: dosage, mode of application and duration, species difference. *J. Molec. Cell. Cardiol.*, **12**, 619

75. Associated Press report – 12 January 1981

76. Smith, A. U. (1961). *Biological Effects of Freezing and Supercooling*. (London: Edward Arnold)

77. Fuller, B. J., Pegg, D. E., Walter, C. A. and Green, C. J. (1977). An isolated rabbit kidney preparation for use in organ preservation research. *J. Surg. Res.*, **22**, 128

78. Pegg, D. E. and Wusteman, M. C. (1977). Perfusion of rabbit kidneys with glycerol solutions at 5 °C. *Cryobiology*, **14**, 168

79. Wusteman, M. C. (1978). Comparison of colloids for use in isolated normothermic perfusion of rabbit kidneys. *J. Surg. Res.*, **25**, 54

80. Bishop, M. C. and Ross, B. D. (1978). Evaluation of hypertonic citrate flushing solution for kidney preservation using the isolated perfused rat kidney. *Transplantation*, **25**, 235

81. Green, C.J. and Pegg, D.E. (1979). Mechanism of action of "intracellular" renal preservation solutions. *World J. Surg.,* **3,** 115
82. Grundmann, R., Strümper, R., Kürten, K., Bischoff, A. and Pichlmaier, H. (1978). Nierenkonservierung durch hypotherme Lagerung nach Collins und Sacks: Der Einfluß von 0–30min warmer Ischämie auf die erreichbare Konservierungszeit. *Arch. Chir.,* **346,** 11
83. Belzer, F.O., Reed, T.W., Pryor, J.P., Kountz, S.L. and Dunphy, J.E. (1970). Cause of renal injury in kidneys obtained from cadaver donors. *Surg. Gynecol. Obstet.,* **130,** 467
84. Keaveny, T.V., Pryor, J.P., White, C. and Belzer, F.O. (1971). Renal vasomotor responses in the agonal period. *Angiology,* **22,** 77
85. Fischer, J.H., Marsen, S., Fabri, P. and Isselhard, W. (1979). Renal energy metabolism during hypothermic storage – comparative experiments on dogs, rats and guinea pigs. *Eur. Surg. Res.,* **11** (suppl. 2) 85
86. Grundmann, R., Landes, T. and Pichlmaier, H. (1972). Hypothermic pulsatile perfusion of dog kidneys. *Transplantation,* **14,** 742.

PART VIII
CRYOPRESERVATION

52
Perfusion of canine kidneys with dimethyl sulphoxide: techniques and toxicity

I. R. HARDIE, L. B. HAMLYN, G. A. BALDERSON,
K. L. GALL and P. W. H. WOODRUFF

Canine kidneys were perfused by gravity flow with cold (0–1 °C) 12.5% w/v Me_2SO in either extracellular (Ringer's) or intracellular (Collins') crystalloid solutions, or in a colloid (5% albumin) solution. Me_2SO was then removed rapidly by flushing with the base solution, or gradually by flushing with solutions containing mannitol to reduce osmotic gradients. One kidney of each pair was bisected, and each half cut into five segments (two poles, dorsal, lateral, medial), which were homogenized and centrifuged. Reference of the supernatant osmolality to a standard curve of Me_2SO osmolality allowed tissue Me_2SO levels to be estimated. The second kidney was autotransplanted, and its function followed by daily serum creatinine estimations.

Subsequently, Me_2SO toxicity was assessed *in vitro* by estimating *p*-aminohippurate (PAH) uptake by cortical slices from kidneys stored at 0, -4 or -6 °C for up to 96 h after perfusion with 12.5% Me_2SO at 0 °C, or 15% Me_2SO at -4 °C, Me_2SO having been washed out after storage by

Table 52.1 Me_2SO levels (% w/v) in kidney after perfusion (mean ± SD)

Perfusate	Cortex	Medulla	Whole kidney
Ringers–12.5% Me_2SO 800 ml	9.8 ± 0.8% (78%*)	10.2 ± 0.6% (81%*)	9.9 ± 0.8% (79%*)
Ringers–12.5% Me_2SO 400 ml	9.2 ± 0.7% (73%*)	9.5 ± 0.5% (76%*)	9.3 ± 0.6% (74%*)
Albumin–12.5% Me_2SO 400 ml	10.1 ± 0.8% (81%*)	7.8 ± 1.3% (62%*)	9.7 ± 1.8% (77%*)
Collins–12.5% Me_2SO 400 ml	9.3 ± 0.6% (74%*)	8.5 ± 0.8% (68%*)	9.4 ± 0.8% (75%*)

* Proportion of perfusate Me_2SO concentration

363

immersion in Collins' solution containing mannitol to serially reduce osmolality. The slice/medium (S/M) ratio of PAH uptake was then determined at 25 °C.

The *tissue levels* of Me_2SO after perfusion are shown in Table 52.1. Ringer's and Collins' solutions gave even distribution of Me_2SO throughout cortex and medulla, and the whole kidney level was not significantly greater after 800 ml than after 400 ml of perfusion. The medullary concentration after Me_2SO–albumin perfusion was significantly lower than the other groups.

Vascular resistance and weight increased gradually during infusion of Me_2SO, Collins' solution causing significantly higher resistance and weight gain than Ringer's solution. The additional 400 ml in group 1 caused a rapid gross increase in vascular resistance. The colloid solution gave minimal change in resistance, which was significantly lower after 400 ml than with the crystalloid solutions. Rapid washout caused dramatic increases in vascular resistance and weight during the first 200 ml, after which resistance fell but significant weight gains continued, Collins' being similar to Ringer's. In contrast, resistance fell with gradual washout, Collins' being more marked than Ringer's solution, with no change in resistance after the second (1500 mosmol) aliquot although some weight gain continued throughout washout in both groups. Vascular resistance and total weight gain were significantly lower with Collins' (group 8) than with Ringer's solution (group 4).

Function after Me_2SO perfusion washout is summarized in Table 52.2. Kidneys of non-survivors showed extensive cortical necrosis; serum creatinines in survivors were not significantly different. There were no deaths in the Collins' groups; serum creatinine in group 7 was significantly higher than in all other groups; group 8 was the most successful, with comparable results to C3 controls, in contrast to the corresponding Ringer's group (group 4).

Longer-term toxicity studies showed a progressive fall in PAH uptake with increased storage. S/M ratios fell to 30% of fresh tissue levels after 72 h in Collins' and Collins'–Me_2SO at 0 °C. However, storage at -4 °C gave S/M ratios at 50% of fresh tissue levels after 72 h. Ringer's–Me_2SO at

Table 52.2 Renal function after Me_2SO perfusion

Perfusate (+ 12.5% Me_2SO)	No.	Survivors	Maximum serum creatinine (mg/dl)*
1. Ringers–800 ml, no w/o	7	5	5.8 ± 4.9
2. Ringers–400 ml, no w/o	7	6	3.7 ± 1.7
3. Ringers–400 ml, rapid w/o	7	4	4.8 ± 1.1
4. Ringers–400 ml, slow w/o	7	0	–
5. Ringers control (400 ml)	7	7	3.3 ± 1.9
6. Collins–400 ml, no w/o	7	7	4.1 ± 2.1
7. Collins–400 ml, rapid w/o	7	7	7.8 ± 4.7
8. Collins–400 ml, slow w/o	8	8	2.6 ± 1.5
9. Collins control (400 ml)	7	7	3.1 ± 2.1

w/o = washout

* Mean ± SD

$-4\,°C$ gave significantly worse results. 15% Me$_2$SO led to 20% reduction in fresh tissue S/M ratios, but storage at both $-4\,°C$ and $-6\,°C$ was associated with slower reduction in viability (S/M ratio after $96\,h = 60\%$ of fresh tissue).

Supercooled storage of whole kidneys was attempted on the basis of these *in vitro* toxicity results. However, six kidneys autotransplanted after $48\,h$ storage at $-4\,°C$ in Collins' - 12.5% Me$_2$SO developed no-reflow and failed to function, with extensive cortical necrosis histologically.

In conclusion, gravity perfusion gave adequate tissue penetration by Me$_2$SO and rapid increase in Me$_2$SO concentration to at least 12.5% was possible. Slow washout minimized the effects on vascular resistance and renal function, an intracellular vector solution giving better perfusion and lower toxicity. However, supercooled storage of whole kidneys at $-4\,°C$ failed due to vascular damage: further study of the vascular effects of Me$_2$SO perfusion and washout is required.

53
Prevention of toxicity from high concentrations of cryoprotective agents*

G. M. FAHY

It has been previously reported that 40% w/v dimethyl sulphoxide (Me$_2$SO) is toxic to rabbit renal cortex, whereas 30% w/v Me$_2$SO is completely non-toxic (chapter 60). The toxicity of 40% Me$_2$SO is a barrier to preservation by the Farrant approach[1], by the high-pressure vitrification approach (chapter 60), and by freezing[2]. However, almost nothing is known about the mechanism of cryoprotectant toxicity or, more importantly, about methods for reducing or preventing this toxicity, especially if one excludes osmotically mediated so-called 'toxicity'.

One possible mechanism for Me$_2$SO toxicity in rat kidney cortex was reported by Baxter and Lathe in 1971[3]. They found that Me$_2$SO more or less specifically activated fructose diphosphatase, leading to a blockade of glycolysis. This activation took place at concentrations just over 30% and peaked at 40–50% Me$_2$SO. It was preventable by acetamide at 1 mol/mol of Me$_2$SO, by urea at 1 mol/4 mol of Me$_2$SO, by formamide at 1 mol/2 mol of Me$_2$SO, and by a pH of 10.65. I now report on a follow-up of some of these observations using rabbit renal cortical slices.

Cryoprotectants were introduced in the presence of Rδ solution, whose composition was given before (chapter 60), except that Ca^{2+} and Mg^{2+} were omitted to avoid variations caused by differing solubilities in the different solutions studied. All of the experiments were carried out at 0 °C. In the first experiment the introduction schedule was: 10% w/v cryoprotectant (CPA), 30 min; 20% CPA, 30 min; 30% CPA, 60 min, and 40% CPA, 40 min. In the second experiment, exposure to 20% CPA was for 60 min and exposure to 30% CPA for 30 min. In both experiments, CPA was removed in 5% steps, 20 min per step, all in the presence of 300 mmol/l mannitol.

The results of the first experiment are shown in Table 53.1. First it can be seen that the current protocol, in which exposure is at 0 °C, is much more

---

* Contribution No. 524 from the American National Red Cross, Blood Services Laboratories.

damaging than the usual subzero protocol (cf. groups A and N). This suggests that any improvements shown in Table 53.1 or 53.2 can be further improved by using subzero temperatures in future experiments. Elevating pH did not help very much. However, including either urea or acetamide in place of some of the Me_2SO resulted in a dramatic improvement in viability. Replacing half of the Me_2SO with propylene glycol (PG) also improved the results slightly, and if the Me_2SO concentration in this mixture was further reduced by replacement with either acetamide (AA) or ethylene glycol (EG), the results were improved further to equal the viability seen with the Me_2SO + urea and Me_2SO + AA groups. This is important because inclusion of PG improves the vitrifiability of solutions (chapter 60). A mixture of 20% EG and 20% PG was not significantly better than 20% Me_2SO + 20% PG. Groups E, I and J show the intense concentration dependence of the Me_2SO–PG mixture; the data for 15% Me_2SO + 15% PG were taken from other experiments (chapter 60). Group K shows, unfortunately, that 20% PG by itself is toxic. This is remarkable in view of the non-toxicity of 15% PG + 15% Me_2SO and suggests that using 15% PG rather than 20% PG might give much better results.

Table 53.1 Prevention of cryoprotectant toxicity: first experiment

Group	Cryoprotectant concentrations (% w/v)	n	K^+/Na^+ *	p	vs.
A	40% Me_2SO	7	1.16 ± 0.15	<0.001	L
B	40% Me_2SO, pH 8.8	6	1.45 ± 0.12	NS	A
C	33.55% Me_2SO + 6.45% U	6	2.78 ± 0.20	<0.001	A
D	22.8% Me_2SO + 17.2% AA	7	3.15 ± 0.35	<0.001	A
E	20% Me_2SO + 20% PG	6	2.02 ± 0.19	<0.01	A
F	11.4% Me_2SO + 8.6% AA + 20% PG	7	2.82 ± 0.23	<0.05	E
G	10% Me_2SO + 10% EG + 20% PG	7	2.79 ± 0.19	<0.05	E
H	20% EG + 20% PG	6	2.48 ± 0.17	<0.001	A
I	17.5% Me_2SO + 17.5% PG	7	3.57 ± 0.33	<0.01	E
J	15% Me_2SO + 15% PG (normal protocol)	5	5.60 ± 0.07	<0.001	I
K	20% PG	6	4.79 ± 0.30	<0.05	J&L
L	Control (no treatment)	7	5.71 ± 0.27	—	—
M	Control + mannitol exposure	6	5.07 ± 0.22	NS	L
N	40% Me_2SO, normal (subzero) protocol	5	2.55 ± 0.14	<0.001	A

Me_2SO = dimethyl sulphoxide; U = urea; AA = acetamide; PG = propylene glycol; EG = ethylene glycol
* K^+/N^+ ratio measured after removal of CPA and 90 min active metabolism at 25 °C

The second experiment is shown in Table 53.2. The results were generally much better than those in Table 53.1 and may be due to the reduced exposure to 30% CPA. Group D even fails to differ significantly from control. The purpose of groups A–F was to find out if adding more AA or urea, or adding both in combination, would help. With the possible exception of group D, extra urea, the viability is the same in all of these groups. Unfortunately, the group D solution is hard to vitrify! The group E solution, however, may vitrify more easily than the group A solution, which is the present standard. Adding 15% PG led to worse results (groups G–I). The next four groups (J–M) appear to show that mutual dilution of CPAs does not help.

Table 53.2 Prevention of cryoprotectant toxicity: second experiment

Group	Cryoprotectant concentrations (% w/v)	n	K^+/Na^+ *	p	vs.
A	22.8% Me$_2$SO + 17.2% AA	5	4.10 ± 0.37	<0.03	N
B	20% Me$_2$SO + 20% AA	5	3.89 ± 0.18	NS	A
C	33.55% Me$_2$SO + 6.45% U	7	3.59 ± 0.24	NS	A
D	30% Me$_2$SO + 10% U	4	4.36 ± 0.46	NS	C&N
E	28.17% Me$_2$SO + 8.6% AA + 3.23% U	7	3.80 ± 0.23	NS	A&C
F	25% Me$_2$SO + 10% AA + 5%U	7	3.87 ± 0.15	NS	B&D
G	15% PG + 15.63% Me$_2$SO + 6.25% AA + 3.12% U	6	3.33 ± 0.09	<0.02	F
H	15% PG + 12.5% Me$_2$SO + 12.5% EG	7	3.20 ± 0.15	NS	G&I
I	15% PG + 8.55% Me$_2$SO + 6.45% AA + 10% EG	6	3.37 ± 0.10	NS	G&H
J	13.3% Me$_2$SO + 13.3% AA + 13.4% PG	7	3.27 ± 0.13	<0.02	B
K	13.3% Me$_2$SO + 13.3% EG + 13.4% PG	6	3.26 ± 0.12	NS	J
L	10% Me$_2$SO + 10% AA + 10% PG + 10% EG	6	3.28 ± 0.20	NS	J&K
M	8% M$_2$SO + 8% AA + 8% PG + 8% EG + 8% glycerol	6	3.59 ± 0.08	NS	J,K,&L
N	Control (no treatment)	5	5.16 ± 0.25	-	-

Me$_2$SO = dimethyl sulphoxide,   AA = acetamide,   U = urea;   PG = propylene glycol; EG = ethylene glycol
* K^+/Na^+ ratio measured after removal of CPA and 90 min active metabolism at 25 °C

These results suggest that CPA toxicity at a total concentration of 40% w/v can be prevented.

References

1. Farrant, J. (1965). Mechanism of cell damage during freezing and thawing and its prevention. *Nature (Lond.), 205,* 1284
2. Fahy, G. M. (1980). Analysis of 'solution effects' injury: rabbit renal cortex frozen in the presence of dimethyl sulfoxide. *Cryobiology, 17,* 371
3. Baxter, S. J. and Lathe, G. H. (1971). Biochemical effects on kidney of exposure to high concentrations of dimethyl sulphoxide. *Biochem. Pharmacol., 20,* 1079

54
Kidney preservation with Me₂SO- and sucrose-containing solutions

R. GRUNDMANN and K. KÜRTEN

The main principle of all preservation methods used in the clinical situation today is that kidney metabolism can be reduced by hypothermia. Therefore, kidneys are normally stored at $+2$ to $+4\,°C^1$. Lower temperatures are not used because of the fear of freezing and, therefore, of damaging the organ. In the experiments presented here we tried to improve the preservation results by a further reduction of metabolism at subzero temperatures. In doing so, freezing of the organ was prevented by the application of two different principles: in one part of the experiments the osmolality of the flush solution was increased by adding sucrose and in the other the penetrating cryoprotectant Me_2SO^2 was used. In detail, the following questions were investigated:

(1) The osmolality of the Euro-Collins flush solution was increased to 770 mosmol/kg by adding sucrose. It was then determined whether freezing of the kidneys at $-2\,°C$ was prevented and how kidneys stored at this temperature functioned after transplantation.

(2) As it was not clear whether the use of a strongly hyperosmolar perfusate would impair function after transplantation, the use of this perfusate at $+4\,°C$ was examined in a control group.

(3) Finally, the function of kidneys stored in Euro-Collins solution containing various concentrations of Me_2SO was measured after storage at $+4\,°C$ and at $-2\,°C$.

Bilateral nephrectomy was performed in mongrel dogs weighing 20–25 kg. After nephrectomy the kidneys were flushed at $+4\,°C$ with the solution in question and then stored for 12–24 h in this solution at $+4\,°C$ or $-2\,°C$. During storage, the temperature was recorded continuously with needle probes and was also about $+4\,°C$ or $-2\,°C$ in the medulla of the kidney. After storage, the kidneys were transplanted to the neck vessels of a recipient animal and function was followed for 6 h after transplantation by PAH and inulin clearances.

A perfusate osmolality of 770 mosmol/kg was found to prevent the

Table 54.1 PAH and inulin clearances (ml/min/100 g kidney weight) after transplantation

| Temperature | Clearance | Euro-Collins | | Hyperosmolar perfusate | | Me₂SO solution | | |
		12 h	24 h	12 h	24 h	0.5 mmol/l 12 h	1.0 mol/l 12 h	1.5 mol/l 12 h
+4°C	PAH	50.2 ± 14.9 (n=6)	14.2 ± 9.3 (n=6)	–	9.08 ± 8.16 (n=8)	72.7 ± 16.61 (n=6)	32.39 ± 25.91 (n=6)	11.83 ± 4.26 (n=6)
	Inulin	8.3 ± 3.6 (n=6)	2.9 ± 2.0 (n=6)	–	3.03 ± 2.33 (n=8)	23.32 ± 4.28 (n=6)	13.74 ± 9.7 (n=6)	2.67 ± 0.67 (n=6)
−2°C	PAH			50.1 ± 21.1 (n=8)	35.9 ± 19.4 (n=6)	16.67 ± 12.53 (n=6)	11.35 ± 9.2 (n=6)	7.69 ± 6.36 (n=6)
	Inulin			13.4 ± 5.5 (n=8)	9.8 ± 5.3 (n=6)	5.14 ± 3.80 (n=6)	3.14 ± 2.32 (n=6)	2.27 ± 1.92 (n=6)

Table 54.2 Composition of the preservation solutions

| | Euro-Collins | Hyperosmolar sucrose perfusate | Me₂SO Euro-Collins solution | | |
			0.5 mmol/l Me₂SO	1.0 mmol/l Me₂SO	1.5 mmol/l Me₂SO
Na⁺ (mmol/l)	10	9	9.64	9.38	8.92
K⁺ (mmol/l)	115	104	110.86	106.72	102.58
Osmolality (mosmol/kg)	375	770	920	1540	2080
Glucose (mmol/l)	194.2	194.2	187.0	180.4	173.1
Sucrose (mmol/l)	–	350.6	–	–	–

kidney freezing at $-2\,°C$. Our results (Table 54.1) did not demonstrate the maximum perfusate osmolality that kidneys can tolerate, but it can be concluded that an osmolality of 770 mosmol/kg was harmless, since kidneys stored in the sucrose perfusate at $+4\,°C$ showed nearly the same function as kidneys stored in Collins' solution. Table 54.1 also demonstrates that kidneys can be stored successfully for at least 24 h at $-2\,°C$ in the sucrose perfusate: the immediate function after transplantation was significantly better than that of kidneys stored for the same period in Collins' solution at $+4\,°C$. Since the same results were obtained by storing kidneys at $+4\,°C$ in the hyperosmolar solution as in Collins' solution, the improvement of kidney function at $-2\,°C$ is due only to the fact that this group of kidneys was stored at a subzero temperature.

In kidneys stored in Me$_2$SO solution at $-2\,°C$, function was reduced compared to the control group, even after 12 h of preservation. The decline of kidney function depended on the concentration of Me$_2$SO: this is even more obvious with kidneys stored at $+4\,°C$. This result cannot be explained by the temperature used, since kidneys stored in the sucrose perfusate at $-2\,°C$ functioned better than, or at least as well as, those in the control group. Nevertheless, kidney function after 12 h storage in the three different concentrations of Me$_2$SO was always better when the kidneys were stored at $+4\,°C$ than at $-2\,°C$.

It must be assumed on the basis of these results that the application of Me$_2$SO resulted in kidney injury[3]. One mechanism could be the increase of intracellular osmolality, in our experiments from 630 to 1100 mosmol/kg (Figure 54.1). In addition, a toxic effect of Me$_2$SO on the renal metabolism is suggested by oxygen consumption measurements made immediately after kidney storage. (To make these measurements, the kidneys were flushed

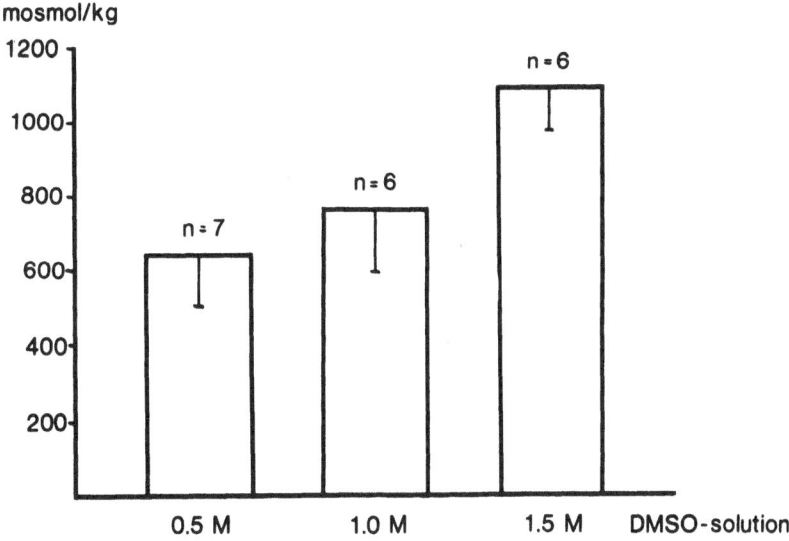

Figure 54.1 Intracellular osmolality after 12 h of preservation at $+4\,°C$

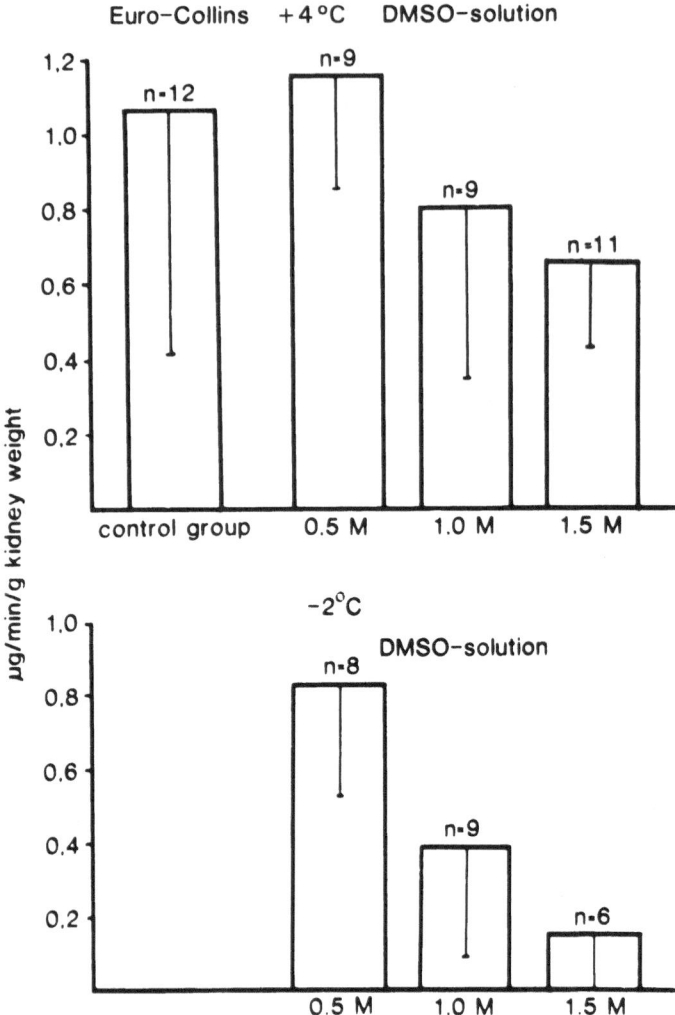

Figure 54.2 Oxygen consumption measured immediately after 12h of storage

with 100 ml of Euro-Collins solution at +4 °C, and the arteriovenous oxygen difference and the renal flow rate were recorded. The renal temperature during flushing was similar in the −2 °C group and the +4 °C group, since both groups were flushed with Euro-Collins solution at +4 °C.) We found that the oxygen consumption of kidneys stored in 0.5 molar Me$_2$SO at +4 °C did not differ from the control group (Figure 54.2), but at −2 °C the oxygen consumption was reduced. At both +4 °C and −2 °C a reduction of the renal oxygen consumption was found which depended on the Me$_2$SO concentration in the storage solution, but it was more marked at −2 °C. It appears that Me$_2$SO blocks renal metabolism, and harms the kidneys in doing so.

In conclusion, successful kidney storage for 24 h is possible at $-2\,°C$ using a hyperosmolar sucrose perfusate, but kidneys stored in Me₂SO solutions do not function as well.

References

1. Collins, G. M., Bravo-Shugarman, M. and Terasaki, P. I. (1969). Kidney preservation for transportation. Initial perfusion and 30 hours' ice storage. *Lancet,* **2,** 1219
2. Karow, A. M. (1979). Cryoprotectants in oxygen perfusion. In Pegg, D. E. and Jacobsen, I. A. (eds.) *Organ Preservation II,* pp. 147–158. (Edinburgh: Churchill Livingstone)
3. Fahy, G. M. (1980). Analysis of 'solution effects' injury: rabbit renal cortex frozen in the presence of dimethyl sulphoxide. *Cryobiology,* **17,** 371

55
Investigation into subzero non-freezing storage of rabbit kidney

D. R. OSBORNE, B. J. FULLER, G. R. ATKINS, V. D. ATTENBURROW,
L. H. NUTT and K. E. F. HOBBS

Successful long-term storage of kidneys at subzero temperatures in the frozen state has never been consistently achieved. An alternative to freezing is the use of high concentrations of penetrating solute to depress the freezing point of tissues[1], but with whole organs there is little information on the benefit, if any, of this approach[2]. In our studies the solute investigated was methanol, which we have found to be rapidly penetrating and non-toxic to mammalian cells under controlled conditions[3].

METHODS

Male albino New Zealand white rabbits (2–4 kg) were used as kidney donors. The animals were sedated (0.4 ml of Hypnorm (Jansen Ltd) given intravenously). Anaesthesia was induced by intravenous infusion of a mixture of Ketamine hydrochloride (Parke Davis Ltd) and zilazine (Bayer Ltd) followed by heparin and mannitol. Through a midline incision bilateral nephrectomy was performed and both renal arteries cannulated immediately (as previously described[4]) before flushing with cold Haemaccel (Hoechst Ltd). The organs were then weighed and either stored in ice or taken to the perfusion apparatus. The apparatus consisted of a programmed liquid nitrogen cooling unit similar to that already described[5]. The programme was set to give a slow cooling rate of 0.4 °C/min and a rewarming rate of approximately 1 °C/min. The perfusion pressure was kept constant at 50 ± 5 mmHg and the whole apparatus controlled and parameters recorded with a computer. The basic perfusate consisted of human serum albumin (HSA) at a concentration of 3 g/l and containing (mmol/l) Na+ 130, K+ 5, Mg2+ 1, Cl− 136, HEPES buffer 10, glucose 5; pH 7.4 at 20 °C.

Kidneys were investigated after:
(A) perfusion with HSA for 3 h at +7 °C;

Table 55.1 Measurements of tissue water content, tissue K^+/Na^+ ratios and perfusate flow rates (for perfused groups only) in kidneys after various storage regimes

	A HSA perfusion (n=5)	B HSA perfusion + 3 molar methanol (n=5)	C Storage at −5°C for 48 h (n=5)	D Ice storage (3 h) (n=10)	E Ice storage (48 h) (n=5)
Tissue water content (g H_2O/g)	3.2 ± 0.5	3.5 ± 0.6	5.6 ± 0.6	2.7 ± 0.8	4.9 ± 1.0
K^+/Na^+ ratio	1.0 ± 0.3	0.6 ± 0.1	0.3 ± 0.1	0.7 ± 0.2	0.3 ± 0.1
Perfusate flows (ml/min/g):					
Initial	1.53 ± 0.04	0.60 ± 0.20	0.63 ± 0.18	—	—
Final	2.26 ± 0.46	0.75 ± 0.30	0.19 ± 0.04	—	—

378

(B) perfusion with HSA plus 3 molar methanol initially at $+7\,°C$ (cooling to $-5\,°C$ and returning to $+7\,°C$ to remove the methanol) (total time 3 h);

(C) perfusion as for group B but with 48 h storage at $-5\,°C$ before returning to perfusion for rewarming and removal of methanol at $+7\,°C$;

(D) storage in ice for 3 h;

(E) storage in ice for 48 h.

After each preservation protocol, one pole of the kidney was freeze-clamped and tissue adenine nucleotides were measured as described previously[4]. Cortical slices, 0.3 mm thick, were prepared for estimation of *para*-aminohippuric acid (PAH) uptake[6]. Samples were also taken for measurement of tissue water, Na^+ and K^+ contents[4].

RESULTS AND DISCUSSION

The values for tissue water content and K^+/Na^+ ratio for each of the groups A to E and the initial and final flow rates for the perfused groups A, B and C can be seen in Table 55.1.

Perfusion with 3 molar methanol resulted in an increased vascular resistance (reduced flow) and some drop in tissue K^+ when compared with HSA perfusion alone. Storage for 48 h at $-5\,°C$ with 3 molar methanol resulted in an increased tissue water content and further K^+ loss. A similar picture was obtained with the 48 h ice-stored group.

The metabolic assessments can be seen in Table 55.2. The kidneys perfused with HSA alone showed the highest TAN, whilst groups perfused with 3 molar methanol (B) and 3 h ice-stored (D) exhibited similar levels. The ratio of the multiphosphorylated nucleotides in the TAN (energy charge) was similar in groups A, B and D. Accumulation of PAH was slightly reduced after perfusion with 3 molar methanol (B) when compared with HSA alone (A), and 3 h ice-storage (D) resulted in a further drop in activity. After 48 h in ice (E) there was a large drop in PAH uptake and in energy charge, whilst storage at $-5\,°C$ resulted in a higher energy charge and significantly improved PAH uptake ($p = 0.001$).

Our results suggest that there is some metabolic protection to be gained by use of protocol C in which kidneys were taken to $-5\,°C$ with 3 molar methanol for 48 h and subsequently reperfused, when compared to 48 h ice

Table 55.2 Values for tissue total adenine nucleotide content (TAN), energy charge $((ATP + \frac{1}{2}ADP)/TAN)$ and PAH uptake in kidney tissues after storage

	A	B	C	D	E
TAN (μmol/g)	11.5 ± 3.1	5.4 ± 2.1	5.7 ± 0.8	5.0 ± 2.9	4.5 ± 0.8
Energy charge	0.7 ± 0.4	0.7 ± 0.1	0.4 ± 0.1	0.7 ± 0.1	0.3 ± 0.1
PAH uptake (slice/medium ratio)	16.2 ± 2.2	13.0 ± 2.6	8.6 ± 2.5	10.2 ± 2.6	3.7 ± 2.0

storage. However there were obviously problems with oedema formation and ion disbalance inherent in this procedure. We have used a simple perfusate for these initial studies and it remains to be seen whether alterations in ion balance, pH and non-penetrating solutes, e.g. mannitol, will result in control of these harmful effects.

Acknowledgement

We gratefully acknowledge the support of the National Kidney Research Fund award to B. J. F.

References

1. Farrant, J. (1965). Mechanism of cell damage during freezing and thawing and its prevention. *Nature (Lond.)*, **205**, 1284
2. Jacobsen, I. A., Kemp, E. and Starklint, H. (1975). Glycerol as a cryoprotectant in subzero preservation of rabbit kidneys. *Cryobiology*, **12**, 123
3. Fuller, B. J., Morris, G. J., Nutt, L. H. *et al.* (1980). Functional recovery of isolated rat hepatocytes upon thawing from − 196 °C. *Cryoletters*, **1**, 139
4. Fuller, B. J., Pegg, D. E., Walter, C. A. *et al.* (1977). An isolated rabbit kidney preparation for use in organ preservation research. *J. Surg. Res.*, **22**, 128
5. Ellis, M. J., Davies, P. W. and Hobbs, K. E. F. (1974). A programmed cooling unit for experimental organ preservation. *Cryobiology*, **11**, 100
6. Cross, R. J. and Taggart, J. V. (1950). Renal tubular transport: accumulation of para-aminohippurate by rabbit kidney slices. *Am. J. Physiol.*, **161**, 181

56
Survival of hepatocytes upon thawing from −196 °C: functional assessment after transplantation

B. J. FULLER, R. J. WOODS, L. H. NUTT and V. D. ATTENBURROW

Increasing experimental evidence suggests that transplantation of isolated hepatocytes might afford a method for treatment of liver insufficiency and correction of some congenital enzyme deficiency diseases[1,2]. The technique has been attempted clinically, although information is scant[2]. Since any clinical application of the method would require large numbers of viable cells at short notice we have investigated methods for cryopreservation of mature isolated rat hepatocytes. We have developed an ectopic autotransplantation model to investigate extended cell survival after cryopreservation because mature hepatocytes exhibit rapid functional deterioration when maintained in culture.

METHODS

Uptake of [99Tc]HIDA (N-[N-(2,6-dimethyl phenyl) carbamoylmethyl] iminodiacetic acid) by hepatocytes

Hepatocytes for HIDA uptake studies were prepared by collagenase perfusion of the liver[3]. [99Tc]HIDA is an agent used clinically for visualizing the biliary tract. It is avidly taken up by hepatocytes *in vivo* and secreted into the bile. The present studies were undertaken to confirm that isolated hepatocytes retained the ability to accumulate the agent. [99Tc]HIDA was generated from reagents supplied by the Radiochemical Centre Ltd. 0.16μCi was added to 5 ml suspensions of hepatocytes (10×10^6 cells) in Leibovitz L15 medium (Gibco Ltd). After 15 min incubation the cells in $6 \times 200 \mu$l samples were separated from the medium by centrifugation through silicone oil[4]. Uptake of [99Tc]HIDA was measured by gamma radiospectrometry and was expressed in nmol/10^6 cells. The measurement was performed on cells incubated at 37 °C, at 0 °C and at 37 °C after plunging to −196 °C.

Preparation of autografts

Male albino Sprague–Dawley rats were anaesthetized with ether, a 70% hepatectomy was performed, and the incision closed. Isolated hepatocytes were prepared from the liver segments by sequential incubation in collagenase solutions. Cells were harvested and purified by centrifugal washes[3]. An average of 15×10^6 live cells were obtained, and reimplanted, suspended in L15 medium, by injection into the splenic pulp of the re-anaesthetized donor. Autografts were produced with cells either (i) freshly-harvested; (ii) plunged directly to $-196\,°C$ and there maintained for $> 2\,h$; (iii) equilibrated with 1.5 molar dimethyl sulphoxide (Me_2SO) before cooling at $2\,°C/min$ as described previously[3] and maintained at $-196\,°C$ for $> 2\,h$ before rapid thawing.

Uptake of [99Tc]HIDA by spleens

An infusion of $2.5\,\mu Ci$ of HIDA was given via the tail veins of rats under ether anaesthesia during 10 min. The spleens were removed after 45 min, along with blood samples, and HIDA was estimated as described above. The results were expressed as (CPM/g spleen) ÷ (CPM/ml blood).

Histology

Samples of spleens were fixed in 10% v/v formol saline and prepared sections were stained (a) by the periodic acid–Schiff method, and (b) with haematoxylin and eosin.

RESULTS AND DISCUSSION

Isolated liver cells were seen to retain the ability to take up HIDA, and this activity was related to the metabolic capacity of the cells. Incubation of cells at 37 °C for 15 min resulted in 0.92 ± 0.27 nmol being accumulated per 10^6 cells ($n=5$), whereas incubation at 0 °C resulted in only 0.08 ± 0.07 nmol being taken up ($n=5$). Cells damaged by plunging to $-196\,°C$ before incubation at 37 °C similarly showed depressed uptake of HIDA (0.17 ± 0.10 nmol/10^6 cells; $n=5$).

Table 56.1 shows the results for the uptake of [99Tc]HIDA by spleens. It

Table 56.1 Uptake of [99Tc]HIDA by spleens expressed as spleen/blood ratio (means ± SD for groups > 6 weeks after transplantation)

A Control, non- transplanted	B Transplanted with cells plunged to $-196\,°C$	C Transplanted with cells cooled at $2\,°C/min$ in Me_2SO	D Transplanted with fresh cells
0.26 ± 0.04 ($n=7$)	0.30 ± 0.01 ($n=4$)	0.59 ± 0.15 ($n=5$)	1.35 ± 0.90 ($n=7$)

can be seen that in control, non-transplanted animals (A) and in transplants performed with lethally frozen cells (B), the spleen/blood ratios were low.

Autografts prepared with fresh cells showed a significantly increased uptake of HIDA when compared with controls (A) or grafts prepared with lethally frozen cells (B) ($p < 0.01$ in each case). Transplants performed using cells cooled at $2\,°C/min$ in 1.5 molar Me_2SO also showed increased splenic uptake ($p < 0.01$ compared with groups A and B), but significantly less than for fresh-cell autografts (D).

The HIDA uptake correlated well with the histological appearance of the spleen. In group D there were areas of large, liver-like cells, many of which were binucleate. These cells were not present in controls (A) or grafts made with lethally frozen cells (B). Spleens transplanted with cells cooled at $2\,°C/min$ (C) showed small patches of cells, but not as numerous as seen in group D.

The splenic autograft model provides a method for locating and assessing hepatocytes many months after transplantation. The hepatocytes appear to maintain the structure and at least some functions attributed to liver cells. The model has allowed us for the first time to demonstrate that at least some of the original population of hepatocytes can be recovered in a functionally viable state after cryopreservation procedures. Sekiguchi et al.[5] did report some histological evidence of survival of cryopreserved liver cells, again using Me_2SO as protectant, in an isograft model but no functional estimations were recorded. We have not been able to establish splenic isografts of hepatocytes, presumably because of rejection even between inbred animals. We feel that splenic autografting of hepatocytes should provide us with an additional tool to investigate the value of different cryopreservation protocols.

Acknowledgements

This work was supported by a grant awarded to B. J. F. from the Special Trustees Endowment Fund of the Royal Free Hospital. We thank Professor K. E. F. Hobbs for advice and guidance during the studies. We are also grateful to Miss C. Tolchard for the typing of this paper.

References

1. Groth., C. G., Arborgh, B., Bjorken C. et al. (1977). Correction of hyperbilirubinemia in the glucoronyl transferase deficient rat by intraperitoneal hepatocyte transplantation. Transplant. Proc., 9, 313
2. Makovka, L., Rotstein, L., Falk, R. et al. (1980). Reversal of toxic and anoxic induced failure by syngeneic, allogeneic and xenogeneic hepatocyte transplantation. Surgery, 88, 244
3. Fuller, B. J., Morris G. J., Nutt L. H. et al. (1980). Functional recovery of isolated rat hepatocytes upon thawing from −196 °C. Cryoletters, 1, 139
4. Baur, H., Kasperek, S. and Pfaff, E. (1975). Criteria of viability of isolated liver cells. Hoppe-Seyler's Z. Physiol. Chem., 356, 827
5. Sekiguchi, S., Kusano, M., Onishi, T. et al. (1978). Cryogenic preservation of isolated hepatocytes in rat. Cryobiology, 15, 724

57
The effect of cryoprotectant concentration on freezing damage in kidney slices*

G. M. FAHY

Cryopreservation of organs will probably require the use of very high concentrations of cryoprotective agents. Unfortunately, there are many indications that cryoprotection is 'sub-colligative' when high cryoprotectant (CPA) concentrations are used, i.e., that as the amount of CPA increases prior to freezing, the amount of freezing tolerated by the system decreases[1-4]. It has been contended that this may represent intrinsic CPA toxicity occurring during freezing[2]. The present results supply more information on this possibility.

Two experiments have been done. In the first, Me_2SO was studied and in the second glycerol was studied. If Me_2SO toxicity is the main cause of freezing injury in Me_2SO-treated kidney slices, then pretreatment with higher concentrations of Me_2SO should have no effect on the injury observed after thawing from a particular temperature, since the Me_2SO concentration at this temperature will be about the same regardless of its concentration prior to freezing. If other factors are significant, then doubling the Me_2SO concentration prior to freezing should dramatically improve recovery. In the case of glycerol, I have tried to find the critical temperature at which freezing injury becomes statistically significant as a function of pre-freeze glycerol concentration. If there is no injury attributable to glycerol, this critical temperature, T_k, should be diagnostic of the mechanism of freezing injury, i.e., it should correlate with the unfrozen fraction of the solution[5], the water content of the solution, etc. Failure to conform to any such prediction would be evidence for cryoprotectant-associated injury.

Slices treated with Me_2SO were prepared and frozen in a base solution of RPS-2 (expressed in mmol/l: dextrose 180; K_2HPO_4 7.2; $NaHCO_3$ 10; reduced glutathione 5; adenine 1; $MgCl_2$ 2; $CaCl_2$ 1, and KCl 28.3; pH = 7.4). Glycerol-treated slices were handled in the presence of either

* Contribution No. 525 from the American National Red Cross, Blood Services Laboratories.

BP-4 (mmol/l: dextrose 5; sodium acetate 10; mannitol 40; NaCl 50; KCl 20; $MgCl_2$ 30; $CaCl_2$ 1, and bovine serum albumin 3% w/v; pH = 7.4) or Rδ solution (chapter 60).

Slices were treated with 15, 20 or 30% Me_2SO for 60 min prior to freezing, except for one 15% group which was treated for 90 min to rule out incomplete permeation prior to freezing. Another 15% group was placed first in 7.5% Me_2SO for 30 min prior to the hour in 15% Me_2SO to rule out pre-freezing osmotic stress which might increase the sensitivity to freezing. Slices treated with 20% Me_2SO or with 20% followed by 30% Me_2SO were placed initially in 10% Me_2SO for 30 min to prevent osmotic stress upon transfer to 20% CPA. CPA removal was done in the presence of 640 mmol/l mannitol as described elsewhere[2]. Treatment with 30% Me_2SO was at $-8\,°C$ and treatment with the other concentrations was at $0\,°C$. The cooling rate used was $1.06 \pm 0.11\,°C/min$ (mean ± SD), and thawing was rapid[2].

Figure 57.1 shows that slices frozen with 15% Me_2SO were injured equally regardless of gradual addition (grad) or 90 min exposure prior to freezing. Slices frozen with 20% or 30% Me_2SO were less injured, but not much less injured, and recoveries for these concentrations were identical. These results suggest that some salt-mediated injury may exist when freezing with 15% Me_2SO, and that removing this injury may allow some recovery from $-50\,°C$, but that most of the injury is still due to Me_2SO toxicity.

Treatment with glycerol was done at a concentration of 300 mmol/l, using 10 min increments (30 mmol/l/min) at $10\,°C$. Removal of glycerol was done the same way, but in the presence of 300 millimolar mannitol. Freezing was at either $< 0.3\,°C/min$ or at $1\,°C/min$, it was done either in

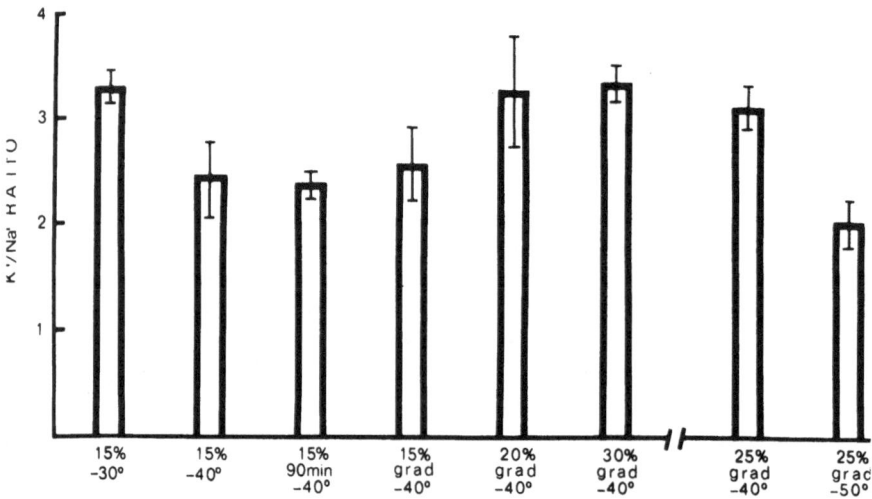

Figure 57.1. Effect of freezing treatment on the ability of rabbit kidney tissue to establish a high K^+/Na^+ ratio after thawing. For details, see text. 'grad' indicates gradual addition of the cryoprotectant. Two bars on the right were from an independent set of experiments

BP-4, Rδ, or 0.95% NaCl base, and thawing was either slow (< 0.5 °C/min) or rapid. The results are shown in Figure 57.2 and do not conform to any reasonable prediction of freezing injury. Unfortunately, the results are equivocal because there was some injury in non-frozen slices treated with 3 molar glycerol, but the lack of dependence of the results on the various treatments and on the degree of injury to the 3 molar controls indicates that the trend in freezing injury is probably meaningful.

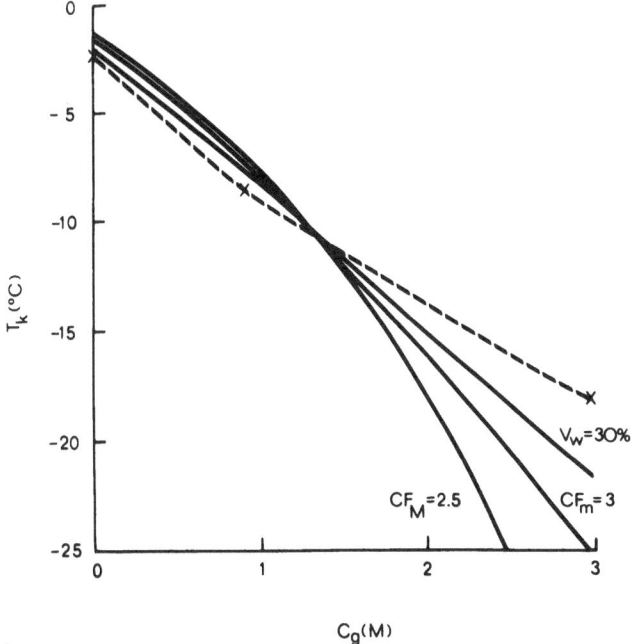

Figure 57.2. Effect of prefreeze glycerol concentration (C_g) on the temperature at which freezing injury becomes statistically significant (T_k) (indicated by x's on the dashed line). The solid curves are theoretical predictions of lethal temperature based on water content reaching 30% of physiologic ($V_w = 30\%$), on the molarity rising by 2.5 times ($CF_M = 2.5$), or on the molality rising by 3 times ($CF_m = 3.0$). The experimental results do not conform to any such theoretical prediction

Cryoprotectants therefore may help to cause freezing injury. Perhaps abolishing toxicity from cryoprotectants will prevent this.

References

1. Fahy, G. M. and Karow, A. M., Jr (1977). Ultrastructure-function correlative studies for cardiac cryopreservation. V. Absence of a correlation between electrolyte toxicity and cryoinjury in the slowly-frozen, cryoprotected rat heart. *Cryobiology*, **14**, 418
2. Fahy, G. M. (1980). Analysis of 'solution effects' injury: rabbit renal cortex frozen in the presence of dimethyl sulphoxide. *Cryobiology*, **17**, 371
3. Rall, W. F., Mazur, P. and Souzu, H. (1978). Physical–chemical basis of the protection of slowly frozen human red cells by glycerol. *Biophys. J.*, **23**, 101

4. Kahn, R. A. (1978). Biochemical changes in frozen platelets. In Greenwalt, T. J. and Jamieson, G. A. (eds.) *The Blood Platelet in Transfusion Therapy,* pp. 167–180. (New York: Alan R. Liss)
5. Mazur, P., Rigopoulos, N. and Weiss, R. (1979). Role of solute composition and concentration *vs.* channel size on slow-freezing injury in human red cells. II Survival *vs.* phase relations. *Cryobiology,* **16,** 587

58
The mechanism of cryoinjury in glycerol-treated rabbit kidneys

D. E. PEGG and M. P. DIAPER

We have previously shown that rabbit kidneys can be equilibrated with 3 molar glycerol at 10 °C, and that after removal of the cryoprotectant they retain sufficient function to support life, and eventually to recover normal creatinine clearances[1]. This result required the slow introduction and removal of glycerol (30 mmol/l/min), and mannitol (111 mmol/l) was present to act as an osmotic buffer. However, Jacobsen, using a similar technique to introduce and remove glycerol, found that such kidneys would not function after cooling at 0.3 °C/min to −80 °C, holding at that temperature for 30 min and rewarming at the same rate: they had a high vascular resistance during deglycerolization, became cyanosed on transplantation, and exhibited interstitial bleeding but no function[2]. Retarding the process of deglycerolization further, or increasing the maximum glycerol concentration, was without avail: even cooling to − 5 °C for 50 min, without freezing, produced damaged kidneys, and storage at this temperature for 120 h gave no post-transplant survivors. These results show that rabbit kidneys glycerolized to 3 or 5 mol/l will not tolerate freezing and thawing under these conditions, and they also suggest that even cooling alone, to − 5 °C, may be damaging. The experiments to be reported here were designed to determine the relative importance of cooling, freezing and solute concentration in this system.

The subject of this study was the kidney, excised with minimal warm ischaemia, from anaesthetized New Zealand White rabbits. Each kidney was flushed with cold WF6 solution at 60 mmHg as previously described[3] and then perfused at 10 °C and 40 mmHg with HP5 perfusate, which contains 1.75 % Haemaccel (Hoechst) and 111 mmol/l mannitol[1]. A 3 molar solution of glycerol in this perfusate has a freezing point of − 8 °C while 6 molar glycerol freezes at − 26 °C. The four experimental groups, each consisting of three to five animals, were designed as follows:

Group 1. Cooling only

Kidneys were glycerolized at 30 mmol/l/min to 3 mol/l, cooled at

0.25 °C/min to -7 °C (1 °C above the freezing point of that solution), were perfused at that temperature for 3 h 30 min, rewarmed at the same rate to $+10$ °C, and deglycerolized as previously described[4].

Group 2. Cooling with solute concentration

Kidneys were glycerolized and cooled to -7 °C as in group 1, but cooling was continued to -25 °C while perfusing continually with a solution of increasing glycerol and salt concentration such that the increase in solute concentration was the same as that produced by freezing the 3 molar glycerol perfusate to -26 °C (i.e. 6 mol/l glycerol and $2 \times$ salts) this was achieved by a time-proportioning gradient mixing apparatus. Kidneys were held at -25 °C for 1 h, and the process then reversed, returning them to 3 molar glycerol at -7 °C and then warming to $+10$ °C at 0.25 °C/min, and deglycerolizing as before.

Group 3. Freezing with glycerol

Kidneys were glycerolized and cooled to -7 °C as in group 1, but cooling was continued to -25 °C without further perfusion. They froze. After 1 h at -25 °C they were rewarmed to $+10$ °C at 0.25 °C/min, and deglycerolized as before.

Group 4. Freezing without glycerol

This group was flushed with WF6 as were the other groups, then perfused with 100 ml of HP5 at 10 °C. They were then cooled to -2 °C in a -15 °C bath, seeded with ice and transferred to a -1.5 °C bath for 1 h. They were finally rewarmed to $+10$ °C and reperfused with HP5 for 15 min.

The total time below $+10$ °C was kept constant at 5 h 40 min in groups 1–3 inclusive. Group 4 provided the same concentration factor for salts as groups 2 and 3 ($\times 2$), and the same time of exposure to these concentrations. Controls consisted of six freshly isolated rabbit kidneys and eight kidneys subjected to the same glycerolization and deglycerolization at $+10$ °C, but without additional cooling. In each case function was measured by the normothermic perfusion assay already described[5] using inulin clearance (C_{IN}) para-aminohippurate clearance (C_{PAH}), fractional albumin leakage ($C_{ALB}/C_{IN} \times 100\%$) and the tubular reabsorption of glucose (T_{GLU}) and sodium (T_{Na}) to indicate function. The results are shown in Figures 58.1–58.4.

Figure 58.1 shows the absolute values of the measured functions in freshly isolated kidneys, and the corresponding values in perfused control kidneys as a percentage of these values (except for protein leakage which is shown as percentage leaking into the urine).

Figure 58.2 shows that cooling, whether to -7 °C without solute concen-

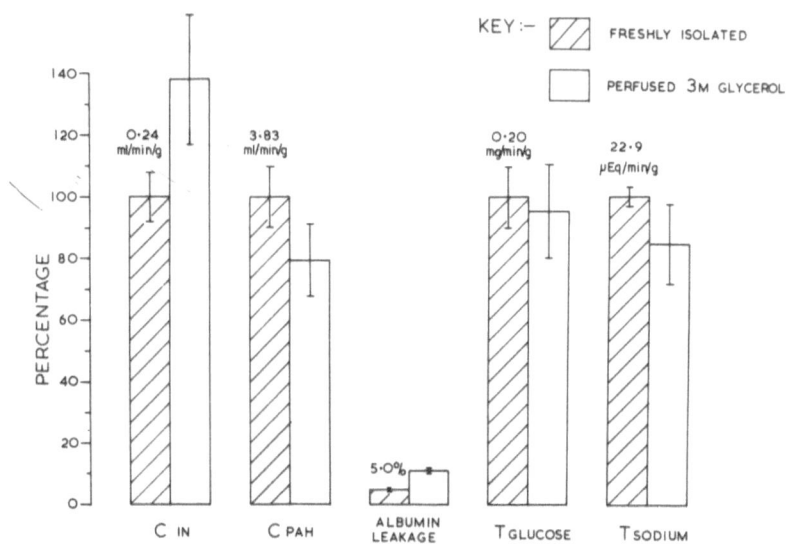

Figure 58.1 Inulin clearance (C IN, PAH clearance (C PAH), albumin leakage, tubular glucose transport (T GLUCOSE) and tubular sodium transport (T SODIUM) in freshly isolated kidneys, and kidneys that had been glycerolized and deglycerolized as previously described

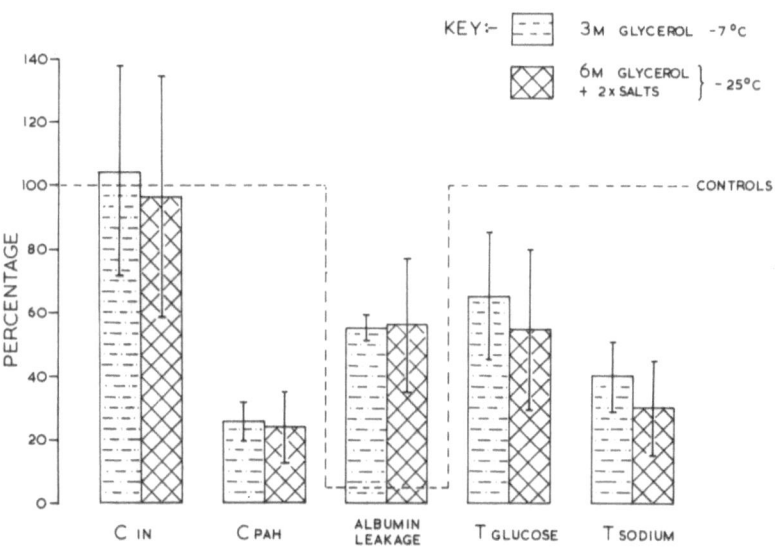

Figure 58.2 The effect of cooling, without freezing, on renal functions, expressed as a percentage of control values. Note the similarity of the effect of cooling to $-7\,°C$ in 3 molar glycerol and to $-25\,°C$ in 6 molar glycerol

tration, or to $-25\,°C$ with a doubling of solute concentration has similar effects: C_{IN} is unaffected, but C_{PAH}, T_{GLU} and T_{Na} are reduced and protein leakage is increased to a considerable degree.

Figure 58.3 shows that freezing, whether at $-1.5\,°C$ in the absence of glycerol or at $-25\,°C$ with an initial concentration of 3 molar glycerol reduces C_{IN}, drastically reduces C_{PAH}, T_{GLU} and T_{Na}, and causes total protein leakage. It should be noted that these conditions both produce a doubling of salt concentration, as does the $-25\,°C$ cooling protocol in Figure 58.2.

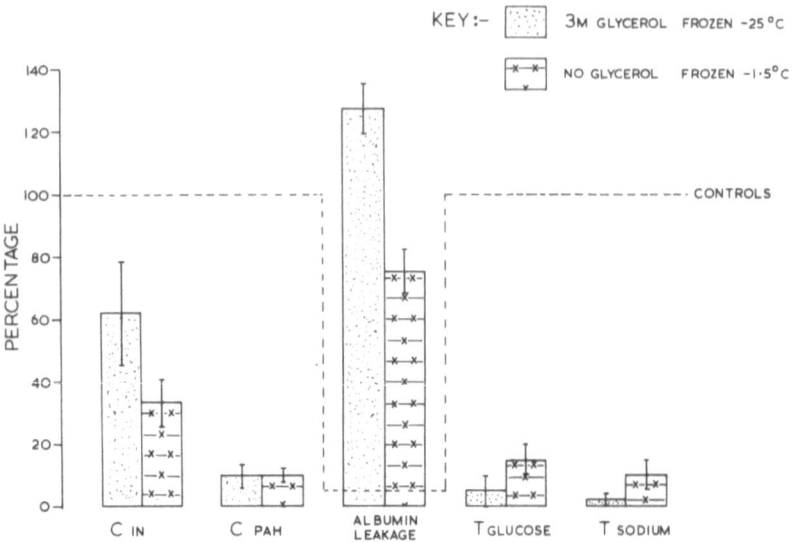

Figure 58.3 The effect of freezing on renal functions, expressed as a percentage of control values. Note that freezing is far more damaging than cooling to the same temperature, and that there is severe damage at both $-1.5\,°C$ without glycerol and $-25\,°C$ with an initial glycerol concentration of 3 mol/l

Figure 58.4 combines groups 1 and 2 (cooling without freezing) and groups 3 and 4 (freezing with different degrees of cooling) and demonstrates that freezing is far more damaging than cooling.

The freezing and solute concentration conditions used in this study were relatively mild, and yet they produced far more damage than would be expected by extrapolation from typical single-cell systems. Increasing the solute concentration to $2\times$ normal had no measurable effect, yet the formation of sufficient ice to double the solute concentration was severely damaging. Reduction in temperature, even in the absence of freezing, was also damaging, but less so than freezing. The location of ice in these experiments remains to be determined, but one could expect that, at such slow cooling rates, it would be extracellular, which raises the possibility that damage may not be cellular at all, but to the extracellular architecture as previously proposed[6]. It was observed that only the two groups of frozen kidneys exhibited a high vascular resistance during the normothermic assay perfusion, which supports this suggestion. We conclude that future research should concentrate upon possible mechanisms of extracellular

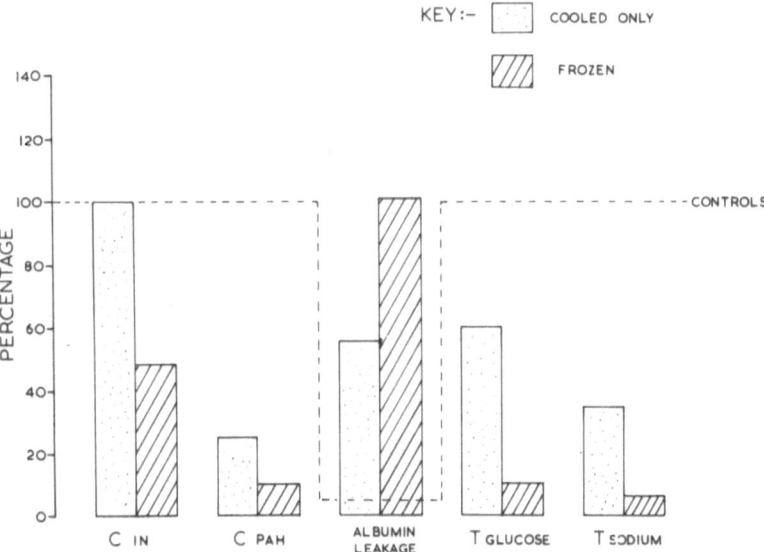

Figure 58.4   The data of Figures 58.2 and 58.3 are combined to emphasize the greater damaging effect of freezing than of cooling

injury, in particular to the vascular system. If these mechanisms can be understood new approaches to organ cryopreservation may become possible.

References

1. Jacobsen, I. A., Pegg, D. E., Wusteman, M. C. and Robinson, S. M. (1978). Transplantation of rabbit kidneys perfused with glycerol solutions at 10 °C. *Cryobiology,* **15,** 18
2. Jacobsen, I. A. (1979). Cooling of rabbit kidneys permeated with glycerol to sub-zero temperatures. *Cryobiology,* **16,** 24
3. Wusteman, M. C., Jacobsen, I. A. and Pegg, D. E. (1978). A new solution for initial perfusion of transplant kidneys. *Scand. J. Urol. Nephrol.,* **12,** 281
4. Pegg, D. E. and Wusteman, M. C. (1977). Perfusion of rabbit kidneys with glycerol solutions at 5 °C. *Cryobiology,* **14,** 168
5. Wusteman, M. C. (1978). Comparison of colloids for use in isolated normothermic perfusion of rabbit kidneys. *J. Surg. Res.,* **25,** 54
6. Pegg, D. E., Jacobsen, I. A., Armitage, W. J. and Taylor, M. J. (1978). Mechanisms of cryoinjury in organs. In Pegg, D. E. and Jacobsen, I. A. (eds.) *Organ Preservation II,* pp. 132–146. (Edinburgh: Churchill Livingstone)

59
Rabbit kidney function *in vitro* following cooling to − 20 °C with glycerol or dimethyl sulphoxide

F. M. GUTTMAN, J. BORZONE and N. B. SEGAL

Limited but sporadic successes in kidney freeze-preservation have been achieved. After freezing to − 50 °C for 15 min in 2.2 molar glycerol, Halasz et al.[1] found 25% of dog kidneys had life-sustaining function. Mundth et al.[2] reported 2 of 14 kidneys survived freezing to − 20 °C with 1.6 molar Me$_2$SO. Dietzman et al.[3] reported function in 2 of over 150 kidneys cooled to − 20 °C for 15 min with 1.6 molar Me$_2$SO. Using 1.4 molar Me$_2$SO and cooling to − 80 °C for 15 min, Guttman el al.[4] found 9 of 17 kidneys could support life. These findings could not be repeated by Pegg et al.[5], or by Guttman himself[6]; however Toledo-Pereyra[7] did obtain survival of 3 out of 10 kidneys frozen to − 80 or − 120 °C using similar techniques but held at the minimum temperature for only 3–5 min. In these experiments the concentration of cryoprotectant was low. The organs were kept at the lowest temperature for a short period, not allowing equilibrium freezing to occur. These experiments were empirical studies using techniques extrapolated from freezing cells in suspension without providing information of the mechanisms operating in whole-organ preservation. By proceeding in a stepwise fashion using an *in vitro* technique of rabbit kidney perfusion to assess function after cryobiological manipulation, we hope to understand more about the freezing process.

METHODS

Details of the normothermic *in vitro* assay techniques for rabbit kidney function have been described[8]. The technical details of the infusion of Me$_2$SO (3 mol/l) and its removal on a 10 °C perfusion apparatus using hypertonic mannitol washout have also been described[9]. In this study we have compared glycerol and Me$_2$SO as cryoprotectants both at 3 mol/l in control studies and after cooling to − 20 °C in a Linde BF4 freezing chamber at a rate of 0.3 °C/min. The cooling was carried out using cold intra-arterial helium, as has been previously described[10]. Thawing was carried out by immersion in a saline bath at 37 °C. There were four groups tested: *group 1:* control – 3 mol/l Me$_2$SO; *group 2:* cooling – 0.3 °C/min – 3 mol/l Me$_2$SO; *group 3:* control – 3 mol/l glycerol; *group 4:* cooling – 0.3 °C/min – 3 mol/l glycerol. There were six rabbit kidneys in each group. Four periods of 15 min were evaluated for creatinine clearance, Na and glucose reabsorption and flow rate.

The results were tested by the method of analysis of variance. Two independent 'blinded' pathologists assessed damage on a scale of no damage, moderate damage, severe damage.

RESULTS AND DISCUSSION

The results are outlined in Table 59.1. The GFR in group 1 was equal to our previous controls established with no cryoprotectant[9]. However, the GFR of the control glycerol group was significantly depressed ($p < 0.01$). This was also true for the two experimental groups ($p < 0.01$). Significant differences in Na reabsorption were also found in groups 2, 3 and 4. This was also true of glucose reabsorption. The two pathologists agreed that the most severe damage was seen in the – 20 °C glycerol group. The control glycerol group had damage ranging from 0 to + + (severe). The control Me$_2$SO group showed no damage whereas the – 20 °C Me$_2$SO group varied from 0 to + with no kidneys showing the severe changes found in some glycerol controls.

Table 59.1 Function measurements

Treatment	Glucose (Reabs. %)	Flow (ml/min/g)	GFR (ml/min/g)	Na (Reabs. %)
Me$_2$SO control	92.63 ± 0.68	6.97 ± 0.52	0.49 ± 0.03	43.96 ± 1.10
Glycerol control	51.13 ± 4.01	3.56 ± 0.27	0.139 ± 0.01	29.84 ± 2.14
Me$_2$SO – 20°	30.42 ± 5.04	5.45 ± 0.50	0.23 ± 0.02	18.34 ± 2.71
Glycerol – 20°	14.43 ± 2.35	3.16 ± 0.15	0.09 ± 0.01	12.72 ± 1.49

The *in vitro* perfusion system has been shown by our studies to be sensitive to minor manipulation and to more severe cryobiological manipulation[8,9]. Pegg and co-workers[11] have been the pioneers in the use of an *in vitro* perfusion set-up. Although the function of the kidneys cooled after treatment with Me$_2$SO or glycerol was impaired, the flow rates through the kidneys were adequate. This indicates that the vascular system has remained intact. The kidneys with high flows also had high urine output. We have worked out the optimal conditions of introduction, equilibration, and removal in this system for Me$_2$SO but we have not established these parameters for glycerol. It is also possible that the choice of such a slow rate of cooling (0.3 °C/min) is not the optimum rate in the rabbit kidney.

Functionally and morphologically glycerol seems to be more harmful even in controls, but this could easily be because of the way we have chosen to introduce and remove the cryoprotectant.

Acknowledgements

This work was supported by Medical Research Council Grant Ma 7077. This is publication no. 82008 of the McGill University – Montreal Children's Hospital Research Institute. We would like to thank Drs J. P. de Chadarévian and R. P. Bolande for the evaluation of histology.

References

1. Halasz, N. A., Rosenfield, M. A., Orloff, M. J. *et al.* (1967). Whole organ preservation. II. Freezing studies. *Surgery,* **61,** 417
2. Mundth, E. D., Defalco, A. J. and Jacobsen, Y. G. (1965). Functional survival of kidneys subjected to extracorporeal freezing and transplantation. *Cryobiology,* **2,** 62
3. Dietzman, R. H., Rebelo, A. E., Graham, E. F. *et al.* (1973). Long term functional success following freezing of canine kidneys. *Surgery,* **74,** 181
4. Guttman, F. M., Lizin, J., Robitaille, P. *et al.* (1977). Survival of canine kidneys after treatment with dimethyl sulphoxide, freezing at – 80 °C and thawing by microwave illumination. *Cryobiology,* **14,** 559
5. Pegg, D. E., Green, C. J. and Walter, C. A. (1978). Attempted canine renal cryopreservation using dimethyl sulfoxide, helium perfusion and microwave thawing. *Cryobiology,* **15,** 618
6. Guttman, F. M., Segal, N. B. and Borzone, J. (1979). Cryopreservation of canine kidneys with dimethyl sulphoxide: further studies. In Pegg, D. E. and Jacobsen, I. A (eds.) *Organ Preservation II,* p. 185. (London: Churchill Livingstone)
7. Toledo-Pereyra, L. H. (1980). Factors involved in successful freezing of kidneys for transplantation. *J. Surg. Res.,* **28,** 563
8. Segal, N. B. and Guttman, F. M. (1979). Function of rabbit kidneys during normothermic in vitro perfusion. *Cryobiology,* **16,** 616
9. Segal, N. B. and Guttman, F. M. (1982). Function of rabbit kidneys *in vitro* at normothermia following equilibration with 3.0 M Me$_2$SO and removal by hypertonic washout at 10 °C. *Cryobiology.* (In press)
10. Guttman, F. M., Khalessi, A., Huxley, B. W. *et al.* (1969). Whole organ preservation. I. A technique for *in vivo* freezing canine intestine using intra-arterial helium and ambient nitrogen. *Cryobiology,* **6,** 32
11. Fuller, B. J. and Pegg, D. E. (1976). The assessment of renal preservation by normothermic bloodless perfusion. *Cryobiology,* **13,** 177

60
Prospects for organ preservation by vitrification*

G. M. FAHY and A. HIRSCH

Although most organized tissues and cell types can be successfully frozen with relatively simple techniques, the heart, the liver, and the kidney have so far uniformly failed to survive freezing to $-80\,°C$. Freezing and thawing set into motion a myriad of complex, simultaneous destructive events, and dealing with these events is a problem which has daunted most organ preservationists. There is, however, an alternative approach to indefinite low-temperature banking of organs.

Vitrification refers to solidification without freezing. Highly concentrated solutions of cryoprotective agents (CPAs) normally solidify into a non-structured, amorphous state upon cooling to sufficiently low temperatures. This solidification occurs at a particular temperature, the glass transition or glass transformation temperature, T_g. At the glass transition there is a more-or-less abrupt arrest of all translational molecular motions such as diffusion, and the solution is said to become a glass. All biological events cease. There is no elevation in electrolyte concentration, no ice crystals to cause mechanical damage or intracellular freezing, no potentially damaging osmotic shifts. There is also no need to worry about finding a cooling rate and a warming rate which are optimal for all of the cell types in the organ. In short, all of the mechanisms which cause freezing injury are avoided except one, namely, exposure to elevated concentrations of CPAs, an event which also takes place during freezing.

Figure 60.1 shows the effect of ethylene glycol concentration on a number of interesting events that take place during cooling[1,2]. The upper curve is the melting point of the solution, T_m. Although water becomes freezable below T_m, it generally does not freeze until some lower temperature is reached, a situation known as supercooling. The lowest temperature a solution can supercool to without freezing is the next curve shown, the homogeneous nucleation temperature, T_h. The lowest curve is T_g, the glass transition temperature. As the concentration of CPA goes up, T_g goes up and both T_m and T_h go down. At a certain concentration of

* Contribution No. 523 from the American National Red Cross, Blood Services Laboratories.

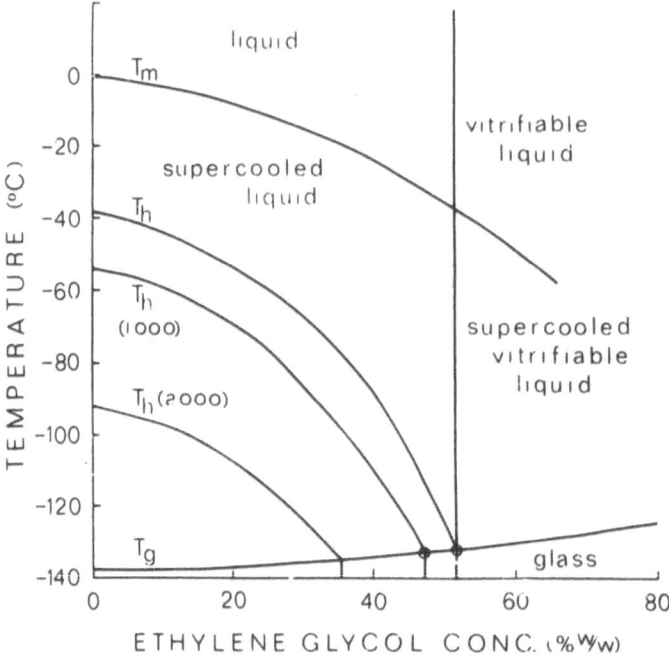

Figure 60.1 Relationship between ethylene glycol concentration and the melting point (T_m), homogeneous nucleation temperature (T_h) and glass transition temperature (T_g). Circles are data points from Table 60.1

CPA, T_h becomes equal to T_g. At this and higher concentrations freezing becomes difficult, and cooling tends instead to vitrify the solution, even if heterogeneous nucleating agents, or freezing catalysts, are present. Any biological system which can be thoroughly equilibrated with such high concentrations of CPA could be vitrified. The only real barrier to organ preservation, therefore, is the magnitude of the concentration of CPA required for vitrification. The required concentration can, however, be lowered by high hydrostatic pressure. High pressures, like cryoprotectants, lower T_m and T_h and slightly elevate T_g^2 and can therefore take the place of a portion of the required cryoprotectant. In Figure 60.1 we have sketched hypothetical T_h curves for 1000 and 2000 atmospheres (atm) of pressure. At 1000 atm we find experimentally (circle) that about 5% less ethylene glycol is required for vitrification. Although we do not know how much ethylene glycol will be needed at 2000 atm, a conservative guess based on this sketch is that it will only be about two-thirds of what is needed at 1 atm. Once the temperature goes below T_g, incidentally, the pressure can be safely released.

We have collected data on the effect of pressure on the critical concentration of CPA required for vitrification (Table 60.1). The results are based on an 8 ml sample cooled at between 3 and 9 °C/min between − 90 °C and

T_g and at about 30–50 °C/min down to -90 °C. The criterion for vitrification was the total absence of visible ice nuclei or, at most, one ice nucleus per sample. Our results show that the least effective CPAs are glycerol and ethylene glycol and the most effective agents are propylene glycol and trimethylamine acetate. The effect of 1000 atm amounts to a reduction in the required concentration of only about 5% w/v cryoprotectant. Nevertheless, our experiments with CPA toxicity suggest that even a small reduction in the necessary concentration for vitrifiction could be crucial. In addition, at 2000 atm the effect is likely to be closer to a 15% w/v reduction in the required concentration. Unfortunately, technical limitations have so far prevented us from doing this experiment.

Table 60.1 The effect of pressure on the vitrifiability of cryoprotectant solutions

| | *Critical concentration for vitrification at* | | | |
| | *1 atm* | | *1000 atm* | |
Cryoprotectant(s)	*(% w/v)*	*(mol/10 mol of water)*	*(% w/v)*	*(mol/10 mol of water)*
Glycerol	65	2.7	60	2.3
Ethylene glycol	55	3.2	49	2.6
DA*	53	2.8	48.5	2.3
Dimethyl sulphoxide	49–50	2.1	44–45	1.7–1.8
PD†	46	1.9	42	1.6
Propylene glycol	43.5	1.8	38.5	1.4
TMAA‡	41	1.1	?	?

* DA = dimethyl sulphoxide plus acetamide, equimolar
† PD = dimethyl sulphoxide plus propylene glycol, equal weights of each
‡ Trimethylamine acetate

We have, however, studied the effect of high pressure on the viability of rabbit renal cortical tissue in the presence and absence of cryoprotective agents, as shown in Figure 60.2. The y-axis is the K^+/Na^+ ratio achieved by the tissue slices after restoration to active metabolism at 25 °C for 90 min and is our index of viability. Control tissue is severely injured by a 20 min, 0 °C exposure to between 7500 and 10000 pounds per square inch (p.s.i.), which is 500–670 atm. Treating the tissue with 30% w/v dimethyl sulphoxide (Me_2SO), 15% w/v Me_2SO + 15% w/v propylene glycol (PG), or 30% w/v PG, however, almost completely protects against exposure to at least 15000 p.s.i., or 1000 atm. This 'baroprotective' effect, unfortunately, was unable to protect against damage at 1500 and 2000 atm (23000 p.s.i. and 29000 p.s.i.). In these experiments, slices were placed into 10%, 20%, and 30% solutions for 30, 60, and 44–52 min, respectively. Removal of CPA was done by exposure to 20% CPA + 150 millimolar mannitol for 60 min, then by exposure to 10%, 5%, and 0% CPA all containing 300 millimolar mannitol, for 20 min each. All procedures were carried out at 0 °C.

Since 1000 atm is safe and is sufficient to vitrify Me_2SO solutions at concentrations close to 40% w/v, we studied the effect of pressure at this

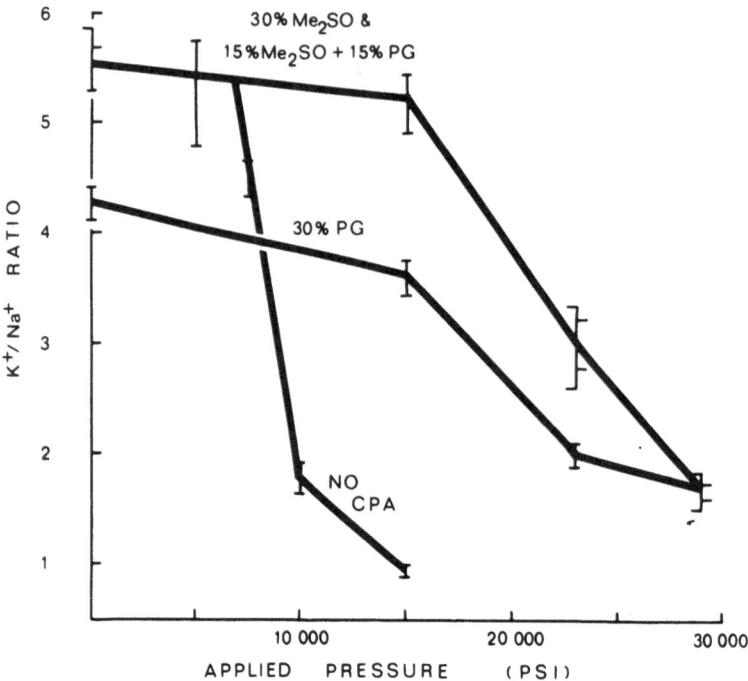

Figure 60.2 Effect of high pressures on kidney slice viability in the presence and absence of cryoprotectants. The base solution used (Rδ solution) consisted of (mmol/l): glucose 180; K_2HPO_4 30; NaCl 10; reduced glutathione 5; $MgCl_2$ 2; adenine HCl 1; $CaCl_2$ to saturation; pH = 8.0

total concentration of CPA (Table 60.2). In these experiments the CPA was added and removed as before, except that treatment with 30% CPA was at −9.5 °C and that 40% CPA was introduced for 5 min at −14 °C and then at −20 °C for the duration of the pressurization/depressurization procedure (total time, 74 min). A 40 min step at −14 °C employing 30% CPA + 150 millimolar mannitol was also used as part of the washout procedure. Unfortunately, even though the pressure was applied at −20 °C to minimize CPA toxicity, exposure to 1000 atm was damaging at this level of CPA. However, exposure to the CPA was damaging in itself, and it is not clear whether the failure of baroprotection was due to the preceding toxicity or to an inherent reduction in baroprotection at concentrations greater than 30% CPA. Recent experiments (see chapter 53) indicate that it may be possibel to abolish CPA toxicity at the 40% level, in which case more favourable results may be possible.

We feel at this point that vitrification should be pursued. The vitreous organ is a simpler system to study than the frozen organ, and the required CPA concentrations are actually less than those produced during organ freezing[3]! Several systems tolerate the high concentrations of CPA required for vitrification[4-7] and, in fact, all cells frozen at just below their optimal cooling rates probably vitrify internally[8], suggesting that vitrification is

Table 60.2 Effects of cryoprotectants and pressure on kidney slice viability

Treatment	n	K^+/Na^+	p^*
Dimethyl sulphoxide, 40% w/v, 1 atm	5	2.55 ± 0.14	—
Same treatment, 1000 atm	3	1.46 ± 0.13	< 0.005
Dimethyl sulphoxide, 30% w/v, plus acetamide, 10% w/v, 1 atm	7	2.62 ± 0.13	—
Same treatment, 1000 atm	6	1.56 ± 0.12	< 0.001
Dimethyl sulphoxide, 30% w/v, plus propylene glycol, 10% w/v	6	2.72 ± 0.18	—
Same treatment, 1000 atm	6	1.84 ± 0.11	< 0.005

K^+/Na^+ refers to the steady-state K^+/Na^+ ratio attained by slices following cryoprotectant removal and return to active metabolism at 25°C for 90 min; mean $\pm$ SEM; n refers to the sample size

* Comparison between pressurized and non-pressurized control slices

generally tolerated. It is physically possible to perfuse kidneys with glycerol or Me$_2$SO at temperatures down to -25 to -30 °C[9-11] and it is possible to avoid cracking of vitreous organs[7,12] during cooling to -196 °C and rewarming to 0 °C (Fahy, unpublished observations). The discovery of baroprotection and possible future enhancement of baroprotection is also encouraging. Organ preservation by vitrification may not be easy to achieve, but it does seem to be within the realm of possibility.

References

1. Rasmussen, D. and Luyet, L. (1970). Contribution to the establishment of the temperature–concentration curves of homogeneous nucleation in solutions of some cryoprotective agents. *Biodynamica,* **11,** 33
2. Kanno, H., Speedy, R. J. and Angell, C. A. (1975). Supercooling of water to -92 °C under pressure. *Science,* **189,** 880
3. Luyet, B. (1969). On the amount of water remaining amorphous in frozen aqueous solutions. *Biodynamica,* **10,** 277
4. Elford, B. C. and Walter, C. A. (1972). Effects of electrolyte composition and pH on the structure and function of smooth muscle cooled to -79 °C in unfrozen media. *Cryobiology,* **9,** 82
5. Farrant, J. (1965). Mechanism of cell damage during freezing and thawing and its prevention. *Nature (Lond.),* **205,** 1284
6. Luyet, B. and Gonzales, F. (1953). Growth of nerve tissue after freezing in liquid nitrogen. *Biodynamica,* **7,** 171
7. Rapatz, G. (1970). Resumption of activity in frog hearts after freezing to low temperatures. *Biodynamica,* **11,** 1
8. Leibo, S. P., McGrath, J. J. and Cravalho, E. G. (1978). Microscopic observation of intracellular ice formation in unfertilized mouse ova as a function of cooling rate. *Cryobiology,* **15,** 257
9. Carruthers, R. K., Clark, P. B., Anderson, C. K. and Parsons, F. M. (1969). Prevention of weight gain and protein loss during perfusion of the rat kidney for storage at -79 °C. *Br. J. Urol.,* **41,** 179
10. Kemp. E., Clark, P. B., Anderson, C. K., Laursen, T. and Parsons, F. M. (1968). Low temperature preservation of mammalian kidneys. *Scand. J. Urol. Nephrol.,* **2,** 183

11. Pegg, D.E. (1979). The mechanism of cryoinjury in glycerol-treated rabbit kidneys. *Cryobiology,* **16,** 618
12. Kroener, C. and Luyet, B. (1966). Formation of cracks during the vitrification of glycerol solutions and disappearance of the cracks during rewarming. *Biodynamica,* **10,** 47

61
General discussion of cryopreservation

ADDITION AND REMOVAL OF CRYOPROTECTANTS: TOXICITY

Karow Dr Fahy, you used two methods of introducing cryoprotectants in your slice experiments (chapter 53). Could you review them more fully?

Fahy Yes, I have found that it is all right actually to transfer the slices directly to 20% cryoprotectant (CPA) for 30 min, and then go straight on to 30% CPA but in all these experiments they were incubated in 10% CPA for 30 min first. In the first experiment I reported, they were then transferred into 20% CPA for $\frac{1}{2}$ h, and then into 30% CPA for 1 h, to make sure they were fully equilibrated at 30% before I went on to 40%. In the second experiment, I let them equilibrate for 1 h at the 20% level followed by only $\frac{1}{2}$ h at 30% CPA, and the results were better. I found in other experiments that incubation in 30% CPA for 2 h causes some deterioration, whereas after 1 h there is no detectable damage, so I think that the total time of exposure at or above 30% CPA, is important.

Karow So the primary difference between the two is the rate of change of concentration.

Fahy I don't want to put it that way. What I would say is that the difference is the total time of exposure to 30% CPA which is greater in the first experiment: everything else is more or less the same.

Guttman What was the temperature you used, Dr Fahy?

Fahy This was all done at 0 °C.

Karow Would you elaborate on your Group N, that you referred to as your 'usual subzero protocol'.

Fahy Yes, in that protocol I load with 10% Me_2SO at 0 °C for 30 min, then with 20% Me_2SO for 1 h. I then transfer the slices to 30% Me_2SO at −8 °C for an additional hour. Forty per cent Me_2SO is introduced for 5 min at −14 °C, after which the temperature is lowered to −20 °C for the duration of the experiment. Removal is done by transfer to 30% Me_2SO plus 150 millimolar mannitol at −14 °C for 40 min, then to 20% Me_2SO plus 150 millimolar mannitol at 0 °C for 60 min, 10% Me_2SO plus 300 millimolar mannitol for 25 min at 0 °C, 5% Me_2SO plus 300 millimolar mannitol for 15 min, 300 millimolar mannitol for 20 min, and then isotonic Rδ solution. I think the difference between the sub-zero results and the 0 °C results reported in chapter 53 is due to the difference in temperature of exposure, and I would expect that the results in chapter 53 would have been better if I had used subzero temperatures. The fact that we are getting K^+/Na^+ ratios of about 4 at 0 °C is quite encouraging, and I would presume that we shall be able to reach 40% CPA all right.

Fuller Since both freezing point depression and cryoprotectant activity are dependent on molar concentration, do you think it is fair to compare CPAs on a w/v percentage basis?

Fahy
That is a good point, but in this case the molecular weights and densities of all the additives are very similar, not the same but close, so the two concentration scales are comparable. In the case of ethylene glycol there is a slightly higher molar concentration for a given w/v concentration than is true of the other agents, but we obtained good results when ethylene glycol was included.

Pegg
Dr Fahy, you are assuming that the results will be better at lower temperatures, but have you actually looked at that?

Fahy
Actually I have, and it has been a bit disappointing; however, I haven't given it what I would call a really fair test. I have loaded up to 30% CPA at 0 °C and then gone down to subzero temperatures with 40% CPA, and this did improve things a bit, but not terribly much. I think that the 30% CPA step probably has to be subzero as well, but I haven't done that experiment yet.

Halasz
We published some studies some years ago on the effect of mixing cryo-protectants, and mixtures clearly had diminished toxicity[1]. The total toxicity was greater than each individual component, but it was less than the sum of the effects of the other cryoprotectants given separately. It is disappointing that you cannot accomplish that in the kidney slice system.

Fahy
Well, if you compare Groups A and E in Table 53.1 in which I compared straight 40% Me_2SO with 20% Me_2SO plus 20% propylene glycol, the result was a slight improvement with the mixture, even though the propylene glycol by itself was mildly toxic at that level. I think we need to do more experiments before we can answer that question.

Gundmann
In our work (chapter 54) we stored kidneys after flushing with different concentrations of sucrose or Me_2SO and we found that it was not possible to store kidneys in solutions with an osmolality greater than 1000 or 1400 mosmol/kg, whether we used sucrose or Me_2SO. So my question is what was the osmolality of the Me_2SO solution Dr Hardie used (chapter 52)?

Hardie
The osmolality of 12.5% Me_2SO is 2750 mosmol/kg and after perfusion with 12.5% Me_2SO we get about 10% Me_2SO in the kidney homogenate. Whether that is actually the intracellular concentration I cannot say, of course.

Fahy
Huggins and Miura[2] found that the dog kidney can tolerate only a 4 times increase over isotonic osmolality in the perfusate as a single step and this correlates with Dr Grundmann's results. Dr Hardie is considerably above that, but this 12.5% Me_2SO limit was also found by Lillihei's group who gave it as a single shot[3,4]: had it been given gradually, the results would probably have been better.

Halasz
That raises a more general question we should discuss, which concerns the administration of cryophylactic agents and the whole question of stepwise versus continuous introduction of cryophylactics. I think that *a priori* one certainly would expect the gradual introduction and elution to be the ideal, but is that truly established?

Pegg
In our own work we have looked only at a single step increase in CPA concentration from zero to 2 molar, and a slow continuous increase to 2–4 molar with glycerol in kidneys[5-7] and in hearts, Dr Armitage and I looked only at a slow continual increase[8]. I think there are excellent theoretical reasons and experimental observations to support the notion that you should remove the cryoprotectant slowly – these are obvious to us all, but there is much less evidence on the question of introduction. In both the kidney and the heart experiments we both increased and decreased the CPA concentrations slowly, and did not look separately at the two phases. One piece of evidence I do recall, however, is from Dr Smith's work on the isolated heart[9], where she certainly showed that there was better recovery of function if the glycerol was added gradually

Harness

rather than in one step. But I would be very surprised if there was any detectable difference between many small steps and a smooth curve.

A student of mine studied the addition of ethylene glycol to rat hearts stepwise in one or three steps, and continuously, and stepwise he killed them.

Armitage

Really, it all depends on the temperature at which the cryoprotectant concentration is changed. In their work on cryophylactic agents in the rat heart[10], Hobbs and Huggins showed that contractile function was retained following single step changes in ethylene glycol concentration from zero to 3 molar and back, but that was done at 37 °C. Assuming that cryoprotectant permeability increases with temperature there will be less of an osmotic problem at 37 °C, but this has to be balanced against the possibility of increased toxicity at higher temperatures.

Grundmann

We have perfused kidneys stored in hyperosmolar solutions from 700 to 1500 mosmol/kg, but when we decreased the osmolality gradually the function was not improved. I think it may be important that the viscosity of the solution is high and this may cause problems with the vascular system.

Guttman

In the experiments described in chapter 59, where we compared the effects of 3 molar glycerol and Me_2SO with and without freezing to -20 °C, we certainly added the CPA slowly but Dr Segal's idea was to carry out the removal in a single step, and I think his idea was unique. He used an *in vitro* rabbit kidney system at 10 °C, and the perfusate for removing the CPA contained no CPA but either 600 or 800 mosmol/kg of mannitol. He found that the perfusion flow rate increased immediately when he switched to the 800 mosmol/kg solution, whereas at 600 mosmol/kg mannitol, it was almost 25 min before the flow rate increased[11]. I think that it is interesting that this system is not noxious at all, although there is no cryoprotectant in the washout fluid and in fact the flow rate seems to be improved over all of the other methods we have used with either glycerol or Me_2SO.

Fahy

We have also done some studies to reduce the rise in vascular resistance that takes place during the deglycerolization of rabbit kidneys and we found that if we used 300 millimolar mannitol, instead of the 100 millimolar that Dr Pegg used, we came close to abolishing that peak. It appears that 400 millimolar mannitol will just about do it, but we have no measurements of the viability of those kidneys yet. In this experiment we used a continuous gradient of glycerol concentration with 300–400 millimolar mannitol present throughout deglycerolization, but it would also be possible to ramp up the mannitol concentration as the glycerol goes down.

Halasz

We have done the same thing as far as propylene glycol washout is concerned, and by using about 300 millimolar mannitol we found very much the same.

Fuller

We did one or two experiments to remove 3 molar methanol by perfusion of 1 molar mannitol, and we found that we could get good vascular resistance but our *in vitro* viability assays were very much reduced. Perhaps our methanol concentrations were too high anyway.

Pegg

Levin has recently published a theoretical study that optimizes the introduction and removal of cryoprotectants with isolated cells[12] and he has some as yet unpublished studies, showing the application of this method to whole organs. His idea is to design a system that prevents any volume changes in all the compartments of the organ during the addition and removal, and to do it in a reasonable length of time, instead of taking hours as we now do. The principle is to remove all the non-permeating solutes from the perfusate, and to perfuse the organ with the CPA solution in water. Now of course the cells will swell, and to prevent that he ramps up the CPA concentration at the correct rate to

300 mosmol/kg above the target concentration and then does a step reduction back to 300 mosmol/kg less of the CPA plus 300 mosmol/kg of salts so that the volumes remain constant. During removal the process is reversed. The theoretical advantage is that osmotic stresses are minimized, and practically there should be a considerable advantage in terms of time. I think it will be very interesting to test this theoretical model experimentally as soon as we have all the relevant data.

Ozaki   Dr Hardie, can you tell us more about the histology, particularly of the vascular system, in the Me$_2$SO perfused kidneys that you transplanted (chapter 52).

Hardie   In those that did not survive, we found extensive cortical necrosis. In the ones that did survive and returned to normal serum creatinines, the histology was pretty normal by light microscopy, and we do not yet have enough electron micrographs to draw any firm conclusions.

Halasz   This raises the question of vascular toxicity of Me$_2$SO. Does anyone have any data on that?

Karow   We have published a study similar to Dr Hardie's[13]. Using an intracellular type of perfusate, rather than a extracellular solution we were unable to demonstrate, by electron microscopy, any alteration in the vasculature of the kidneys perfused with the Me$_2$SO under favourable conditions.

Pearson   Cultured vascular cells, that is endothelium and smooth muscle, in common with many other mammalian cell types, freeze perfectly well in 10% Me$_2$SO, so any harmful action is not a function of toxicity to the cell[14].

Fahy   That agrees with the results of studies on intact vessels published by Barner et al.[15].

Hardie   On the other hand that does not exclude the possibility of endothelial cell swelling as you remove the Me$_2$SO, which could produce a microvascular obstruction, which would then cause the no-reflow phenomenon, exactly as we see.

Pegg   I think that perhaps some experiments that we reported were responsible for the notion that there is a specific toxic effect of Me$_2$SO on the microvascular system. I think there is no doubt that, in the particular model we used, Me$_2$SO produces a form of vascular damage which is not seen with either glycerol or ethylene glycol, and that is a stripping of the endotheial cells from the basement membrane, so that they are loose in the lumen and then embolize[5]. But that was a particular model where the CPA concentration was increased in one step from zero to 2 molar in each case, and we used an 'extracellular' perfusate containing dextran. I would hesitate to predict that the same phenomenon would occur with Me$_2$SO in a different system, but it certainly happened in that one.

Guttman   I neglected to mention in my paper (chapter 59), that the solution we used as a carrier for Me$_2$SO (and glycerol) was Fahy's RPS solution with glutathione and adenine.

Halasz   Has anybody any data on the effect of methanol on blood vessels; does it cause problems of blood flow subsequently?

Green   I have done the very simple experiment of washing out rabbit kidneys at 4 °C with 3 molar methanol, storing them for 1 h, and when I put them back in the rabbit, they did not reflow. There was immediate vascular damage in that situation.

Pegg   Dr Osborne, when you introduced methanol you observed a reduction in flow (chapter 55). Do you think this was an osmotic effect? Did you see a corresponding weight change? It is usually assumed that methanol has roughly the same permeability as water, but if so, you would not expect it to have any osmotic effect, and the vascular resistance change must have another cause.

Osborne	We did not weigh the kidneys continuously, so we do not know what happened when the methanol got in. I think that the increased vascular resistance may just be an effect of the hypothermia, but we do not know.
Fuller	Methanol does have an osmotic effect – we have found that in other more controlled studies.
Guttman	I just want to refer to the feeling that some people have that Me_2SO is very toxic. I do not think it is, and this is supported by some recent studies where it has been used *in vivo* clinically to 'clean out' amyloid deposits[16]. It has also been shown to prevent immune complex deposition in an animal experimental model (Kaplan, B., personal communication). So really I do not think it should be thought of as 'toxic'.
Frödin	I would just add that we use Me_2SO clinically locally in the bladder to treat Hunner's cystitis.

PERMEATION OF CRYOPROTECTANTS

Fischer	Dr Fahy, do you know how much time was needed to achieve equilibration between your slices and the medium?
Fahy	Yes, I have measurements for 15% Me_2SO and equilibration was almost complete after $\frac{1}{2}$ h. An extra hour gave a little more permeation, but not very much. In the experiments I described in chapter 53 we may not have had total permeation, in the sense that the cells may have been partially shrunken still, but the intracellular concentration of Me_2SO is going to be the same as the extracellular concentration because of the osmotic withdrawal of water. As far as vitrifying the organ is concerned (chapter 60) that is just fine, so long as the shrinkage of the cells does no damage. I have done studies in which slices were weighed after loading with different concentrations of Me_2SO and they weighed between 85 and 90% of their control weight, so any possible shrinkage is limited. As a matter of fact, if you do the same experiment with the control slices they tend to weigh slightly less too, because of some loss of surface material in the course of manipulations. Slices loaded with 3 molar glycerol were at 85% of their initial weight, but so were non-glycerolized, manipulated control slices. Although I am not sure if I have total permeation, I think I am close.
Pegg	I would like to make the point that there is a problem in using osmolality measurements to determine whether or not there is equilibration of Me_2SO concentration, as for example, Dr Hardie did (chapter 52) because all you need is water movement to get the same osmolality throughout the organ, and that happens very rapidly indeed. Equality of osmolality does not mean that the substance has permeated. Also, it is not correct to refer to a tissue osmolality measurement as 'intracellular osmolality' and really we must pay more careful attention to this. That does not mean that these measurements are not of interest; it is just a question of interpretation. In fact I think it is very interesting that Dr Hardie did not find equilibration of osmolality between his Me_2SO perfusate and the kidney tissue. You may remember some experiments we did a long time ago with a step increase of Me_2SO, glycerol and ethylene glycol in perfused rabbit kidneys[5], where we found that in spite of its slower diffusion and greater viscosity, glycerol gave complete osmotic equilibration whereas Me_2SO did not. With our more recent method of increasing and decreasing glycerol concentration slowly we get virtually 100% equilibration, as measured by a chemical glycerol assay[17]. Would Dr Hardie agree that the reason for this is likely to be incomplete perfusion of the tissue with the Me_2SO perfusate?

Hardie	Yes, that's one explanation, and we should look more accurately into the precise Me_2SO levels we have got in the tissue. But I do think that the problem may well be incomplete perfusion, particularly with the vascular resistance changes we see.
Harness	I believe that in red blood cells, Farrant did show that he obtained the same Me_2SO concentration inside and outside the cells. But really it is the chemical potential you should be considering: that has got to be the same inside and outside the cell, and once it is, you have nothing to pull any more Me_2SO into the cell.
Pegg	Farrant actually found the Me_2SO space in red cells to be less than the water space[18], and Elford found that the same was true of smooth muscle, at least at $-7\,°C$[19]. Whether you interpret this as non-solvent water, changes in water activity or whatever, it is a fact that there may be a fraction of the cell water that appears to be inaccessible to Me_2SO. So that is a possibility we should remember with kidneys as well.
Frödin	Dr Guttman, I believe you observed a difference in Me_2SO equilibration between the cortex and the medulla. What conclusion do you draw from that?
Guttman	I think the flow must be greater through the medulla, and that is why we get a more rapid exchange. Perhaps we would have seen the difference more strikingly if we had done our studies in the first hour. Equilibrium was reached in the medulla at 60 min but not in the cortex. However it was complete in the cortex also at 75 min.
Pegg	The same as the water space? Our findings and Dr Hardie's suggested incomplete equilibration with Me_2SO.
Guttman	Yes, it was the same as the water space in our experiments[20].
Karow	From an osmotic standpoint it might be attractive to have equilibration of Me_2SO concentration between the intracellular and extracellular space, but it may not be necessary to have cryoprotectant in the intracellular space for it to exert a cryoprotective effect[21]. However, if it is desired to achieve intracellular permeation then I would point out that we have demonstrated that Me_2SO can be administered to dog kidneys and rabbit kidneys at temperatures as high as $37\,°C$, with relatively innocuous consequences[22]. This should facilitate equilibration between the intra- and the extracellular spaces, and this technique is certainly available.

SUBZERO PRESERVATION WITHOUT FREEZING

Karow	I am puzzled by Dr Grundmann's experiments (chapter 54). There were two storage periods, 12 and 24 h, and I do not understand why you were looking at Me_2SO in kidneys stored at relatively high temperatures of $+4\,°C$ and $-2\,°C$ for these long periods of time. In my own laboratory we have measured Me_2SO toxicity at 10, 25 and $37\,°C$, but only for the short periods of time, 60–90 min, that would be needed to get Me_2SO into the kidney and remove it again for cryopreservation purposes[22]. Of course, during cryopreservation, the Me_2SO is going to be in the kidney for a long period of time, but that is at a deep subzero temperature, which is going to essentially eliminate toxicity. So I really do not see the point of studying toxicity for 12–24 h at $+4\,°C$ or $-2\,°C$.
Grundmann	The point of these experiments was that we wanted to store kidneys at subzero temperatures to see if that would improve preservation, but that is possible only if we prevent freezing; for example, when we stored kidneys with 0.5 molar Me_2SO at $-6\,°C$ they froze, and after only 12 h the kidneys did not function at all on transplantation. We chose the times of 12 and 24 h because after longer than 24 h, the function of the kidneys decreased still further and the results were already significant at

12 h. In fact, these kidneys did function after 12 h preservation, much better than if I had frozen them in the same Me₂SO concentration. The point is that if these methods are to be useful for clinical practice, they must be at least as good as Euro-Collins' solution.

Guttman I agree with Dr Karow. Firstly, there is already ample evidence that prolonged contact at -2, or $+4\,°C$ with a cryoprotective agent is probably not going to work, and Dr Grundmann's evidence that 12 h is better than 24 h supports this: if he repeated his experiment at 6 h, he would find that Me₂SO is not toxic at all. We need maybe 3 or 4 h, but we don't need 24 h to get the cryoprotectant in so that we can take an organ down to very low subzero temperatures. The concern is for preservation for weeks, months and years, not days.

Grundmann If you only want to get the Me₂SO into the cells then it doesn't need even 3 h. We have measured the intracellular osmolality and already between 1 and 3 min, we had almost the same intracellular osmolality as after 1 h; this means that Me₂SO penetrates the cells very rapidly. But it was not the point of my experiments simply to prepare the kidneys for cryopreservation, and if I wanted to store kidneys for only 6 h I could do it with Ringers' lactate solution: I was trying to prolong the preservation time by these methods.

Pegg I must repeat the points I have already made concerning osmolality measurements (page 409). First if you measure tissue osmolality you should call it that, not intracellular osmolality. Secondly, osmotic equilibrium is established by water movement, which is very rapid, not by the much slower movement of solute, and consequently equal osmolality does not mean that the CPA has penetrated.

Kemp But Dr Grundmann, I thought you reported better function in kidneys preserved at $-2\,°C$ with the sucrose solution, than with Collins' solution at $+4\,°C$.

Grundmann Kidney function decreases logarithmically with the time of preservation in all types of hypothermic storage, and it was the same with the sucrose solution at subzero temperatures. The kidneys stored in the hyperosmolar sucrose solution at $-2\,°C$ for 48 h, showed a very low PAH clearance but they were functioning at about the same level as kidneys stored in Collins' solution at $+4\,°C$ for the same time.

Frödin When did you measure the PAH clearances?

Grundmann We measured PAH and inulin clearances throughout the first 24 h after preservation, and there was no difference between the clearances done in the first 2 h and the last 2 h. The data in chapter 54 were from the 6 h measurements. Of course, I cannot say that a kidney which has a low clearance will not improve several days later but the point of the model is just to compare the state of preservation by a standard measurement of function in the different groups.

Collins I think there is a point in Dr Grundmann's efforts to use cryophylactic agents to prolong preservation by storing unfrozen kidneys at subzero temperatures, and while doing that it may be possible incidentally to learn something about the toxicity of these agents at both subzero and close-to-zero temperatures. However, an important basic difference between using sucrose and Me₂SO is that when the kidney is reimplanted none of the sucrose will have entered the cells whereas Me₂SO will have done so. Unless steps are taken to wash it out, I would expect a kidney equilibrated with, for example, 1.5 molar Me₂SO, to yield very poor function. I think that a useful extension of your experiment would be to slowly wash out the Me₂SO prior to reimplantation, and then perhaps the results would be better.

Jacobsen I also think that one of the main weaknesses of Dr Grundmann's experiment is the removal of the cryoprotectant, because the damage he observed could easily be explained by osmotic problems due to intra-

	cellular Me_2SO. I would like to add that we have done similar experiments with glycerol, and removed it slowly as we have done in other experiments[7]. We found that after 50 min of exposure to subzero temperatures and glycerol, the kidneys were fine, but after 3 days or 5 days they did not work at all[23]. So I am not too convinced that this is a pathway for the future.
Halasz	We have some data at 24 h, that fills in the gap between 50 min and 3–5 days, and about half of those worked and half did not. So that was not a practical advantage, and actually the technique is not that much simpler than freezing.
Fahy	I would like to mention that we have done some glycerol storage of tissue slices at $-8\,°C$ and it was definitely better than storage at $0\,°C$: we found a K^+/Na^+ ratio of 5 on day zero and of 3 on day 10 of storage, which is at least respectable. So I think there is some potential to this technique but it has to be done carefully. Maybe the key to improving the results with whole organs may be to use a non-damaging method of introducing and removing the cryoprotectant, or perhaps to use a different cryoprotectant. Me_2SO, for example, increases membrane permeability more than glycerol, and this may cause some problems.
Grundmann	I must agree of course that the Me_2SO was not washed out completely in my experiments, but we found that it was not possible, even by flushing 3 or 4 times with 100 ml of Euro-Collins' solution, to get the tissue osmolality back to normal. However, when these kidneys were transplanted and then homogenized 6 h later, the tissue osmolality had come back to about 400 mosmol/kg, so I think there is nothing better to wash out with than blood.
Collins	I am not sure that blood flow is the best way to wash it out, because if the kidney is damaged, blood will not flow through those parts of the kidney where washout is needed.

CRYOPRESERVATION: MECHANISMS OF CRYOINJURY

Fuller	I want to make the point that the viability of liver parenchymal cells (chapter 56) has been lost by $-25\,°C$, and the extrapolation from single-cell systems that Dr Pegg discussed (chapter 6) is very dependent on the cells you are referring to. I think we have been looking at the wrong cells in the past.
Pegg	Dr Fuller, have you looked at a wide range of cooling and warming rates with your liver cells?
Fuller	Yes, it was in our earlier study[24], but all the results were bad.
Guttmann	I was fascinated by Williams' recent paper[25] concerning the roles of cell shrinkage and high electrolyte concentration in cryoinjury. By using valinomycin he loaded red cells with a very high electrolyte concentration, and showed that it was not the electrolyte concentration but rather the amount of cell shrinkage that produced injury. It seems that Meryman's minimum cell volume hypothesis probably does explain freezing damage, and I am wondering if our problem in organ preservation is also volume changes while adding and removing the cryoprotectants.
Fahy	Could I ask Dr Pegg about the kidneys he cooled to $-7\,°C$ in 3 molar glycerol (chapter 58)? They were damaged, but were they perfused or were they simply left at $-7\,°C$?
Pegg	They were perfused.
Fahy	Then there is a possibility that there was a perfusion injury, that the vascular endothelium was more fragile at $-7\,°C$ and that the perfusion was damaging even though in normal circumstances it would not be.
Pegg	Yes, that is possible, although if perfusion were more damaging at lower

temperatures, I would expect the group perfused at $-25\,°C$ to be even more damaged, but it was not. I should add that the $-7\,°C$ group was continuously perfused to make it comparable with the group that was permeated with increasing glycerol concentration as the kidneys were cooled from $-7\,°C$ to $-25\,°C$.

Fahy I might mention that Dr Takahashi in our laboratory has seen super-cooling injury in some systems and he found that it can be prevented by the addition of very low concentrations of Me_2SO.

Armitage With the rabbit heart, perfusion with 3 molar ethylene glycol at between -1 and $-3\,°C$ was no more damaging than perfusion at $+10\,°C$[26]. That was close to the freezing point of the perfusate, but we saw no evidence of vascular damage at the lower temperature.

Fahy It could be a strictly thermal effect, or it could be dependent on an effect on the cryoprotectant, for instance ethylene glycol is a good deal less viscous than glycerol, so the viscosity of 3 molar glycerol at $-7\,°C$ must be a good deal higher than the viscosity of 3 molar ethylene glycol at $-3\,°C$. The greater viscosity might be more hazardous to the vascular system.

Jacobsen Dr Pegg, how did you thaw the frozen kidneys?

Pegg By conduction: they were contained in a test tube that was immersed in a bath that warmed at $0.25\,°C/min$. There was very little temperature gradient at that rate.

Fahy We did an experiment similar to Dr Pegg's $-1.5\,°C$ freeze (see chapter 58), in which we got whole blood coming down the ureter when we connected the kidney back into the circulation. That was with only a three times increase in salt concentration, but when we freeze kidney slices, we can go to -2, or $-2.5\,°C$ before the injury even becomes statistically significant. So there is a mechanical injury, but I think that it may not be necessary to totally eliminate ice; it may depend on where the ice is. It is intriguing to consider the possibility that gas perfusion, as Dr Guttman has been using it for so many years, might just remove freezable liquid from the glomerular tufts and other vessels in the organ, and this might change the results considerably.

Jacobsen I want to support that idea. We have looked at the histology of rabbit kidneys after freezing to $-80\,°C$, and the main problem seems to be rupture of the glomerular capillaries, because all the bleeding is into the tubular system, and there is very little blood outside in the interstitial space. So I agree with you; it all depends on where the ice is.

Fahy I have done some freeze substitution studies which appeared to indicate that mechanical injury from ice does take place in the glomerulus. I think that agrees well with Dr Jacobsen's observations, and others in the literature[27].

Armitage In the rabbit heart we found that selenomethionine improved the tolerance of myocardial cells to freezing injury, but the vascular response during removal of the cryoprotectant and the subsequent flow distribution in the hearts still indicated severe vascular damage[28]; the structural integrity of the vasculature may well be one of the primary sites of freezing damage.

Halasz That leads to a realted question, which is whether freezing diminishes the viability of all the cells, or does it eliminate one population of cells and allow another population to remain? I have a hunch that in freezing it is a population effect, rather than attenuation of the functional capacity of all the cells. This may also be important in relation to viability testing because the surviving population may be able to carry out some functions but not others.

Jacobsen I would like to describe some very preliminary results we have just obtained with the freezing of whole rabbit kidneys. We have already reported that kidneys equilibrated with 3 molar glycerol, and cooled to

−80 °C at 0.3 °C/min have a very high vascular resistance after thawing and removal of the glycerol[23]. We subsequently thought that 0.3 °C/min might be too rapid so we cooled at 0.1 °C/min down to −15 °C, and kept the kidneys there for 3 h and then cooled at 1 °C/min to −80 °C. After 4 h we rewarmed at 1 °C/min up to −20 °C, and then at 0.1 °C/min to +5 °C. After this we deglycerolized in the usual way, and the immediate post-thaw vascular resistance was almost identical to the pre-freeze resistance, and it did not increase as much during subsequent perfusion as it did in the previous experiments. So we seemed to have less damage in this experiment, but there was another factor, which is that by accident we used 2.3 molar glycerol instead of 3.0 molar glycerol: perhaps the very slow cooling avoided intracellular ice, but it could equally well be due to the lower glycerol concentration. We cannot tell yet but I think that there might be some further possibilities along these lines.

Frödin
I want to comment on the use of the term 'vascular resistance', in such experiments. If something goes through the renal artery, but some of it passes into the extracellular space, and then out of the kidney, the resistance is not all 'vascular', it is partly in the interstitium. Certainly you are measuring a resistance but be careful if you call it 'vascular'.

Halasz
Flow resistance perhaps?

Collins
Or perhaps we should express vascular resistance in terms of cannulated venous effluent, rather than the total collected effluent from the kidney.

Jacobsen
I also tried to repeat the same experiment with 3 molar glycerol, using the very slow interrupted cooling holding the kidney at −15 °C. That did not work at all. I then decided to try a lower holding temperature, that would freeze the same amount of ice in 3 molar glycerol as we did in 2.3 molar glycerol at −15 °C, and that did not work either. I think that these results may add some support to the idea of damage by cryoprotectant concentration during freezing.

Armitage
In our studies of freezing in rabbit hearts protected with ethylene glycol, it appeared that the major cause of injury was the increase in cryoprotectant concentration caused by freezing[26]. However, there are certain aspects of the way those experiments were done that might be relevant. To mimic the change in cryoprotectant concentration that occurred during freezing, the hearts were first equilibrated with 3 molar ethylene glycol slowly at +10 °C but the concentration was then increased from 3 molar up to 6 molar at −1 °C, *as a single step*. It actually took about 15 min for the ethylene glycol to get into the heart, but that rate of change of CPA concentration may itself have caused some damage. It wasn't done as rigorously at in Dr Pegg's experiments with kidneys (chapter 58), when he increased the cryoprotectant concentration slowly during cooling, following the solute concentration determined by the phase diagram. However, the result still provides indirect evidence of cryoprotectant damage during freezing.

Pegg
Dr Fahy, do you know whether the addition of urea or acetamide to reduce the toxicity of cryoprotectants has any effect on the cryoprotection they provide?

Fahy
Yes, that's a burning question. Presumably the phase diagram relationships will be different, but I have taken the position that part of the problem with freezing is that it concentrates the cryoprotectants until they reach damaging levels, so that if the damaging level is higher as a result of these additives, then we ought to have better results after freezing. But I do not have any experimental data I am prepared to talk about yet.

Pegg
Can I ask Dr Fahy what mechanisms of injury he considers likely other than cryoprotectant toxicity, in his studies of freezing injury in kidney slices (chapter 57).

Fahy

Unfortunately there is a certain amount of contradiction in the data relevant to that. I would like to be able to say that in my 3 molar glycerol experiments the injury I observed, which would not be predicted from your experiments showing 6 molar glycerol to be non-toxic, is due to mechanical injury from the ice, but I have done other experiments that show that mechanical injury to kidney cells is not apparent after freezing in Me_2SO solutions[29]. With glycerol however, it may be a different story. If you freeze granulocytes in glycerol, they are killed right where the ice comes into contact with the cell, but if you freeze them in Me_2SO this does not happen (Takahashi, T., unpublished data). It may be that there is some strange interaction between the membrane and ice which is modulated by what you add as the cryo-protectant. That is such a strange idea that I hate to fall back on it. On the other hand Olien thinks that plant cells stick to ice. Also, I now recall that I once treated kidney slices with 6 molar glycerol and $2\times$ salts at $-20\,°C$ for 5 min in the absence of freezing with no apparent injury, so maybe the 'ice effect' really is the answer. If this is the case, it would provide a reconciliation between my results and yours. You could still regard the extra injury in my experiments as a harmful effect of glycerol, although 'toxicity' might not be the best word for it. I would also like to make the comment that my findings agree closely with Dr Guttman's results: there is some injury to the kidney treated with 3 molar glycerol (and in fact Dr Guttman used the same perfusate that I used as a carrier) and if you then cool to $-20\,°C$ you have injured kidneys. So there is very good correspondence there. Furthermore, based on my tissue slice work with Me_2SO , I would expect better results with Me_2SO than with glycerol at $-20\,°C$, and Dr Guttman finds that as well.

Halasz

We used to talk a lot about carrier solutions for introducing cryopro-tectants, but now Dr Fahy uses several totally different salt solutions as carriers, and it makes no difference whatsoever.

Fahy

Actually, it does make a difference, but not to the temperature at which injury takes place. It does make a difference to how much damage there is prior to freezing, and I think that it is quite significant; Elford and Walter[30] showed also that it can be very crucial what carrier is used for the cryoprotectant.

Armitage

In the heart we found the best recovery of function, albeit minimal function, with a calcium-free carrier[26]. However, we only compared freezing with a fairly high calcium concentration (4.8 mmol/l) with zero calcium ion concentration in the perfusate, so I do not know whether a sub-physiological level might have been better.

Fahy

I think that in other systems calcium is proven to improve the results after freezing and thawing.

Halasz

If calcium has anything to do with the cytoarchitecture, then it might be an extremely important component to look at. It seems to be involved in the tolerance of the cell to volume change, and I think this needs to be explored.

Fahy

Dr Guttman, was the glyercol added at the same rate as the Me_2SO in your experiments (chapter 59)?

Guttman

Yes. We not only added the glycerol at the same rate that we had established as optimal for Me_2SO, but we also washed it out at the rate we had established as optimal for Me_2SO. So that is a very valid criticism of our work. The rationale and approach on which our experi-ments are based is the feeling that if we can get to $-20\,°C$ with no damage, and keep kidneys there for say, 2 h, we might then be able to cool to a much lower temperature, following the two-step cooling approach used by Farrant for single cells[31].

Fuller

The only glimmer of hope that we have with parenchymal liver cells, Dr

415

Grundmann	Guttman, is the two-step method with $-20\,^{\circ}C$ as the holding temperature. However, we have to use very rapid cooling to get to that intermediate temperature, so it is not applicable to whole organs, unfortunately.

Grundmann   Dr Guttman, do you think that with your method it is possible to store the kidneys at $-20\,^{\circ}C$ for 12 h, with PAH and inulin clearances identical to kidneys stored at $+4\,^{\circ}C$ by conventional methods of hypothermic storage? If you do not have at least the same function as hypothermic storage, I do not see the value of this technique.

Guttman   Let me explain. The purpose is to try to find a technique that gives good function of kidneys that have been at $-20\,^{\circ}C$ for 1 h, and then to go down to $-80\,^{\circ}C$ or perhaps to $-196\,^{\circ}C$, not for 12 h but for weeks. That is the aim.

Collins   One quite different thing that interests me about Me_2SO is that low concentrations might have a protective effect against free radicals (see chapter 4).

Armitage   Where do you think we go from here, Dr Pegg?

Pegg   If our conclusion is correct, that even a small amount of ice formation is damaging, then it seems to me that we have to reduce the amount of ice formed either to a harmless quantity or to zero. That means that we have to use higher concentrations of cryoprotectant and to avoid osmotic problems and any other forms of toxicity. Maybe Dr Fahy's interesting idea of producing vitrification is the way that it will go, but that also requires very high concentrations of cryoprotectant, so the next step is the same in either case.

Guttman   Yes, I agree with Dr Pegg: we do need methods of introducing high levels of cryoprotectant and avoiding ice formation.

Jacobsen   I think that we also have to do a lot of rethinking on what is rapid and what is slow cooling and warming in this situation. As I have already suggested, it might very well be that $0.1\,^{\circ}C/min$ in an organ is rapid cooling in terms of producing intracellular ice. Another factor is that although extracellular ice may be non-damaging in cell suspensions, ice formation in the extracellular space of the organ could well be damaging, and certainly recrystallization during slow rewarming is probably very harmful indeed. I think that our own experience of vascular damage during freezing and thawing may point in that direction[23].

Pegg   While we are talking about cooling and warming rates, I would like to report some experiments which we have just completed looking at the cell packing effect (see chapter 6). This is an effect whereby, under some circumstances, cells that are frozen and thawed at a high packing density suffer greater damage than cells frozen in the more commonly used dilute suspensions[32]. This interests us because one of the attributes of organs is a high packing density[33]. Our experiments were to determine the effect of cooling and warming rates on the haemolysis of human red cells frozen to $-196\,^{\circ}C$ in 2 molar glycerol. At a packed cell volume (PCV) or haematocrit of 2% there was a wide range of cooling and warming rates, which gave > 90% survival. These results were very similar to those of Miller and Mazur[34]. When we increased the PCV to 75% we were still able to obtain > 90% survival but only within a very much smaller range of cooling and warming rates. With relatively slow rates, around 0.1–$1.0\,^{\circ}C/min$, where we had a high survival with 2% cells, we obtained only ~50% survival with a PCV of 75%. Now of course kidneys are not red cells, but it may be significant that we have been looking at cooling and warming rates with kidneys where the packing effect is very marked with red cells. The important point is that in addition to cryoinjury itself being affected by cooling and warming rate, so is this additional secondary effect. I would like to underline

	what Dr Jacobsen has implied, that we really don't have any idea what rates we ought to be using to warm and cool whole organs.
	A further point that can be deduced from these results is that, in this sytem, if the cooling rate is less than 100 °C/min, then the packing effect is independent of cooling rate and is dependent on warming rate. This suggests, contrary to what I said in the meeting at Odense[33], that if we extrapolate to organs we ought to be thawing rapidly and not slowly. When the cooling rate exceeds 100 °C/min the effect is more or less independent of warming rate but is dependent upon cooling rate. I think the findings fit in quite nicely with the proposal that the mechanism of this effect is the production of intracellular ice nuclei at fast cooling rates, and that these then recrystallize during slow warming but not during fast warming.
Fahy	Those are fascinating results; one would expect that if you extended the cooling rate to still slower rates, you would get another peak of survival by avoiding intracellular ice completely, and then you would not need to thaw so quickly. I would just mention that I have done some calculations from data in the literature for rabbit proximal tubules[35,36]. There are estimates of the surface area and the hydraulic conductivity of the cells, and the values are simply huge, since the primary function of the cells is reabsorbing water. The result is that the proximal tubule ought not to freeze intracellularly under any reasonable conditions, unless the system is altered very strongly by cryoprotectants. What happens to other cell types in the kidney is not clear, but maybe we can focus onto those critical cell types that might be responsible for injury from intracellular ice in the whole organ, and eliminate some of the others.
Pegg	I certainly agree that we should look at even slower cooling rates than we have been, and I might also mention that we did in fact find a second peak of survival in a study of the effect of cooling rate and warming rate on tissue culture cells[37]. This of course was quite separate from the packing effect, but certainly supports the idea that we should look at even slower cooling.
Harness	How did you get such fast cooling rates? Did you have a thermometer in the middle of the cells to measure it?
Pegg	The cooling and warming conditions in those experiments were exactly the same as those used by Miller and Mazur[34]. We used $100\,\mu l$ samples and the temperature was measured with a thermocouple. The fastest cooling rate was ~850 °C/min.
Guttman	The final thing I would like to say is this: many people have said, 'There is no consistent success with organ freezing.' Perhaps I am an optimist, but I would rather say, 'There has been some sporadic success!'

TECHNIQUES FOR ASSESSING VIABILITY

Fahy	I liked Dr Fuller's HIDA assay system for hepatocytes (chapter 56): the standard deviations are pretty high, but if you do enough experiments you can control that. It is rather similar to a lot of the earlier work done in England by Smith and her co-workers[9] in which the assay was histological preservation after transplantation. I think that this is more rigorous than an acute viability assay, in which you might get poor results initially, but recovery might be possible.
Halasz	Dr Fuller, is HIDA excreted by a glucuronide addition process?
Fuller	HIDA is excreted by the same carrier system as bilirubin, which is glucuronidated. The exact metabolic route for HIDA remains to be elucidated.
Halasz	So it would look at enzymatic activity, which might be somewhat differ-

Fuller	ent from measurements of protein synthesis as an indicator of injury? Yes, it is different from the protein synthesis. We believe that our test measures the ability of the cell to take up the agent.
Frödin	Many people reporting organ preservation experiments, for example Dr Pegg (chapter 58), refer to glomerular filtration rate (GFR) as a *function*, but I would like to ask, what is the function that is measured by the GFR in those situations?
Pegg	We should call it inulin clearance, because that is what we measured. I can perhaps just add that our philosophy is to use a variety of tests of function, and when they all show changes in the same direction, we feel justified in saying that function has changed in that direction.
Frödin	That may be so, but the only thing you measure with GFR is that something can pass from the vascular system into the pelvis; that is the only thing you measure.
Ross	Yes, I think it might be critical also in the isolated normothermically perfused kidney, that the clearance of inulin may not be a very good measure of GFR. I suppose that when the results of preservation experiments are better, we shall then have to come back and check that what we are measuring actually is GFR. There is clearly an inulin leak in damaged kidneys (Hostetter, T., Trout, J., Ross, B. and Brenner, B., unpublished data) but if you were to use a labelled dextran technique[38], you may find that you have got a better result than you expect, because that is the way round it works.
Rijkmans	Dr Guttman, did you transplant any of the kidneys you had perfused *in vitro* to assess viability (chapter 59)? For example, did control kidneys, perfused *in vitro*, still have life-sustaining function?
Guttman	Yes, we have implanted some control kidneys after 3 h on our *in vitro* perfusion machine, but none of the animals has survived. That of course is a vital requirement to establish the validity of this system: if we cannot do that then there is some factor that is missing, and we may require a much more complicated system. The final judgement has to be reimplantation.
Halasz	What do you think the problem was? Were these technical problems? If so, I don't know whether you necessarily have to say that the system does not work.
Guttman	They were not technical problems, but we tested only half a dozen.
Pegg	I am not sure why you should try to transplant kidneys after normothermic perfusion. Dr Green and I have studied the transplantation of rabbit kidneys perfused at 37 °C with the albumin/dextran mixture, and they were fine after 1 h, but only one survived out of eight after 2 h normothermic perfusion[39]. With Dr Fuller and Dr Walter we looked at the ultrastructure of kidneys perfused with the whole range of normothermic perfusates and demonstrated severe vascular endothelial injury after 2 h with most of them[40,41]. I think this is really the problem; the vascular system is damaged by the normothermic perfusion, and when they are transplanted they become black, and leak red cells. I really do not think it is a valid test of the viability assay to transplant the kidneys afterwards.
Halasz	We have done the same thing with dog kidneys after they have been on a Nizet perfusion system with dilute blood; after 1 h we get about half of them to support life, but after 2 h nothing ever works.
Karow	I think that *in vitro* normothermic perfusion studies provide a valid prediction of post-transplant function. Drs Fuller, Pegg and Green, several years ago, compared the *in vitro* results in rabbit kidneys with the results after transplantation, and found that the physiological *in vitro* test did provide important and significant correlates[41,42]. Similarly, we conducted a series of rabbit kidney studies in which we used simple *in vitro* assessment, and subsequently we treated dog kidneys in

exactly the same way as the rabbit kidneys, except that they were tested by autologous reimplantation, and these kidneys performed as predicted by the preceding physiological measurements on rabbit kidneys *in vitro*[22].

Collins There may be one particular circumstance in which the *in vitro* studies will not correlate, and that is after freezing. Here the cells may be well preserved, and show excellent function *in vitro* but if the vascular system is destroyed, the organ will not function.

Pegg I cannot imagine that anybody would claim that *in vitro* perfusion tests will always correlate with transplantation absolutely. Clearly these tests do not reveal exposure of thrombogenic surfaces inside the vessels which will lead to loss of the organ after it has been transplanted. On the other hand, these assays do not just look at cell function. If, for example, there is back-leakage of substances which are being pumped into the nephron, then that will show up on our system, and that would not be something wrong with the cells, but a disturbance of the intercellular relationships. So I would suggest that normothermic perfusion assays certainly provide data closer to transplantation than simple cell or tissue systems, but ultimately they can never be more than a screening method for transplantation.

Halasz Dr Pegg, I don't think you have to apologize for normothermic perfusion to that extent! I think that what it gives us is several tiers of assessment. We have unicellular systems like Dr Fuller's hepatocytes, then Dr Fahy's tissue slices where we also look at intercellular connections, and then the *in vitro* bloodless system where we have some, but not all, of the vascular components, and finally we have the *in vivo* system. Having several tiers of evaluation is a benefit, not a disadvantage, and it certainly saves a lot of money.

References

1. Halasz, N. A and Orloff, M. J. (1964). New freeze-protecting compounds and their screening. *Surg. Forum,* **15,** 214
2. Huggins, C. E. and Miura, T. (1968). Tolerance of perfused canine kidneys to hypertonic salt solution. In Norman, J. C. (ed.) *Organ Perfusion and Preservation,* p. 71. (New York: Appleton-Century-Crofts)
3. Kubota, S., Graham, E. F., Crabo, B. G., Lillehei, R. C. and Dietzman, R. H. (1974). Influence of DMSO distribution upon renal function following freezing and thawing. *J. Surg. Res.,* **16,** 582
4. Rebelo, A. E., Graham, E. F., Crabo, B. G., Lillehei, R. C. and Dietzman, R. H. (1974). Surgical preparations, perfusion techniques, and cryoprotectants used in successful freezing of the kidney. *Surgery,* **75,** 319
5. Pegg, D. E. (1972). Perfusion of rabbit kidneys with cryoprotective agents. *Cryobiology,* **9,** 411
6. Pegg, D. E. and Wusteman, M. C. (1975). The function of rabbit kidneys following perfusion with 2-molar glycerol at 5 °C. *Proceedings of the 14th International Congress of Refrigeration,* Moscow
7. Jacobsen, I. A., Pegg, D. E., Wusteman, M. C. and Robinson, S. M. (1978). Transplantation of rabbit kidneys perfused with glycerol solutions at 10 °C. *Cryobiology,* **15,** 18
8. Armitage, W. J. and Pegg, D. E. (1978). Cryoprotection of rabbit hearts. In Pegg, E. E. and Jacobsen, I. A. (eds.) *Organ Preservation II.* (Edinburgh: Churchill-Livingstone)
9. Smith, a. U. (1961). *Biological Effects of Freezing and Supercooling.* (London: Edward Arnold)
10. Hobbs, K. E. F. and Huggins, C. E. (1969). Investigation of the effects of cryophylactic agents on the isolated rat heart at 37 °C. *Cryobiology,* **6,** 239
11. Segal, N. B. and Guttman, F. M. (1981). Function of rabbit kidneys *in vitro* following perfusion with 3 M Me_2SO, and hypertonic washout. *Cryobiology* (In press)

12. Levin, R. L. and Miller, T. W. (1981). An optimum method for the introduction or removal of permeable cryoprotectants: isolated cells. *Cryobiology*, **18**, 32
13. Jeske, A. H., Fonteles, M. C. and Karow, A. M., Jr (1974). Functional preservation of the mammalian kidney, III. Ultrastructural effects of perfusion with dimethylsulfoxidse (DMSO). *Cryobiology*, **11**, 170
14. Coriell, L. L. (1979). Preservation, storage and shipment. In Jakoby, W. B. and Pastan, I. H. (eds.) *Methods in Enzymology Cell Structure*, **58**, p.29. (New York: Academic Press)
15. Barner, H. B. (1965). The vascular lesion of freezing as modified by dimethylsulfoxide. *Cryobiology*, **2**, 55
16. Editorial (1980). Treatment of renal amyloidosis. *Lancet*, **1**, 1062
17. Pegg, D. E. and Robinson, s. M. (1978). Flow distribution and cryoprotectant concentration in rabbit kidneys perfused with glycerol solutions. *Cryobiology*, **15**, 609
18. Farrant, J. (1972). Human red cells under hypertonic conditions: A model system for investigating freezing damage. 3. Dimethylsulfoxide. *Cryobiology*, **9**, 131
19. Elford, B. C. (1970). Non-solvent water in muscle. *Nature (Lond.)*, **227**, 282
20. Segal, N. B. and Guttman, F. M. (1981). Kinetics of permeation of Me_2SO during rabbit kidney perfusion *in vitro*. *Cryobiology*. (In press)
21. Shlafer, M. (1981). Pharmacological considerations in cryopreservation. In Karow, A. M. Jr and Pegg, D. E. (eds) *Organ Preservation for Transplantation*, pp. 182-183. (New York: Marcel Dekker)
22. Karow, A. M., Jr, Wiggins, S., Carrier, G. O., Brown, R. and Matheny, J. L. (1979). Functional preservation of the mammalian kidney. V. Pharmacolinetics of dimethyl sulfoxide (1.4 M) in kidneys (rabbit and dog) perfused at 37, 25 or 10 °C followed by transplantation (dog). *J. Surg. Res.*, **27**, 93
23. Jacobsen, I. A. (1979). Cooling of rabbit kidneys permeated with glycerol to subzero temperatures. *Cryobiology*, **16**, 24
24. Fuller, B. J., Morris, G. J., Nutt, L. and Attenburrow, V. D. (1980). Functional recovery of isolated rat hepatocytes upon thawing from − 196 °C. *Cryoletters*, **1**, 139
25. Williams, R. J. and Shaw, S. K. (1980). The relationship between cell injury and osmotic volume reduction: II. Red cell lysis correlates with cell volume rather than intracellular salt concentration. *Cryobiology*, **17**, 530
26. Armitage, W. J. and Pegg, D. E. (1979). The contribution of the cryoprotectant to total injury in rabbit hearts frozen with ethylene glycol. *Cryobiology*, **16**, 152
27. Jacob, S. W., Owen, O. E., Collins, S. C. and Dunphy, J. E. (1958). Cryobiology. *Surg. Forum*, **9**, 802
28. Armitage, W. J., Matthes, G. and Pegg, D. E. (1981). Seleno-DL-methionine reduces freezing injury in hearts protected with ethanediol. *Cryobiology*, **18**, 370
29. Fahy, G. M. (1980). Analysis of 'solution effects' injury: rabbit renal cortex frozen in the presence of dimethyl sulfoxide. *Cryobiology*, **17**, 371
30. Elford, B. C. and Walter, C. A. (1972). Effects of electrolyte composition and pH on the structdure and function of smooth muscle cooled to − 79 °C in unfrozen media. *Cryobiology*, **9**, 82
31. Farrant, J., Walter, C. A., Lee, H. and McGann, L. E. (1977). Use of two-step cooling procedures to examine factors influencing cell survival following freezing and thawing. *Cryobiology*, **14**, 273
32. Pegg, D. E. (1981). The effect of cell concentration on the recovery of human erythrocytes after freezing and thawing in the presence of glycerol. *Cryobiology*, **18**, 221
33. Pegg, D. E., Jacobsen, I. A., Armitage, W. J. and Taylor, M. J. (1979). Mechanisms of cryoinjury in organs. In Pegg, D. E. and Jacobsen, I. A. (eds.) *Organ Preservation II*, p.132 (Edinburgh: Churchill Livingstone)
34. Miller, R. H. and Mazur, P. (1976). Survival of frozen–thawed human red cells as a function of cooling and warming velocities. *Cryobiology*, **13**, 404
35. Fahy, G. M. (1981). Analysis of 'solution effects' injury: cooling rate dependence of the functional and morphological sequelae of freezing in rabbit renal cortex protected with dimethyl sulfoxide. *Cryobiology*, **18**, 550
36. Welling, D. J. and Welling, L. W. (1979). Cell shape as an indicator of volume re-absorption in proximal nephron. *Fed. Proc.*, **38**, 121

37. Akhtar, T., Pegg, D. E. and Foreman, J. (1979). Effect of cooling and warming rates on the survival of cryopreserved L-cells. *Cryobiology,* **16,** 424

38. Myers, B. D., Chui, F., Hilberman, M. and Michaels, A. S. (1979). Transtubular leakage of glomerular filtrate in human acute renal failure: *Am. J. Physiol.,* **237,** F319

39. Pegg, D. E. and Green, C. J. (1973). The functional state of kidneys perfused at 37 °C with a bloodless fluid. *J. Surg. Res.,* **15,** 218

40. Fuller, B. J. (1974). The functional assessment of fresh and preserved rabbit kidneys by isolated bloodless perfusion. *PhD thesis,* CNAA, p. 80

41. Fuller, B. J., Pegg, D. E., Walter, C. A. and Green, C. J. (1977). An isolated rabbit kidney preparation for use in organ preservation research. *J. Surg. Res.,* **22,** 128

42. Fuller, B. J. and Pegg, D. E. (1976). The assessment of renal preservation by normothermic bloodless perfusion. *Cryobiology,* **13,** 177

Index

423